THIRD EDITION

Stuttering

AND OTHER FLUENCY DISORDERS

FRANKLIN H. SILVERMAN

MARQUETTE UNIVERSITY
MEDICAL COLLEGE OF WISCONSIN

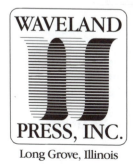

WAVELAND

PRESS, INC.

Long Grove, Illinois

For information about this book, contact:
   Waveland Press, Inc.
   4180 IL Route 83,Inc.
   Long Grove, IL 60047-9580
   (847) 634-0081
   info@waveland.com
   www.waveland.com

Table 1-2, p. 25. Reprinted from *The Onset of Stuttering: Research Findings and Implications*, by Johnson, W. and Assoc. © 1959. Permission granted by University of Minnesota Press.

Table 2.1, p. 60. Reprinted from St. Louis, K. O. and Hinzman, A. R., "Studies of Cluttering: Perceptions of Cluttering by Speech-Language Pathologists and Educators," *Journal of Fluency Disorders*, Vol. II, p. 131–149 (1986), with permission of Elsevier.

Table 4-1 (p. 109), table 4-2 (p. 110), figure 6-2 (p. 196), and various excerpts. Reprinted from *The Nature of Stuttering* by Van Riper, Charles, © 1982. Permission granted by Prentice Hall, Inc.

Contents

Preface   vii

Introduction: The "Why" of this Book   **1**

1   Normal and Abnormal Speech Disfluency   **5**
Instructional Objectives   5
What Are Moments of Speech Disfluency?   7
Four Disorders that Yield Moments of
  Abnormal Speech Disfluency   9
Other Disorders Reported to Have a
  Stuttering-like Symptom   16
When Are Moments of Speech Disfluency
  Symptoms of a Fluency Disorder?   20
Fluency Disorders as Impairments,
  Disabilities, and Handicaps   29
Assignments   31

**2   Symptomatology and Phenomenology of
Fluency Disorders**   **33**
Instructional Objectives   33
Symptomatology and Phenomenology of Stuttering   34
Symptomatology and Phenomenology of Cluttering   59

Symptomatology and Phenomenology of
  Neurogenic Acquired Stuttering   61
Symptomatology and Phenomenology of
  Psychogenic Acquired Stuttering   63
Assignments   64

3   The Person Who Has a Fluency Disorder   67

Instructional Objectives   67
The Person Who Stutters   69
The Person Who Manifests Cluttering   89
The Person Who Manifests Neurogenic Acquired Stuttering   91
The Person Who Manifests Psychogenic Acquired Stuttering   92
Assignments   93

4   Onset and Development   95

Instructional Objectives   95
Onset of Stuttering   96
Development of Stuttering   104
Onset and Development of Cluttering   112
Onset and Development of Neurogenic Acquired Stuttering   113
Onset and Development of Psychogenic Acquired Stuttering   114
Assignments   115

5   Etiology   117

Instructional Objectives   117
How Have Fluency Disorders Been Explained Historically?   118
Schemes for Categorizing Hypotheses about Stuttering   129
Is the Cause of Stuttering Physiological or Psychological?   131
What Factors Cause One Child to Be More
  at Risk for Stuttering than Another?   132
Why Do People Begin to Stutter?   138
Why Do People Continue to Stutter?   157
To What Extent Is Stuttering Learned Behavior?   159
Is Stuttering Truly a Disorder of Speech?   161
Is the Mystery of Stuttering Solvable?   164
Etiology of Cluttering   165
Etiology of Neurogenic Acquired Stuttering   166
Etiology of Psychogenic Acquired Stuttering   166
Assignments   166

6   Evaluation: Principles and Methods   169

Instructional Objectives   169

Reasons for Evaluating Speech Fluency   170

An Overview of the Evaluation Process   173

Cultural Considerations   175

Determining Whether a Client Has a Fluency Disorder   176

Determining Whether the Client Is at Risk
  for Stuttering or Developing a Stuttering Overlay on
  Another Fluency Disorder   179

Determining the Type of Fluency Disorder   179

Identifying the Behaviors in the Set that
  Defines a Client's Fluency Disorder   181

Answering Questions   186

Assessing Motivation   203

Making a Prognosis   206

Reasons for Not Scheduling Therapy
  for a Client Who Has a Disorder   209

Communicating Questions,
  Answers, and Recommendations   211

Assignments   212

7   Intervention: Principles, Goals, and Strategies   213

Instructional Objectives   213

"Do No Harm"   216

The Therapeutic Relationship   222

Cultural Considerations   224

Establishing Goals   225

Selecting and Implementing Intervention Strategies   231

Selecting and Implementing
  Intervention Strategies for Cluttering   262

Selecting and Implementing Intervention Strategies
  for Neurogenic Acquired Stuttering   266

Selecting and Implementing Intervention Strategies for
  Psychogenic Acquired Stuttering   268

Self-help for Stuttering and Other Fluency Disorders   269

Assessing/Documenting Therapy Outcome   271

Assignments   271

8 Preventing Stuttering   275

Instructional Objectives   275

Cultural Considerations   276

Preventing Stuttering in Young Children   276

Preventing Stuttering from Becoming a
Disability and/or a Handicap   279

Preventing Overlays of Stuttering on
Other Fluency Disorders   280

Can Cluttering, Neurogenic Acquired Stuttering, and
Psychogenic Acquired Stuttering Be Prevented?   281

Appendices   283

References   329

Name Index   353

Subject Index   359

Preface

This third edition, like the first two, presents the topics that usually are addressed in stuttering and fluency disorder courses. Its purpose is to provide upper-division undergraduate and masters-level graduate students as well as working clinicians with information they need to be helpful to persons who have these disorders. The material on stuttering has been updated and the material on cluttering, neurogenic acquired stuttering, and psychogenic acquired stuttering has been expanded and integrated into the chapters on symptomatology, etiology, development, evaluation, and management. A chapter has been added on the prevention of stuttering as an impairment, a disability, a handicap, and an overlay.

I have also added instructional objectives at the beginning of each chapter in the third edition to facilitate students and instructors in meeting the requirement of ASHA's KASA initiative to both define and document training programs in speech-language pathology.

I don't believe that it's truly possible to understand the symptomatology and management of a disorder and the effect it can have on people's lives merely by reading about the disorder. You have to encounter, through simulations and other types of experiences, various aspects of it. The simulations and other types of experiential assignments in each chapter can increase your understanding of the symptomatology of fluency disorders, their management, and the attitudes of children and adults who have them.

The abnormal behaviors exhibited by all children and adults who have a particular fluency disorder are not the same. Clinicians need a structure, therefore, for evaluating/describing behaviors that define the stuttering problems of their clients. They also need one for differentiating stuttering from normal disfluency and other fluency disorders. An approach that provides such structures is described in this book. Also provided are "wordings and structures" abstracted from evaluation reports by experienced clinicians that can be helpful when preparing such reports (Appendix A); a list of organizations and Internet resources to use in networking as well as in accessing any specific, clinically relevant information about fluency disorders and help in coping with them (Appendix B); and a number of tasks and questionnaires for describing aspects of a client's fluency disorder and his or her reactions to it (Appendix C).

Clinicians also need a structure for establishing therapy goals and developing intervention strategies for achieving them. An approach that provides such a structure is described in this book. This approach takes into consideration why the clinician believes a client is behaving in a particular way. Considerable stress is placed on the principle that the approach a clinician uses to modify a behavior should be based on his or her assumption (hypothesis) about the reason(s) a client exhibits it.

Throughout the book, I used the terms "stutterer" and "person who stutters" interchangeably. While the latter is currently regarded as being more "politically correct" than the former, few persons who stutter (including myself) object to the label stutterer, nor does its use appear to result in a more negative perception of persons who stutter than does the latter (Dietrich, Jensen, & Williams, 2001; St. Louis, 1999). I used "stutterer" whenever I felt "person who stutters" would make a sentence sound awkward.

I've documented some concepts with comments (lightly edited to preserve confidentiality) from participants in an on-line self-help/support group (STUTT-L@LISTSERV.TEMPLE.EDU) for persons who have a fluency disorder. I refer to the support-group members as STUTT-L participants.

Authorities do not agree about the etiology of stuttering. Some view it as completely physiological (genetic), some as completely psychological, and some (including myself) as a combination of the two. Both contemporary and historical theories of its etiology are discussed in this book. However, like all authors of books on stuttering, I have beliefs about this that influence both the amount of space devoted to discussing individual theories (and topics related to them) and how certain studies are interpreted. To judge the credibility of my points of view, you will need information about my background and experience with stuttering. I have taught courses dealing with stuttering for more than 30 years and have treated children and adults who have the disorder for more than 40 years. I was a research associate in the Stuttering Research Program at the University of Iowa and have authored or coauthored more than 50 papers on the topic of stuttering. Most were published in the *Journal of Speech and Hearing Disorders*, the *Journal of Speech and Hearing Research*, and the *Journal of Fluency Disorders*. I have served as an editorial consultant for papers dealing with fluency disorders for these and other journals, and for three years I was associate editor of the *Journal of Speech and Hearing Research*, with responsibility for the editorial processing of all papers submitted on these disorders. For several years I facilitated a self-help/support group for persons who stutter that was affiliated with the National Stuttering Association. Finally, I have had more than 60 years of personal experience with stuttering, as I have stuttered since early childhood.

It is impossible to give credit to all of the sources from which the concepts presented in this book have been drawn. The book is the product of many years of experience in helping myself and others to cope with fluency disorders, as well as reading about and discussing fluency disorders with students and colleagues. Thus, although I cannot credit this or that concept to a particular person, I can say "thank you" to all who have helped: my students at Marquette University, my mentors (particularly, Drs. Wendell Johnson and Dean Williams), my clients, and my fellow participants in self-help/support groups whose comments, questions, and criticisms through the years have helped me to clarify my own ideas.

Franklin H. Silverman

Introduction
The "Why" of this Book

I've been coping with stuttering for more than 60 years and have helped others to do so for more than 40 years. I've learned a lot about both what is and is not likely to be helpful to someone who stutters or has another fluency disorder. The sources from which my knowledge has come include my own experience, that of my clients, and that of other speech-language pathologists. My intent in this book is to share with you what I've learned by providing you with practical information you'll need (particularly if you're a beginning clinician). Your goal should be to *help* persons who stutter, are at risk for doing so, or have another fluency disorder, as well as to minimize the risk of *harming* such persons.

Many persons who stutter or have another fluency disorder believe that they didn't benefit from the therapy they received from a speech-language pathologist, or—worse yet—were in some way harmed by it. While their negative evaluation probably isn't valid in some cases, in others it undoubtedly is. Fortunately, it's relatively easy to minimize the risk of harming clients who stutter or have another fluency disorder. Information needed to do so is provided in chapter 7.

The best way to cope with stuttering is to prevent it. There are ways that can help you to prevent many (perhaps most) preschoolers from developing the disorder. Information is also available that can help you to prevent some older children who stutter from becoming disabled and handicapped by the disorder. It is also possible to help

1

prevent some persons who have another fluency disorder from developing a stuttering overlay. This information, and practical recommendations for implementing it, appear in chapter 8.

There are four major fluency disorders: stuttering, cluttering, neurogenic acquired stuttering, and psychogenic acquired stuttering. In order to be helpful to someone who has a fluency disorder, you'll need basic information about the symptomatology, phenomenology, etiology, and development of such disorders. This information, as well as how to help clients cope with their disorders, is provided in chapters 1 through 5.

A second type of information is needed to determine whether a client actually has a fluency disorder. You'll have to be able to determine, for example, whether the sound and syllable repetitions of a preschool-age child are the beginning of a stuttering disorder or merely normal disfluency behavior. A misdiagnosis can have disastrous consequences for a child and his or her family, particularly if you misdiagnose normal childhood syllable repetition as the early onset of stuttering (see chapter 5). Furthermore, a client can have more than one fluency disorder, so you'll have to be able to identify the type(s). Since each of them has a different etiology, a misdiagnosis is likely to result in a client receiving inappropriate therapy. Information on maximizing the likelihood of accurately making these determinations (i.e., diagnoses) appears in chapter 6.

A third type of information that you'll need to be helpful to such clients is required to define meaningful goals for therapy. Specifically, you'll need to identify the aspects of a client's speaking behavior and/or attitude, which, if modified, would result in a reduction in his or her level of disability and/or handicap. You must be able to identify changes the client can make that would significantly improve the quality of his or her life. You also must know how to facilitate such changes once you have identified them. Chapter 7 addresses these issues.

If a client isn't highly motivated to achieve a particular goal, he or she is unlikely to make the investment needed to achieve it. A fourth type of information you'll need on various techniques for assessing clients' motivation to achieve specific goals appears in chapter 6.

The fifth type of information you'll need is a knowledge of techniques for assisting your fluency clients to achieve their goals—techniques that can facilitate their behavior being modified. The term *behavior* in this book includes what ordinarily are referred to as attitudes and feelings. We usually become aware of a person's attitudes and feelings through his or her verbal and other behavior. When working with an older child or adult who has a fluency disorder, you can help the client reduce the degree of disability and severity of handicap caused by the disorder, as well as reducing the severity of the impairment itself. These topics are presented in chapter 7.

The final type of information that you'll need is knowledge of how a client's cultural background could affect what would be the "best practices" for managing his or her disorder. Some relevant practical considerations are discussed in chapters 6, 7, and 8.

This book is intended to serve as a starting point for your exploration of stuttering and other fluency disorders. The amount of clinically relevant literature on these disorders, particularly stuttering, is huge. A listing of sites on the Internet and organizations that can provide access to this literature appears in Appendix B.

I'll end by admitting that the "why" of this book is partially personal. I've been training clinicians to help persons who have (or are at risk for developing) fluency disorders for almost four decades. I'd like to continue being helpful by sharing the knowledge and experience I've gained over the years. If my readers are able to implement some of my recommendations, my endeavor will have been rewarded.

1

Normal and Abnormal Speech Disfluency

INSTRUCTIONAL OBJECTIVES

By the end of this chapter, you should be able to:

▸ Describe the seven types of disfluency behaviors.

▸ Define the four major fluency disorders: stuttering, cluttering, neurogenic acquired stuttering, and psychogenic acquired stuttering.

▸ Define five conditions that may precipitate abnormal disfluency: acquired stuttering following laryngectomy, stuttering-like behavior in manual communication, stuttering-like behavior when playing wind instruments, malingered stuttering, and spastic dysphonia.

▸ Specify 14 criteria for differentiating between abnormal and normal disfluency.

▸ Describe the four types of disfluency that are most likely to be found in the speech of persons who stutter or have another fluency disorder.

▸ Specify the relationship between chronological age and the degree of risk for beginning to stutter.

▸ Describe how amount of "abnormal" disfluency is related to the mental age of children who are cognitively challenged (i.e., mentally retarded).

▸ Specify how a client's habitual speaking rate may help to diagnose his or her type of fluency disorder.

▸ Argue that there is and isn't a viable genetic cause for a fluency disorder.

▸ Indicate how frequencies of disfluency of children who stutter are similar to and different from those of their normal speaking peers.

▸ Indicate how the durations of the disfluency of children who stutter are similar to and different from those of their normal-speaking peers.

▸ Describe behaviors evinced by persons while being disfluent that indicate they're being tense.

▸ Describe possible impacts of one's awareness of and concern about moments of disfluency.

▸ Describe behaviors referred to as secondary symptoms, or secondaries, that sometimes accompany moments of disfluency.

▸ Specify how the strength of a person's desire to avoid being disfluent can affect the amount he or she is disfluent.

▸ Describe how expecting a child to begin to stutter can cause a child to begin to stutter.

▸ Specify at least two motivations for malingering a fluency disorder.

▸ Describe each of the four fluency disorders as impairments, disabilities, and handicaps.

I subscribe to a listserv on the Internet, to which clinicians, stutterers, and their families contribute (STUTT-L@LISTSERV.TEMPLE.EDU). (This listserv, incidentally, is an "open" one that welcomes students who are majoring in speech-language pathology.) Following is an e-mail excerpt that expresses a theme I've encountered many times previously from this listserv.

> As a stutterer and the parent of a first grader who stutters I have to chime in here. I definitely believe that an SLP who is not qualified to treat stuttering can do more harm than good. Many don't even have a clue about what emotional baggage comes with stuttering. Don't get me wrong, I am not anti-therapy. But I demand expertise.

My primary objective in this book is to provide you with a portal to access what you need to know about stuttering and other fluency disorders in order to be helpful, not harmful, to persons who have one or more fluency disorder(s).

Our focus in this chapter will be on speech disfluency—both normal and abnormal. We'll begin by considering the kinds of hesitations that can occur during moments of speech disfluency. Next, I'll present an overview of the four main disorders that have abnormal hesitations as an aspect of their *symptomatology* (i.e., stuttering, cluttering, neurogenic acquired stuttering, and psychogenic acquired stuttering) and then briefly describe several other disorders that have a stuttering-like symptom. Following this, I'll indicate a number of crucial factors for assessing the normality of a client's hesitation phenomena. Next, we'll consider the impact that a fluency disorder can have on a person and on his or her family from the three perspectives advocated by the World Health Organization (WHO)—as an impairment, as a disability, and as a handicap. Finally, you'll be given an assignment that will enable you to experience, from each of these perspectives, what it's like to have a fluency disorder.

WHAT ARE MOMENTS OF SPEECH DISFLUENCY?

If you compare the content of a written version of a speech to its content when someone reads it aloud, you're likely to find at least a few examples in the latter version of *moments of speech disfluency*. They may include interjections of syllables (such as "uh" or "um"), repetitions of the initial syllables of words or of entire words, and/or corrections of mispronunciations or misreadings of words or phrases. If the speaker was not regarded by the audience as having a fluency disorder, few (if any) persons in the audience would be likely to consider these behaviors abnormal. On the other hand, if the speaker was thought to have a fluency disorder, at least a few such moments of speech disfluency would be likely to be regarded as abnormal by at least a few of those present. Consequently, judgments of the normality of moments of speech disfluency are affected by both the *mouth of the speaker* and the *ear of the listener*. Some factors that affect such judgments are discussed in the next section.

The types of hesitation phenomena that can occur during moments of disfluency (singly or in combination) have been categorized in several ways by linguists and speech-language pathologists. The categorization scheme that has been used most often by speech-language pathologists, developed by Wendell Johnson and his associates at the University of Iowa (Johnson, 1961; Johnson & Associates, 1959; Williams, Silverman, and Kools, 1968), consists of the following categories:

- *Part-word repetitions.* These are sound and syllable repetitions. They occur most often at the beginnings of words and almost never at the ends of words. The number of times a particular sound or syllable is repeated can be relatively high, although it is usually only once or twice. The repetitions may be accompanied by audible and/or visible signs of tensing. Level of awareness of their occurrence can be relatively high or relatively low. Although the repetitions may be voluntary, they usually are involuntary.

- *Word repetitions.* These are repetitions of an entire word, in most cases a single-syllable word. While a word may be repeated a relatively large number of times, it is usually repeated only once or twice. Like part-word repetitions, they may be accompanied by audible and/or visible signs of tensing, may be voluntary or involuntary, and may vary with the degree to which the speaker is aware of their occurrence.

- *Phrase repetitions.* These are repetitions of units consisting of two or more words. Such units usually are repeated only once or twice. They may be accompanied by audible and/or visible signs of tensing, may be voluntary or involuntary, and may vary with how aware the speaker is of their occurrence.

- *Interjections of sounds, syllables, words, and phrases.* These sound units, which occur between words, usually do not perform a linguistic function in messages—that is to say, the denotative meanings of messages usually are not affected by their presence. Examples are "um" and "you know." They may be accompanied by audible and/or visible signs of tensing, they may be voluntary or involuntary, and the speaker may or may not be aware of their occurrence.

- *Revisions–incomplete phrases.* This category includes instances in which the speaker becomes aware of making an error and corrects it. The error may be in how a word was pronounced or may be related to the meaning of the word(s) that were said. Also included are instances in which the speaker begins an utterance but obviously does not complete it.

- *Disrhythmic phonations.* These are disturbances in the normal rhythm of words. The disturbance may be attributable to a prolonged sound, an accent or timing that is notably unusual, an improper stress, a break (usually between syllables), or any other speaking behavior not compatible with fluent speech. Included here are phenomena that some investigators have referred to as "broken" words (e.g., "I am g—oing to the store"). Disrhythmic phonations may be accompanied by audible and/or visible signs of tensing, may be voluntary or involuntary, and may vary with the degree to which the speaker is aware of their occurrence.

- *Tense pauses.* These phenomena occur between words, part words, and interjections. They consist of pauses in which there are barely audible manifestations of heavy breathing or muscle tightening. The same phenomena within a word would place the word in the category of disrhythmic phonation. Tense pauses vary with how aware the speaker is of their occurrence.

A type of hesitation phenomena that linguists refer to as *unfilled pauses* was not included in the final version of Johnson's scheme. During these abnormally long pauses between words, there are no audible manifestations of heavy breathing or muscle tightening. Johnson initially included this category but subsequently dropped it when he discovered that such pauses could not be identified as reliably as the other types of hesitation phenomena. Another change that Johnson made in the final version of his scheme was to combine the categories of revision and incomplete phrase. He combined the categories because his judges were unable to differentiate between them reliably. Specifically, they were unable to agree with each other sufficiently well about whether the words that immediately followed an incomplete phrase were a revision or a change of thought.

FOUR DISORDERS THAT YIELD MOMENTS OF ABNORMAL SPEECH DISFLUENCY

The four major disorders for which the presence of abnormal hesitation phenomena (speech disfluency) is a necessary condition for diagnosis—stuttering, cluttering, neurogenic acquired stuttering, and psychogenic acquired stuttering—are defined in this section. All four are discussed in detail throughout the book.

Stuttering

Stuttering, which is the most frequently occurring of these disorders, usually has its onset in early childhood between the ages of two and five. There is no consensus regarding its etiology (see chapter 5).

There is disagreement about how the term *stuttering* should be defined. Almost all definitions mention repetitions of sounds and syllables and prolongations of speech sounds, and almost all mention difficulty in beginning to say words. That is, the person knows what he or she wants to say but has to "strain" to say it. This type of abnormal speech disfluency has been referred to as *stammering*. The following extract illustrates how authorities once attempted to differentiate stammering from stuttering.

> Formerly, authorities tried to differentiate between stuttering and stammering by saying, for example, that stuttering was a physical

and stammering a psychological defect; that stuttering was a rapid repetition of one sound (c-c-c-cat) and stammering was an inability to produce voice; that stuttering was a halt on consonants and stammering was a halt on vowels; or, again, that stuttering was a disorder met with only in young children which developed into stammering if incorrectly treated. (Boome & Richardson, 1931, p. 7)

The term stammering is now rarely used in the United States because the hesitations associated with it are thought to have the same etiology (or etiologies) as stuttering-type sound and syllable repetitions (Van Riper, 1982).

Before we examine some definitions of stuttering, we will consider several reasons why there are differences in how it is defined. One is that those who did the defining attended to (or "abstracted") different attributes of the behavior (Johnson, 1946). When you describe an event, you talk about those attributes you consider significant. Two people viewing an event (in this case, stuttering) are unlikely to abstract the same attributes of it and are therefore unlikely to describe it in the same way. This is illustrated by the fable of the six blind men and the elephant:

> Six blind men who attempted to describe an elephant came up with six different descriptions. They differed in part because they had observed (felt) different parts (attributes) of the animal. However, even if they had observed (felt) the same thing, they likely would have "abstracted" (attended to) different aspects of the experience and, hence, still would have come up with different descriptions. (Johnson, 1958, p. xii)

Since each blind man felt a different part of the elephant, he only described one attribute of it (e.g., its trunk, its tail, or its ears); however, all their definitions contained some "kernel of truth." Likewise, those who have tried to define stuttering have not necessarily attended to (abstracted) the same aspects (attributes) of it—hence, their definitions are different.

Another reason why definitions of stuttering differ is that some are partially or wholly based on hypotheses about its etiology. Rather then *describing* stuttering they try to *explain* it. Wendell Johnson (1958), for example, defined stuttering as an "anticipatory, apprehensive, hypertonic avoidance reaction." Coriat (1931) defined it as "a psychoneurosis caused by the persistence into later life of early pregenital oral nursing, oral sadistic, and anal sadistic components." Brutten and Shoemaker (1967) defined it as "that form of fluency failure that results from conditioned negative emotion."

Now that we have considered a few of the reasons why definitions of stuttering tend to differ, we will attempt to glean the kernel of truth from several of them. This discussion is intended to lay a foundation for developing an intuitive understanding of the symptomatology and phenomenology of the disorder.

Some definitions of stuttering deal only with audible aspects of speaking behavior. The following are representative of such definitions:

- Stuttering is a deviation in the ongoing fluency of speech, an inability to maintain the connected rhythms of speech. (Van Riper, 1982, p.11)

- There is a consensus that repetitions and prolongations are necessary and sufficient for the diagnosis of stuttering to be made. (Andrews et al., 1983, p. 227)

The kernel of truth in these definitions is that the stutterer does exhibit a disturbance in the ongoing rhythm or fluency of speech. He or she repeats, prolongs, or both. However, normal speakers—both children and adults—also repeat and prolong. In fact, some persons who are regarded by themselves and others as normal speakers repeat and/or prolong sounds more frequently than some who are regarded by themselves and others as stutterers (see Johnson, 1961; Johnson & Associates, 1959; Silverman, 1974). Such definitions are inadequate, therefore, for differentiating *moments of stuttering* from normal speech prolongations and repetitions. They also are inadequate for determining whether a person, particularly a preschool-age child, is beginning to stutter. Normal-speaking preschool-age children, for example, repeat sounds, syllables, and words (particularly single-syllable ones) a great deal (Johnson & Associates, 1959).

Definitions that deal solely with audible aspects of speaking behavior are inadequate for a second reason. They do not allow the differentiation between stuttering and other fluency disorders.

Following are three somewhat more complex definitions of stuttering:

- Stuttering occurs when the forward flow of speech is interrupted by a motorically disrupted sound, syllable, or word, or by the speaker's reactions thereto. (Van Riper, 1982, p. 15)

- Disorders in the rhythm of speech in which the individual knows precisely what he wishes to say, but at the time is unable to say it because of an involuntary, repetitive prolongation or cessation of a sound. (World Health Organization, 1977, p. 202)

- Stuttering is the involuntary disruption of a continuing attempt to produce a spoken utterance. (Perkins, 1990a, p. 376)

The first of these definitions considers not only the audible disruptions in the forward flow of speech, but also the speaker's reactions to them. Perhaps one of the most significant ways that stutterers' speech hesitations differ from those of normal speakers is that stutterers tend to react to theirs and normal speakers do not (Bloodstein, 1987). Stutterers react to their abnormal disfluencies with fear and embarrassment and try to minimize (avoid) them. One of the most successful strategies they can use for this purpose is not talking, particularly when stuttering is anticipated. When a stutterer doesn't speak, he or she doesn't stutter! While reducing verbal output minimizes stuttering, it also interferes with communication, thereby adversely affecting interpersonal relationships.

The second, which is a definition used internationally because it was promulgated by the World Health Organization, includes the fact that the abnormal repetitions and prolongations exhibited by stutterers are *involuntary*. This is considered by some to be the most invariant fundamental characteristic of the disorder. The inclusion of this word is essential for differentiating the disfluencies of stuttering from normal disfluencies, for the following reason:

> If the essence of clinical stuttering is in the involuntary aspect of disfluency, and not in its overt form, then the question arises whether or not a particular disfluency is stuttered or normal. If normal, the presumption seems to be that it is a manifestation of linguistic uncertainty, and therefore is a characteristic shared by all speakers. If stuttered, the disfluency presumably is a motor speech blockage, an atypical abnormal form of disfluency. (Perkins, 1983a, p. 247)

The third of these definitions, like the second, stresses the involuntary nature of stuttering but also defines the disorder from the stutterer's perspective rather than that of the listener. According to Perkins (1990a):

> Stuttering is a problem of *involuntary* disruption of a word the speaker is otherwise attempting to utter, rather than the resulting acoustic event, which is what the listener perceives. . . . Because all types of disfluency characteristic of stuttering also occur as nonstuttered disfluency, the listener can only guess which is which. . . . From the stutterer's vantage point, however, the judgment is categorical: Involuntary blockage either has or has not occurred to some degree. If it has not occurred, then what sounds like stuttering to the observer would not feel like stuttering to the speaker. The reason that this distinction is categorical is because the proposed definition posits that loss of control of the ability to voluntarily continue a disrupted utterance is the essence of stuttering. If the disruption is not involuntary to some degree, then it is not a stuttered disfluency. Moreover, the stutterer would not react to it with apprehension, struggle, or avoidance as if it were stuttered. (p. 376)

The following comment by a STUTT-L participant reinforces Perkins's argument that it is necessary to consider the stutterer's perspective when defining stuttering:

I do not care whether or not I outwardly stutter. I care that I inwardly stutter. It is easy to think that the inner experience comes from the outer speech problem—but I am convinced that it is the other way around. I have no interest in learning controlled fluency, any more than I would be interested in perfecting avoidance and being a closet stutterer. My goal is to make myself inwardly free. And for me—I do not pretend to speak for anyone else—my stuttered speech is the outer manifestation of an INNER blockage.

For commentaries on Perkins's definition see Bloodstein (1990), Ingham (1990a), Perkins (1990b, 1991), Siegel (1991), and Smith (1990b).

We will consider next the "standard definition" proposed by Wingate (1964), which is more complex than the previous ones:

> The term "stuttering" means: I. (a) disruption in the fluency of verbal expression, which is (b) characterized by involuntary, audible, or silent repetitions or prolongations in the utterance of short speech elements, namely: sounds, syllables, and words of one syllable. These disruptions (c) usually occur frequently or are marked in character and (d) are not readily controllable. II. Sometimes the disruptions are (e) accompanied by accessory activities involving the speech apparatus, related or unrelated body structures, or stereotyped speech utterances. These activities give the appearance of being speech-related struggle. III. Also, there not infrequently are (f) indications or reports of the presence of an emotional state, ranging from a general condition of "excitement" or "tension" to more specific emotions of a negative nature such as fear, embarrassment, irritation, or the like. (g) The immediate source of stuttering is some incoordination expressed in the peripheral speech mechanism; the ultimate cause is presently unknown and may be complex or compound. (p. 498)

This definition, which is among the most frequently cited, provides additional information about moments of stuttering. It can be gleaned from this definition that some moments of stuttering are partially or completely silent. They do not consist of sound prolongations or repetitions. However, there may be audible sounds associated with tension when they occur between words. Such pauses between words for this reason have been labeled *tense pauses* (Williams, Silverman, & Kools, 1968). There may also be visible signs of tensing—particularly in the facial area—during these pauses.

It also can be gleaned from this definition that moments of stuttering may occur frequently, but not on every word. Even the most severe stutterer says some words fluently. This suggests both that the functioning of stutterers' speech mechanisms is adequate for speaking fluently at least some of the time and that they know how to do so.

A third such kernel of truth is that they may exhibit secondary symptoms. These are described elsewhere in this chapter. A final kernel that can be gleaned is that stuttering is frequently accompanied by an emotional state. Listeners may be aware of this state, or it may be experienced solely by the stutterer. The emotional state may be one of fear, anxiety, tension, shame, embarrassment, or some combination of these. While speaking, a stutterer may evince both tension and embarrassment: he or she may communicate tension by voice quality and embarrassment by not maintaining normal eye contact while stuttering (Atkins, 1988; Tatchell et al., 1983). It has not been unequivocally established whether these emotional states are associated with the cause of or are a result of stuttering.

Cluttering

Cluttering, or tachyphemia, is a disorder that begins during childhood and is thought by some to have a genetic basis (Myers & St. Louis, 1992). It is reported to have been first differentiated from stuttering in 1830 by Colombat (Weiss, 1964). The disorder has received considerably more attention in European than in American literature (St. Louis & Rustin, 1992). In fact, until fairly recently most of those who wrote about it in the American literature were Europeans. According to Daly (1986):

> American speech-language pathologists have not, largely, accepted cluttering as a clinical entity, nor have they incorporated information about cluttering into their clinical decision-making processes. Although considerable literature on cluttering exists, American authors treat the problem of cluttering in a most cursory manner. Typically, only a paragraph or two are devoted to this ill-understood disorder. Many authors omit any mention of cluttering. (p. 156)

During the past few decades cluttering has received more attention in the English-language literature than it had previously (e.g., Daly, 1986, 1993a).

Unfortunately, like stuttering, there is no universally agreed-upon definition for this disorder. One of the most accepted (judging by the frequency with which it has been referred to in papers on cluttering) appears to be that of Weiss (1964):

> Cluttering is a speech disorder characterized by the clutterer's unawareness of his disorder, by a short attention span, by disturbances in perception, articulation and formulation of speech, and often by excessive speed of delivery. It is a disorder of the thought processes preparatory to speech and based on a hereditary disposition. Cluttering is a verbal manifestation of Central Language Imbalance, which affects all channels of communication (e.g., reading, writing, rhythm, and musicality) and behavior in general. (p. 1)

Weiss, then, views cluttering as one manifestation (symptom) of a generalized disturbance in language functioning—one "tip" of a submerged iceberg.

Daly's definition of cluttering (1993b) describes in more detail the speech and language-processing disturbances of persons who have the disorder:

> Cluttering is a disorder of both speech and language processing that frequently results in rapid, disrhythmic, sporadic, unorganized, and often unintelligible speech. Accelerated speech (or tachylalia) is not always present, but impairments in formulating language almost always are. . . . Those who clutter confuse their listeners with incomplete and awkward sentences, false starts, sound sequencing errors, and word-retrieval problems. Their garbled speech is confounded by a lack of clarity of inner language formulation. Equally frustrating for clinicians are the absence of self-awareness and unconcerned attitude of many clients who clutter. Their self-monitoring skills for speech and social situations are deficient. (p. 7)

Neurogenic Acquired Stuttering

A number of case descriptions of stuttering acquired during childhood and adulthood following damage to the central nervous system have appeared in the literature. Most of these pertain to persons who had no history of stuttering and whose onset of the disorder (which was usually sudden) was associated with a neurological event. A few of them pertain to persons who experienced a recurrence or worsening of childhood stuttering following brain damage. The neurological events with which the onset of their stuttering was associated included strokes, head trauma, extrapyramidal diseases, tumors, dementia, drug usage, anoxia, and cryosurgery (Helm-Estabrooks, 1986). Their disorder is referred to as neurogenic acquired stuttering, stuttering associated with acquired neurological disorders (SAAND), neurogenic stuttering, acquired stuttering, neurological stuttering, neurological disfluency, cortical stuttering, or stuttering of sudden onset.

Psychogenic Acquired Stuttering

A number of reports of stuttering acquired during adulthood at least partially as a reaction to acute or chronic psychological disturbances have appeared in the literature. These are reports of persons who did not have a childhood history of stuttering and the onset of their disorder—which was usually sudden and could not be accounted for solely on the basis of central nervous system damage—appeared to be associated with some form of psychological stress (Helm-Estabrooks & Hotz, 1998; Roth, Aronson, & Davis, Jr., 1989). One young man, for example, suddenly began to stutter after his ship received a direct missile hit during the Korean conflict (Dempsey & Granich, 1978). Another suddenly began doing so during an acute anxiety attack (Wallen, 1961), and a third is reported to have started stuttering when his marriage began to experience difficulty (Attanasio, 1987). In some cases, the presence of psychopathology was established through performance on the Minnesota Multiphasic Personality Inventory (MMPI) (Roth et al., 1989).

OTHER DISORDERS REPORTED TO HAVE A STUTTERING-LIKE SYMPTOM

In this section we'll briefly consider several other disorders that have a stuttering-like symptom. Descriptions of them are included mainly for purpose of completeness. They will not be discussed extensively in this book.

Acquired Stuttering Following Laryngectomy

There is evidence that suggests stuttering may be acquired following a laryngectomy. Rosenfield and Freeman (1983) have described two cases in which this presumably occurred. The first was of a 71-year-old-man who claimed to have stuttered for one year following a laryngectomy performed at age 59. The second was of a man who was still stuttering when contacted by the authors:

> C.M. had also been a fluent speaker prior to his laryngectomy. He is 67 years old, right-handed, and has stuttered since his surgery at age 63. There is no family history of stuttering. He has used a Western Electric electrolarynx for more than 3 years. He exhibited disfluencies including multiple-, whole- and part-word repetitions, interjections, and occasional prolongations. He demonstrates struggle behaviors and experiences extreme frustration associated with the disfluency problem. He was independently judged by two experienced speech pathologists to be a stutterer. (Rosenfield & Freeman, 1983, p. 266)

Since these, to my knowledge, are the only reports of this type of fluency disorder, it is probably a relatively rare phenomenon. However, it apparently is not unusual for laryngectomized patients to be highly disfluent at the early stages of relearning speech (Freeman & Rosenfield, 1982).

Stutter-Like Disfluencies in Manual Communication

Many persons who are severely speech impaired because they are deaf, mentally retarded, or autistic use manual communication (signing) alone or in combination with speech. The simultaneous use of both is referred to as "total" communication. There have been a few reports of persons with these disorders who exhibit stutter-like disfluencies while signing (Liles, Lerman, Christensen, & St. Ledger, 1992; Montgomery & Fitch, 1988; Silverman & Silverman, 1971). The types of stutter-like disfluencies observed in manual communication include part-word repetitions, word repetitions, and prolongations. For the persons reported on who used "total" communication, the signing disfluencies were sometimes accompanied by speech disfluencies and at other times not.

While it appears quite likely that there is a fluency disorder that can affect manual communication, its prevalence, symptomatology, etiology, and management are uncertain. Fortunately, it appears to be quite rare: Montgomery and Fitch (1988) identified only 12 cases in the 9,930 hearing-impaired students they surveyed.

It is not particularly surprising that users of manual communication can develop a fluency disorder. Certainly, conditions that result in neurogenic acquired stuttering and psychogenic acquired stuttering could as easily affect the musculature of the upper extremities as that of the mouth. Many of the conditions that have been hypothesized to cause stuttering could also do so. These would include hypotheses that view stuttering as an anticipatory-struggle behavior or as resulting from demands exceeding capacities (see chapter 5).

Wind Instrument Stuttering

There have been two case reports of stuttering-like behavior occurring during the playing of a wind musical instrument. One involved the flute (Silverman & Bohlman, 1988) and the other the French horn (Meltzer, 1992). Both persons were stutterers. Meltzer (1992) described the stuttering-like behavior on the French horn as follows:

> . . . a blocking of the flow of sound as a result of closure and tightening in the throat and a breakdown in coordination of tonguing movements. The frequency of occurrence varied, increasing under conditions of fatigue, stress, anticipation, speed, and the need to maintain a high standard of performance. (p. 260)

Since playing a wind instrument uses the same muscle groups as does speech—respiratory, laryngeal, and oropharyngeal—it is not particularly surprising that whatever causes stuttering could also interfere with playing a wind instrument. How might a musician who has such a disorder be helped? The case report by Meltzer (1992) suggests that he or she may benefit from stuttering therapy.

Both the prevalence of such disorders and whether a person who does not stutter can develop one are uncertain. There is a little anecdotal evidence which suggests that nonstutterers can develop them (Meltzer, 1992).

Malingered Stuttering

Speech pathologists have been asked by courts to provide expert testimony about whether a person really has a fluency disorder or is malingering (Shirkey, 1987; Bloodstein, 1988). Shirkey (1987), for example, was asked to provide such testimony about a 33-year-old man accused of a series of sexual assaults on children, whose defense in a previous arrest had been that as a stutterer he could not have committed the crimes because none of the victims stated that their attacker stuttered. Bloodstein (1988) was asked to provide testimony about a man in his early thirties accused of armed robbery whose defense was that, being a stutterer, he could not have said fluently; "This is a stickup. Get down on the floor and don't make a move or I'll blow your head off." In both cases it was concluded that the suspect probably was a stutterer because his "moments of stuttering" varied in a manner that was consistent with what had been reported in the literature.

Identifying Malingering

Establishing "beyond a reasonable doubt" that a person is malingering a fluency disorder is likely to be quite difficult, particularly if the person has read the stuttering literature and is knowledgeable about conditions under which stuttering varies. Malingering should always be considered a possibility if a client is likely to benefit in some way from this diagnosis. The benefit might be financial compensation from the person who it is claimed caused the disorder, or eligibility for financial aid (e.g., for vocational rehabilitation), or special consideration in hiring because of it. Malingering a fluency disorder could also be a way to discredit witness identification if witnesses to a crime reported that the person who committed it was a fluent speaker.

Unfortunately, there are no established guidelines for determining whether a person is malingering a fluency disorder. Consequently, the approach suggested here may not be the best—most effective—one. First determine whether the age of onset, symptomatology, and phenomenology of the fluency disorder claimed is consistent with what is known about the disorder. If they are not consistent with what is known, it is likely that the client does not have the disorder. On the other hand, if they are consistent with what is known about the disorder, there are two possibilities: one, the client has the disorder; or two, the client has read enough about the disorder to simulate it. You can ask the client what he or she has read about the disorder. If the client claims to have read nothing about the disorder, you might want to express concern about some aspect of the symptomatology he or she evinced or reported that is not consistent with what is known about it. The malingering client may be thrown off guard and insist that it is consistent with the symptomatology of the disorder, thereby demonstrating knowledge of the literature.

Spastic Dysphonia (Spasmodic Dysphonia)

The focus in this chapter thus far has been on what are usually labeled as fluency disorders. Might there be others that are not usually labeled as such? A number of comments in the literature suggest that there is such a disorder—spastic dysphonia.

Spastic dysphonia has been referred to by clinicians as "stammering of the vocal cords and laryngeal stuttering" (Aronson, 1973) and the resultant speech has been labeled "disfluent" by listeners (Silverman & Hummer, 1989). Persons who have spastic dysphonia (specifically, adductor spastic dysphonia) evince "a repeated blockage of phonation by spasms of the adductor muscles of the larynx, resulting in an intermittently strangled, choked utterance" (Bloodstein, 1984, p. 204). The severity of their problem appears to vary on a situational basis. According to Boone (1987):

> The patient may experience a normal voice in some situations, such as talking to a cat, repeating a memorized verse, or singing. It is no wonder that spastic dysphonia has been described as "laryngeal stutter". . . with the faulty voice varying in severity according to how the speaker views the listener. The more critical the communicative act, such as giving one's name to a ticket seller on the telephone, the more likely it is that the laryngeal tightness will occur and the voice will be shut off. (p. 285)

Persons with this disorder also speak normally when reading in chorus, speaking to children, and speaking when no listener is present (Arnold, 1959) and to demonstrate the adaptation effect—that is, the number of strain-strangle syllables decreases significantly during successive readings of a passage (Salamy & Sessions, 1980).

The symptomatology and phenomenology of stuttering and spastic dysphonia seem similar. Both disorders are characterized by intermittent disturbances in the ability to control the musculature of the speech mechanism (particularly that of the larynx) in the manner necessary to produce fluent speech. Also, the severity of both disorders varies on a situational basis. In fact, both stuttering and spastic dysphonia appear to increase and decrease in severity under the same conditions.

The etiology of spastic dysphonia, like that of stuttering, has not been definitely established. Some writers regard it as being primarily neurological, possibly the result of some degenerative process in the central nervous system. The fact that its onset is during middle age, and that some persons with the disorder exhibit neurological abnormalities, could be construed to support their position. Others regard it as psychological, and the fact that its onset appears to be related to some psychological trauma and that persons with it can at times speak normally appears to support their position. More writers regard its etiology as psychological rather than neurological (Bloodstein, 1984).

While the symptomatology, the phenomenology, and possibly the etiology of stuttering and spastic dysphonia seem to be similar, their age of onset and their relative frequencies of occurrence among males and females are not. As we have previously noted, most cases of stuttering have their onset in early childhood, while most cases of spastic dysphonia begin during middle age. And while stuttering tends to occur far more often in males than in females, spastic dysphonia does not. In fact, several authors (see Arnold, 1959) have reported that it occurs more often in females than in males.

WHEN ARE MOMENTS OF SPEECH DISFLUENCY SYMPTOMS OF A FLUENCY DISORDER?

The presence of hesitation phenomena in the speech of a child or adult may or may not indicate that he or she has a fluency disorder. While all of them can be symptoms of a fluency disorder, some are more likely to be than others.

Decisions about whether hesitation phenomena are normal or symptoms of a fluency disorder can be difficult to make reliably. This is particularly likely to be the case for preschool-age children. The reason is that many (perhaps most) children between the ages of two and five go through a phase in their language development where they repeat sounds, single-syllable words, and the first syllable of multisyllable words a great deal. Children who are beginning to stutter also do so. A mistake in diagnosis here can have serious consequences—either keeping a child from receiving appropriate intervention or, perhaps worse yet, precipitating stuttering (see chapters 5 and 8).

A number of factors can influence the likelihood of at least some of the hesitation phenomena in a person's speech being regarded as symptoms of a fluency disorder. These include:

- the types of hesitation phenomena

- the person's chronological age

- the person's mental age

- the person's speaking rate

- the presence of neurological or psychological trauma that could have precipitated a fluency disorder

- the belief that a person has a genetic predisposition for a fluency disorder

- the frequency at which particular types of hesitation phenomena occur

- the longest durations for individual moments of hesitation (i.e., disfluency)

- the amount of tension usually accompaning the hesitation phenomena that are considered abnormal

- the person's awareness of and concern about hesitation phenomena in his or her speech
- the presence of "secondaries" while moments of disfluency are occurring
- the person's motivation to avoid being disfluent
- the predisposition of a person's listeners to regard some of his or her hesitation phenomena as symptoms of a fluency disorder
- the person's motivation to "fake" a fluency disorder

Some of the ways that each of these have been shown to affect judgments about the normality of hesitation phenomena are discussed below.

The Types of Hesitation Phenomena

Some types of hesitation phenomena (disfluencies) are more likely than others to be considered symptoms of a fluency disorder. Those that are probably most likely to be considered symptoms of a fluency disorder are *tense pauses, part-word repetitions, single-syllable word repetitions*, and *dysrhythmic phonations*. Of these four types of hesitation phenomena, only tense pause is almost never observed in the speech of normal speakers. The presence of instances of the other three types of hesitation phenomena in the speech of persons who don't have a fluency disorder (particularly preschool-age children) is far from rare.

The Person's Chronological Age

The more frequently the four types of hesitation phenomena mentioned above occur in a person's speech, the more likely he or she is to be regarded as having a fluency disorder. These phenomena tend to occur more often in the speech of preschool children than in that of older children and adults. Consequently, preschool-age children tend to be at greater risk of having these types of hesitation phenomena considered symptoms of a fluency disorder than are older children or adults.

The Person's Mental Age

The amount of syllable repetition concomitant to language development appears to vary as a function of mental age. For children whose cognitive development is in the normal range, the peak tends to occur somewhere between the ages of two and five. For children who are mentally retarded, however, it tends to occur later. Frequent syllable repetition in a preschooler is probably less likely to be considered a symptom of a fluency disorder than is the same amount of syllable repetition in the speech of an elementary-school-age child. Consequently, children who are cognitively impaired may be at greater risk for having their normal syllable repetitions (that are a concomitant of their language development) labeled stuttering than children who are not so impaired.

The Person's Speaking Rate

If a person habitually speaks at a very rapid rate, is very disfluent while doing so (e.g., has large numbers of part-word repetitions), and appears to be unaware of both speaking excessively rapidly and being excessively disfluent, he or she may have the disorder that has been labeled both *cluttering* and *tachyphemia* (described earlier in this chapter). The term cluttering focuses on a perceived lack of organization in the person's speech and the term tachyphemia its excessive rate.

An excessively slow speaking rate can also be associated with abnormal disfluency, even though none is heard. A person who stutters, for example, may purposefully speak at a very slow rate because doing so enables him or her to avoid at least some moments of stuttering. When a person who stutters purposefully speaks in a nonhabitual manner (e.g., at an abnormally slow rate), he or she is likely to stutter less severely. This type of coping strategy, unfortunately, tends to lose its effectiveness when the nonhabitual way of talking becomes habitual (see chapter 2).

The Presence of Neurological or Psychological Trauma that Could Precipitate a Fluency Disorder

Abnormal disfluency can be precipitated by events that result in neurological damage and/or psychological trauma. While both children and adults can evince abnormal disfluency for these reasons, it is more common for adults to do so than for children. If the event that precipitated the abnormal disfluency is a neurological one, the client probably will be diagnosed as having *neurogenic acquired stuttering*. If the event that precipitated the abnormal disfluency is psychological, the client probably will be diagnosed as having *psychogenic acquired stuttering*.

The Belief that a Person Has a Genetic Predisposition for a Fluency Disorder

A person who is assumed to have a genetic predisposition for a fluency disorder is probably at greater risk than otherwise for having some of the hesitation phenomena in his or her speech labeled abnormal. Following are two reasons why they may be so labeled:

- They are abnormal. The etiology of cluttering is widely assumed to be genetic, and many speech-language pathologists believe that genetic factors contribute to the etiology of at least some cases of stuttering. There is a history of stuttering in the families of many persons who have the disorder (see chapter 5).

- They are normal, but listeners assume that they are abnormal. Labeling them as such, incidentally, may actually cause the speech of these persons to become abnormal (see the discussions of the diagnosogenic theory in chapters 5 and 8).

The Frequency at which Hesitation Phenomena Occur

The more frequently hesitation phenomena occur, the more likely they are to be labeled abnormal. Be aware, however, that frequency alone may not be a particularly good indicator of whether such phenomena are normal or abnormal. There is, for example, overlap between persons labeled stutterers and those labeled nonstutterers for frequencies of most types of hesitation phenomena, particularly at the preschool-age level. Representative data on the frequency of occurrence of hesitation phenomena in the spontaneous speech of preschool, elementary school, and adult male stutterers and nonstutterers are presented in tables 1-1, 1-2, and 1-3. The same types of data are reported in all three tables. The only differences are the age levels of the subjects from whom speech samples were elicited and whether data were reported for tense pause. For a particular type in a particular group, the *lowest index* is the frequency of disfluencies per 100 words spoken by the subject who had the fewest occurrences; the *highest index* is the frequency found in the subject who had the most occurrences; Q_2 (the median) is the frequency exceeded by 50 percent of the subjects; Q_1 is the frequency exceeded by 75 percent of the subjects; and Q_3 is the frequency exceeded by 25 percent of the subjects.

These data indicate that among preschoolers (table 1-1), elementary schoolers (table 1-2), and adults (table 1-3), the "typical" person (the one designated by Q_2) who stutters is disfluent more often than his or her "typical" nonstuttering peer. For all three age groups, the median disfluency frequency in "all categories" for the stutterers exceeded that for the nonstutterers. This finding should not be particularly surprising, since excessive disfluency is almost universally considered a defining characteristic of stuttering.

Although the typical stutterer is disfluent more often than the typical nonstutterer, there is overlap between the groups. That is, there are persons who are not regarded by themselves or others as stutterers, yet who hesitate more often than persons who are regarded by themselves and others as being stutterers. Twenty-five percent of the elementary school nonstutterers, for example, hesitated more often than 25 percent of the elementary school stutterers (see table 1-2): that is, the frequency exceeded by 25 percent of the nonstutterers (6.1) was greater than that for 25 percent of the stutterers (4.2). This same trend also was evinced by the preschoolers and adults.

Table 1-1   Range and quartile distribution of the frequency indices of disfluency (number of disfluencies per 100 words) for each of the six disfluency (hesitation) types and for all types combined for 68 young male stutterers (MS) and 68 matched young male nonstutterers (MN). The majority of the subjects in both groups were *preschoolers*. The values for Q_1 and Q_3 are interpolations from the decile distribution in which the data are reported.

Disfluency Category and Group	Lowest Index	Quartiles			Highest Index
		Q_1	Q_2	Q_3	
Interjections					
MS	0.0	1.6	2.9	4.9	15.2
MN	0.0	1.0	2.0	4.6	12.7
Part-Word Repetitions					
MS	0.0	1.2	3.1	6.8	36.6
MN	0.0	0.1	0.6	0.8	2.4
Word Repetitions					
MS	0.0	2.2	3.2	5.8	14.8
MN	0.0	0.4	1.0	1.6	4.6
Phrase Repetitions					
MS	0.0	0.4	1.0	1.7	7.1
MN	0.0	0.1	0.5	0.9	2.5
Revisions–Incomplete Phrases					
MS	0.0	0.5	1.1	2.5	6.9
MN	0.0	0.6	1.1	2.3	8.8
Disrhythmic Phonations					
MS	0.0	0.1	0.6	1.9	20.0
MN	0.0	0.0	0.0	0.2	2.0
All Categories					
MS	3.3	9.5	13.6	24.5	46.5
MN	0.6	3.8	7.1	10.2	18.3

Source: From Johnson & Associates, 1959, p. 206.

Let's now consider the hesitation phenomena individually (see tables 1-1, 1-2, and 1-3). There is considerable overlap between the groups of stutterers and of nonstutterers for four types: word repetitions, phrase repetitions, revisions–incomplete phrases, and interjections. For part-word repetition and disrhythmic phonation, the overlap between the groups isn't as great as for the others.

Durations for Individual Moments of Hesitation (i.e., Disfluency)

Speakers not only differ in how often they are disfluent, but also in how long their moments of disfluency tend to last. For example, speak-

Table 1-2 Range and quartile distribution of the frequency indices of disfluency (number of disfluencies per 100 words) for each of the seven disfluency (hesitation) types and for all types combined for 56 elementary-school male stutterers (MS) and 56 matched elementary-school male nonstutterers (MN).

Disfluency Category and Group	Lowest Index	Quartiles			Highest Index
		Q_1	Q_2	Q_3	
Interjections					
MS	0.0	0.0	0.0	0.2	3.2
MN	0.0	0.0	0.0	0.1	2.2
Part-Word Repetitions					
MS	0.0	1.0	1.9	5.3	21.2
MN	0.0	0.4	0.9	1.7	4.7
Word Repetitions					
MS	0.0	0.0	1.0	3.1	12.5
MN	0.0	0.0	0.4	0.9	1.8
Phrase Repetitions					
MS	0.0	0.0	0.0	1.0	3.2
MN	0.0	0.0	0.0	0.9	2.3
Revisions–Incomplete Phrases					
MS	0.0	0.0	1.0	2.1	4.2
MN	0.0	0.9	1.5	3.0	6.1
Disrhythmic Phonations					
MS	0.0	0.0	0.5	1.5	40.0
MN	0.0	0.0	0.0	0.6	3.0
Tense Pauses					
MS	0.0	0.0	0.0	0.0	5.6
MN	0.0	0.0	0.0	0.0	0.6
All Categories					
MS	0.0	4.2	7.3	13.7	80.0
MN	0.0	2.6	3.5	6.1	16.7

Source: From Silverman, 1974.

ers differ in the maximum number of times they tend to repeat words and part-words and in the maximum number of seconds their disrhythmic phonations tend to last.

The "typical" (median) stutterer's word and part-word repetitions and dysrhythmic phonations tend to last longer than those of the "typical" (median) nonstutterer (Johnson, 1961; Johnson and Associates, 1959). However, there appears to be some overlap between stutterers and nonstutterers with regard to how long their longest moments of disfluency tend to last. Some nonstutterers, particularly preschoolers, occasionally repeat sounds, syllables, and single-syllable words more

Table 1-3   Range and quartile distribution of the frequency indices of disfluency (number of disfluencies per 100 words) for each of the six disfluency (hesitation) types and for all types combined for 50 adult male stutterers (MS) and 50 matched adult male nonstutterers (MN). The values for Q_1 and Q_3 are interpolations from the decile distribution in which the data are reported.

Disfluency Category and Group	Lowest Index	Quartiles			Highest Index
		Q_1	Q_2	Q_3	
Interjections					
MS	0.0	3.0	7.2	15.0	71.6
MN	0.0	1.4	2.6	6.8	15.3
Part-Word Repetitions					
MS	0.0	1.9	4.2	9.5	52.2
MN	0.0	0.0	0.2	0.4	1.2
Word Repetitions					
MS	0.0	1.3	3.1	5.3	13.5
MN	0.0	0.3	0.6	1.2	2.5
Phrase Repetitions					
MS	0.0	0.3	0.9	1.9	5.5
MN	0.0	0.0	0.2	0.6	1.3
Revisions–Incomplete Phrases					
MS	0.0	0.9	1.2	2.1	32.0
MN	0.3	0.7	1.2	2.1	5.6
Disrhythmic Phonations					
MS	0.0	0.0	0.7	4.0	37.4
MN	0.0	0.0	0.0	0.0	1.0
All Categories					
MS	4.6	12.6	22.6	40.3	135.8
MN	0.7	3.4	6.6	9.3	19.9

Source: From Johnson, 1961, p. 10 & 14.

than four times (Silverman, 1972b). Some stutterers rarely, if ever, make such repetitions more than once or twice. Similar overlap exists between groups for the duration of sound prolongations. It would then appear that the presence of occasional words and part-words that are repeated a relatively large number of times and/or occasional disrhythmic phonations that are relatively long, by themselves, would not allow persons who stutter to be differentiated reliably from their normal-speaking peers.

The Degree of Tension while Being Disfluent

A speaker may appear relatively relaxed while being disfluent or may produce audible and/or visible signs of tensing during at least some of his or her disfluencies. Such tensing can be manifested in a number of ways (singly or in combination), including tense pauses, audible tension (strain) evinced in the voice while speaking, abnormally rapid rates of syllable repetition, audible manifestations of irregularities in breathing, and visible manifestations of excessive tensing of muscle groups in the speech mechanism and elsewhere.

Frequently evincing a significant degree of tension while being disfluent appears to differentiate persons who stutter (or who are at risk of developing stuttering) from their normal-speaking peers (Bloodstein, 1987; Starkweather, 1987; Van Riper, 1973). It also appears to differentiate stuttering from cluttering, neurogenic acquired stuttering, and psychogenic acquired stuttering. A significant degree of tension isn't a usual concomitant of the disfluency of persons who have one of these three disorders.

Awareness of and Concern about One's Hesitation Phenomena

While a person's awareness of and concern about hesitation phenomena in his or her speech provide some support for the conclusion that he or she has a fluency disorder or is at risk for developing one, the opposite is not necessarily true. Children who are beginning to stutter usually are neither aware of nor concerned about the syllable repetitions and other hesitation phenomena in their speech. Furthermore, persons who evince cluttering appear to have little or no awareness of either their excessive speaking rate or the resultant disfluency.

Secondary Symptoms ("Secondaries") Accompanying Moments of Disfluency

Moments of disfluency in the speech of stutterers frequently are accompanied by movements (gestures) not needed for producing the phonemes in the message. These extraneous movements sometimes are referred to as *secondary symptoms* or *secondaries*. Such movements can involve the musculature of the speech mechanism, the head and neck, and the extremities and also can involve utterances of sounds, words, or phrases that are not a part of the message being communicated. Examples of movements involving the speech mechanism would be pressing the lips together when attempting to produce phonemes that are not bilabials and attempting to speak with inadequate breath support. Examples involving the head and neck would be closing the eyes and moving the head back. Those involving the extremities would be swinging an arm or tapping a foot. Examples of extraneous sounds, words, or phrases would be single or multiple productions of a vowel such as the schwa, a word such as "well," or a phrase such as "it is." Such utterances may be devices that the stutterer uses to keep from stuttering or has used in the past for this purpose and, although no longer working, have become a habitual part of this person's stuttering behavior.

Secondary symptoms rarely accompany moments of disfluency in the speech of persons whose fluency disorder is cluttering, neurogenic acquired stuttering, or psychogenic acquired stuttering. When persons having one of these fluency disorders do evince secondary symptoms, the reason may be that stuttering has been overlaid on their original disorder—for example, their abnormal moments of disfluency may be precipitated by both stuttering and cluttering (Freund, 1966).

The Strength of the Person's Desire to Avoid Being Disfluent

Desiring to avoid being disfluent can increase stuttering severity. (Stutterers tend to stutter most when they want to stutter least!) It can also place a person (particularly a child) at risk for developing the disorder (see chapters 5 and 7). Consequently, reports or observations of increases in disfluency at times when a client strongly desires to avoid being disfluent would be consistent with a diagnosis of stuttering. Some situations in which a client may be so motivated are described in chapter 2.

Some persons whose disorder is cluttering tend to become *more fluent* when they desire to speak well (Weiss, 1964). Their increase in fluency appears to be related to a reduction in speaking rate.

A desire to avoid being disfluent appears to have little, or no, impact on the hesitation phenomena of persons whose disorder is neurogenic acquired stuttering or psychogenic acquired stuttering, unless an overlay of stuttering is present.

A Predisposition to Expect Some Hesitation Phenomena to Be Symptoms of a Fluency Disorder

The adage "Seek and ye shall find" is applicable here. If, for example, there were a history of stuttering in a family, the syllable repetitions of a young child born into that family would more likely be labeled (and reacted to as) stuttering by his or her parents than would be the case otherwise. This is thought to explain at least partially why there is a history of stuttering in the families of some persons who stutter (see the discussion of the diagnosogenic theory in chapter 5).

This factor does not appear to affect judgments about the normality of hesitation phenomena in the speech of persons whose disorder is cluttering, neurogenic acquired stuttering, or psychogenic acquired stuttering.

The Person's Motivation to "Fake" a Fluency Disorder

There have been a few reports of persons faking a fluency disorder (Shirkey, 1987; Bloodstein, 1988). Whenever a client is involved in a situation (e.g., civil or criminal litigation) from which he or she would benefit by having some of his or her hesitation phenomena certified as being abnormal, the possibility of malingering should be considered.

FLUENCY DISORDERS AS IMPAIRMENTS, DISABILITIES, AND HANDICAPS

The World Health Organization (WHO) has advocated a framework for assessing the impacts of disorders on those who have them and their families in three ways—as impairments, as disabilities, and as handicaps. Impairments are "losses or abnormalities of body function and structure"; disabilities are "limitations of activities"; and handicaps are "restrictions of participation" (Boyce, Broers, & Paterson, 2001, p. 3). I'll be using this WHO framework for organizing our discussion of ways in which a fluency disorder can affect a client and his or her family. It's useful to view the impacts of disorders in these three ways because doing so increases the likelihood that we'll identify therapy goals, other than reducing abnormal disfluency, that would best serve the client and/or members of his or her family.

Fluency Disorders as Impairments

The *abnormality in body function* that fluency disorders yield can be an abnormally high frequency of the kinds of hesitation phenomena found in the speech of persons who do not have a fluency disorder, or the presence of hesitation phenomena that would rarely, if ever, be found in the speech of such persons (e.g., tense pauses or "broken" words), or both of these. It would also include, in the case of cluttering, an abnormally rapid speaking rate.

Elimination of the "abnormality" (i.e., the fluency disorder) would only sometimes eliminate the disability and the handicap associated with it. That is, a reduction in the severity of the stuttering or other abnormal disfluency wouldn't necessarily result in an equivalent reduction in the amount of disability or handicap. The reduction in disability and handicap could be either greater or less than what would be anticipated. There can, in fact, be a significant reduction in disability and/or handicap with no reduction in impairment! Some implications of a less-than-perfect relationship between these three variables for the management of fluency disorders are discussed in chapter 7 and elsewhere in the book.

Fluency Disorders as Disabilities

The activity that fluency disorders limit (i.e., interfere with) is communication. Their interference with communication can range from minimal to severe. An example of minimal interference would be the speaker being negatively stereotyped, but he or she would rarely (if ever) have difficulty making himself or herself understood. An example of interference at the severe end of the continuum would be the speaker having considerable difficulty making himself or herself understood. Be aware, however, that persons who have a fluency disorder—even a relatively severe one—are rarely completely unable to make themselves understood through speech.

It sometimes is possible to lessen a "limitation of activities" (i.e., the disability) from a fluency disorder. As an example, some persons who stutter severely are limited in their ability to communicate by telephone. They can lessen this limitation to their activities by, at least occasionally, using their state's telecommunication relay service (Silverman, 1999b).

Fluency Disorders as Handicaps

Fluency disorders can *restrict participation* in activities and, thereby, cause persons who have them to be handicapped. A restriction on participation in an activity may be imposed by somebody other than the person who has the disorder or by the person himself or herself. More often than not, the latter is partially or completely the cause. In other words, it is the person's attitude, not the person's disability, that restricts his or her participation in activities. The handicap is self-imposed!

For example, while persons who have a fluency disorder may have reality-based reasons for avoiding certain vocations or avocations, most of those fields avoided by persons with whom I've worked were ones in which they probably could have performed competently judging, in part, by the success of others who have such disorders. These fields include medicine, nursing, law, teaching, politics, sales, social work, theater, sports, business administration, writing, and speech pathology. Some persons who were very successful in their fields despite having a fluency disorder were King George VI of England, Winston Churchill, V. I. Lenin, Theodore Roosevelt, Washington Irving (author), George Washington, Charles Lamb (author), Charles Darwin, Moses, Aesop, Virgil, Aristotle, Demosthenes, and Napoleon the First. Other prominent persons with fluency disorders include Michael Ramsey (one hundredth Archbishop of Canterbury), Mel Tillis (country-western singer), Lewis Carroll (author), Marilyn Monroe (actress), Clara Barton (founder of the Red Cross), Somerset Maugham (author), Moses Mendelssohn (eighteenth-century Jewish philosopher), Annie Glenn (wife of U.S. Senator and astronaut John Glenn), Carly Simon (composer-performer), and John Updike (author).

The correlation (relationship) between the severity of the impairment and disability from a fluency disorder and the severity of the handicap resulting from it is far from perfect. Some persons for whom the degree of impairment and disability are minimal are far more handicapped by their disorder than are some for whom the degree of impairment and disability is severe. Some implications for the management of fluency disorders of this less-than-perfect relationship between degree of handicap and degree of impairment and disability are discussed in chapter 7 and elsewhere in the book.

ASSIGNMENTS

Stuttering Simulation

This chapter has introduced you to fluency disorders. To develop a deeper understanding of the impact that having this disorder can have on a person, I recommend that you simulate stuttering in at least three situations and observe the effect it has on communication, how other people react to you, and how you feel about their reactions.

How typical are the experiences of persons who simulate stuttering when compared to those of persons who actually have the disorder? Judging by feedback I have received from hundreds of students who have done this assignment and others (see Ham, 1990a; Hulit, 1989; Leahy, 1994; Rami, Kalinowski, Stuart, & Rastatter, 2003), they tend to be quite representative. This conclusion is also based both on my experiences as a stutterer and on those of persons with fluency disorders whom I have treated.

Identification of Hesitation Phenomena

Watch a videotape of a person who has a fluency disorder reading a passage, and on a copy of the passage mark each word on which a hesitation phenomenon occurred, indicating the type. Have a fellow student (or some other person) also do this task. How well do your judgments agree? Why are there disagreements? Is your identification and cataloging of hesitation phenomena reliable enough for clinical purposes?

Delayed Auditory Feedback

While the simulation assignment described above provides insight into how people react to persons who have fluency disorders and how those who have them are likely to react to their reactions, it does not provide insight into what it is like to be unable to speak fluently. One way that you can gain this insight is to speak while your auditory feedback is being delayed. The instrumentation used for this purpose is a special audiotape recorder that plays back through headphones what a person says a fraction of a second (usually approximately 0.2

seconds) after he or she says it. Most normal speakers experience some disruption in their speech fluency when they attempt to speak under this condition. As well as you can describe them in words, what are your reactions to not being able to control your fluency—that is, to speak fluently?

Autobiography

Another way that you can gain some insight into how stuttering and other fluency disorders can affect a person's life is by reading autobiographical articles and books, such as those by Johnson (1930) and Tillis and Wager (1984).

Depiction of Persons Who Have a Fluency Disorder in the Arts and Literature

One way to gain a little insight into how persons who have a fluency disorder are viewed in a particular culture is to observe how they are portrayed in the arts and literature of that culture. Characters who have them appear in novels, children's books, movies, dramas, popular songs, and operas (Anderson, 1994; Benecken, 1994; Silverman, 1997a; Trotter & Silverman, 1976). For a listing of some of the novels in which they appear, see Trotter and Silverman (1976). How are persons who have a fluency disorder depicted in the arts and literature of your culture? Has the manner in which they are depicted changed during the course of this century? If you feel that it has changed, how so?

2

Symptomatology and Phenomenology of Fluency Disorders

INSTRUCTIONAL OBJECTIVES

By the end of this chapter, you should be able to:

- Describe several common variations in the symptomatology of fluency disorders.
- Define the term "moment of stuttering" and state several ways that this concept can be utilized clinically.
- Describe 11 observable behaviors that can occur during moments of stuttering.
- Specify nine characteristics of words that can cause the nonrandom distribution of moments of stuttering.
- Describe the expectancy (anticipation) phenomenon.
- Describe 19 conditions under which stuttering severity decreases at least temporarily.
- Describe 12 conditions under which stuttering severity increases at least temporarily.
- Define the term *secondary behavior* (symptom) and describe at least four that can accompany moments of stuttering.
- Describe physiological anomalies during respiration, phonation, and articulation that could affect moments of stuttering.
- Describe self-perception (psychological) concomitants of moments of stuttering.

> ▸ Describe essential aspects of the symptomatology and phenomenology of cluttering.
> ▸ Describe essential aspects of the symptomatology and phenomenology of neurogenic acquired stuttering.
> ▸ Describe essential aspects of the symptomatology and phenomenology of psychogenic acquired stuttering.

A necessary condition for someone to be diagnosed as having a fluency disorder is for there to be hesitation phenomena in their speech, all or some of the time, that are not considered normal by the person doing the diagnosing. This chapter focuses on a number of attributes of the hesitation phenomena and other abnormal behavior evinced by persons who have one or more of the following disorders: stuttering, cluttering, neurogenic acquired stuttering, or psychogenic acquired stuttering. This information is needed both to establish which fluency disorder(s) a client has and to be maximally helpful to him or her (see chapters 6 and 7).

It's important while reading this chapter to keep in mind that the symptomatology of a particular fluency disorder is not the same for all persons who have it. Nor will the symptomatology of a client's fluency disorder and his or her reaction to it necessarily remain the same over time. This lack of sameness was conveyed rather well, metaphorically, by a STUTT-L participant:

> Stuttering is something we are given to work with in our lives, and what each person does with it is unique to them and appropriate for them. Give a hundred people a blank canvas and a palette of paints and you'll get a hundred different paintings. Give a hundred people stuttering to deal with and you get a hundred different ways that it is displayed, felt, experienced, fought, embraced, worked with, and accepted. Pretty neat.

More information is available about the symptomatology and phenomenology of stuttering than of any of the other fluency disorders. Therefore, the amount of such information presented here is greater than that presented about any of the other fluency disorders.

SYMPTOMATOLOGY AND PHENOMENOLOGY OF STUTTERING

Few stutterers, if any, stutter on all the words they say (see Johnson, 1961; Johnson & Associates, 1959; Silverman, 1974). While speech-language pathologists agree that almost all stutterers appear at times to be saying some words and utterances fluently, they often disagree on the percentages of words on which stuttering occurs in particular speech samples (see Cordes & Ingham, 1994, for a review of the literature on the identification and measurement of moments of stuttering). Those who attempt to determine these percentages from audiotape recordings may identify fewer moments of stuttering than those who derive them from videotapes, introspective reports, and various types of physiological recordings.

We will refer in this section to periods of time during which stuttering appears to be occurring as *moments of stuttering*. These periods are also referred to as stutterings, instances of stuttering, stuttering events, and stuttering blocks. They are regarded by stutterers as being involuntary. Their duration can range from slightly less than one second to several minutes. It is sometimes difficult to specify the exact duration of moments of stuttering because of uncertainty about where they begin and end. There is wide variability from stutterer to stutterer with regard to the behaviors that occur during these moments (Starkweather, 1987). While one could argue that the moment of stuttering continues to be an accepted entity (judging by the frequency with which it has been referred to in recent papers published in the *Journal of Fluency Disorders* and other professional and research journals), there are data that suggest that for some stutterers periods of speech between moments of stuttering may contain perceptible or physiological abnormalities (van Lieshout, Peters, Starkweather, & Hulstijn, 1993). The degree of abnormality that was observed in most of these studies was relatively small (McClean, 1990).

Not all stutterers have moments of stuttering that can be detected by listeners. Some who have relatively mild cases can conceal their stuttering by substituting words for those on which they expect to stutter and/or by using other avoidance techniques. Nevertheless, such closet stutterers can be significantly disabled and handicapped by their disorder. As a STUTT-L participant commented:

> What do closet stutterers do when they stutter? Nothing. They don't stutter. They avoid, they live in fear, they have a complex inner life of feeling and emotion that they themselves do not fully understand (as do we all!). I had a close friend who was a closet stutterer, who NEVER stuttered but lived in CONSTANT FEAR OF BEING FOUND OUT. I never heard him stutter for the first four YEARS I knew him. He had unusual, creative, distinctive speech patterns—that's what everyone's impression of him was. Nobody knew he had a stuttering problem. The one and only time I heard him stutter, he was reading aloud before a group of people and stuttered on the one word, WEPT. Then he kept reading. As soon as he was finished he got up and quietly left—I learned later that he went home in anguish, crying. I believe the inner experience of covert stuttering for some people is greatly underestimated.

The section begins with descriptions of those behaviors that occur during moments of stuttering that can be seen and/or heard by a listener. Next, conditions that influence the location (loci) and frequency of moments of stuttering are described. Finally, the moment of stuttering is described from two other perspectives—physiological and introspective.

Why is it necessary to view the moment of stuttering from several perspectives in order to understand it? Because by doing so one can obtain a more complete description. As the fable about the six blind men and the elephant in chapter 1 demonstrates, the description of a phenomenon (such as the moment of stuttering) is determined in large part by the perspectives from which it is viewed.

Observable Behaviors Occurring during Moments of Stuttering

A number of types of behavior that can be seen and/or heard occur during moments of stuttering. Some of these are hesitation phenomena that also occur in the speech of normal speakers (see chapter 1). Our focus in this section will be on the occurrence of such behaviors during moments of stuttering.

Sound, syllable, and word repetitions

One of the behaviors of which listeners are likely to be aware is repetition of sounds, syllables, and words (particularly single-syllable ones). These are observable in the speech of young children who are beginning to stutter as well as in that of persons in their seventies who have stuttered all their lives (Johnson, 1961; Johnson & Associates, 1959). Most repetitions occur on the initial syllables of words and almost never occur on their final syllables (Lebrun & Van Borsel, 1990; Stansfield, 1995). The number of times a sound, syllable, or word is repeated (the number of units of repetition) by most stutterers is usually five or fewer (Van Riper, 1982). The person may appear relatively relaxed while repeating or relatively tense. Children are more likely than adults to appear relaxed while repeating (Bloodstein, 1987). If the person is tense while repeating, one or more of the sounds during each repetition may be prolonged or otherwise spoken disrhythmically (Van Riper, 1982).

Disrhythmic phonations

As mentioned in chapter 1, this phenomenon includes any disturbances in the normal rhythm or timing of elements in words other than sound and syllable repetitions (Williams, et al., 1968). Hence, this is a within-word rather than a between-word phenomenon. It is also a "wastebasket" category because it includes all the abnormalities in timing and rhythm that occur during production of words that are not repetitions. The two most frequently occurring behaviors in this category are prolongations and "broken" words (pauses within words that usually occur between syllables).

Prolongations usually occur on the initial sounds of words and almost never on the final sounds (Bloodstein, 1987). While they can last almost any length of time, most are less than five seconds (Sheehan, 1974). They may begin with a complete, or almost complete, blockage of airflow though the articulators (Van Riper, 1982). (Because of this blockage, moments of stuttering containing them sometimes are referred to as "blocks.") Such blockages are particularly likely to occur during the production of plosive sounds and often are accompanied by visible tensing in muscle groups that are not directly involved with respiration, phonation, or articulation. While such tensing can occur in almost any muscle group, it usually involves the musculature of the face and neck. For example, a stutterer may tightly close his or her eyes during such a blockage.

Abnormal pauses within words—usually between syllables—are referred to as *broken words* (Johnson, 1961). Most pauses tend to be shorter than five seconds. They may be silent or the person may produce some sound during them. If they are not silent, the sounds produced may or may not be the ones in the next syllable of the word. During such pauses, there is often observable tensing of muscle groups (particularly in the facial area) that are not directly involved with respiration, phonation, or articulation

Tense pauses

These are abnormally long pauses between words, during which sound caused by tensing of muscles in the speech mechanism, particularly the larynx, is evident (Williams, et al., 1968). They usually occur before words in which the person appears to be having difficulty saying (initiating breath flow for) the initial sound. The duration of these pauses is usually less than five seconds, and the tensing associated with them may be evident visually as well as auditorily. It may, in fact, be more evident visually than auditorily.

The mechanism underlying these pauses appears to be the same as that underlying broken words. With both, pauses tend to occur because the person is having difficulty saying (initiating breath flow for) the next sound.

Incomplete phrases

These are utterances that a person begins but does not complete. An example would be the statement, "I want a . . . ." (Johnson, 1961). Incomplete phrases occur in the speech of both normal speakers and stutterers (Johnson, 1961). However, they sometimes occur in the speech of stutterers for a reason that would not apply to the speech of normal speakers—such as the avoidance of stuttering (Van Riper, 1982). If a stutterer feels himself or herself beginning to block or anticipates blocking in an utterance, he or she may decide not to complete the utterance. While doing so may avoid the stuttering, it could confuse the listeners.

Interjections of sounds, syllables, words, or phrases

All speakers occasionally interject into their utterances sounds, sylla-bles, words, and phrases that do not appear to affect the meaning (Johnson, 1961). Examples would be "um," "er," and "you know." Some types of interjection are referred to as *filled pauses*. Interjecting these can be a strategy for holding a listener's attention while deciding what to say next. Some stutterers also use interjections as a device to avoid stuttering (Van Riper, 1982). By interjecting a sound, syllable, word, or phrase before attempting to say a word on which they expect to stut-ter, they believe they can reduce the severity of their stuttering on it. Such interjections are referred to as *starters* (Van Riper, 1982).

Revisions

When speakers realize that they have made an error, they are likely to correct it, particularly if they believe that not doing so could cause their message to be misunderstood (Johnson, 1961). Some stutterers tend to avoid revising errors if they believe that they are likely to stut-ter while doing so (Silverman & Williams, 1973). In addition, some of them use revision as a device to reduce the severity of the stuttering. When they begin to stutter on a word they do not complete it, but instead substitute a synonym they think they can say more fluently (Van Riper, 1982).

Abnormal speaking rate

There are several reasons why stutterers may have relatively slow speaking rates. One is the act of stuttering itself. Since stuttering blocks consume time, their presence obviously reduces speaking rate. Another reason why they may speak relatively slowly is to reduce the severity of their stuttering. Some stutterers tend to stutter less severely when they speak slowly (Bloodstein, 1987). Other stutterers use an abnormally rapid speaking rate as a device to avoid stuttering. They appear to believe that if they pause they are likely to stutter more severely (Van Riper, 1982).

Abnormal loudness or pitch level

One occasionally encounters a stutterer whose speech is usually abnormally loud or soft or whose voice is abnormally high- or low-pitched for his or her age and sex. While these behaviors may not be related to the person's stuttering, they may be devices that he or she is purposefully using to reduce stuttering severity (Van Riper, 1982).

Tensing of muscle groups uninvolved with speech production

Tensing of muscle groups that are not involved with respiration, pho-nation, or articulation may occur during moments of stuttering (Van Riper, 1982). Such tensing may or may not be visually obvious. Visually observable movements (i.e., gestures) associated with such tensing include closing the eyes and moving the head backward. An example that would not be visually obvious (without special instrumentation) would be tensing of the musculature of the ear, particularly that of the tympanic membrane.

While authorities agree that such tensing occurs, they do not agree on the reasons for it. One hypothesis is that the person is either currently using it as a device to reduce stuttering severity or has used it in the past for this purpose and, although it no longer works, it has become an habitual component of the person's moments of stuttering (Wingate, 1964; Brutten & Shoemaker, 1967).

Use of gestures
Some evidence exists that adult stutterers tend to gesture less and include less detail in their gestures during moments of stuttering than they would otherwise (Shenker, Mayberry, Scobble, Grothe, & White, 1994).

Distribution of Moments of Stuttering in the Speech Sequence
Moments of stuttering are not distributed randomly in the speech sequence. They are more likely to occur at some locations (loci) than at others (Brown, 1945). A location in this context can be a word or a syllable within a word.

Why is it important that moments of stuttering are more likely to occur on words possessing certain attributes than on others and on some syllables of words than on others? The main reason is that this phenomenon tends to make some explanations (theories) for the etiology of stuttering more plausible than others. Those who propose theories for the etiology of stuttering must explain how they would account for what is known about the phenomenology of the disorder if they want their theories to be taken seriously. Since the approaches clinicians use for managing stuttering should be influenced by their beliefs about its etiology (Williams, 1968), the presence of such phenomena could have clinical as well as theoretical implications.

While stuttering tends to occur on certain words and at certain locations within words more often than would be expected by chance, it is important to remember that it can occur on any word and at any location within a word. Some of the characteristics (attributes) of words and syllables that have been shown to influence the loci of moments of stuttering are described below.

The position of a word in an utterance
Moments of stuttering are considerably more likely to occur at some word positions in utterances (sentences) than at others. They occur more often on the first, second, or third words of utterances than

would be expected by chance—that is, if their distribution based on this attribute were random (Brown, 1945). This is true for both school-age and adult stutterers during both oral reading and spontaneous speech (Wingate, 1982). Word position, incidentally, is the only attribute discussed in this section that does not appear to influence the distribution of hesitations in the speech of normal speakers in the same way as it does the speech of stutterers (Silverman & Williams, 1967; Williams, Silverman, & Kools, 1969b). Hence, the tendency to be considerably more disfluent at the beginning of an utterance than at other positions in the utterance appears to be a characteristic of stuttering rather than of disfluency in general.

Do the sentences on which stuttering tends to occur on the first three words differ from others? There is some evidence (Gaines, Runyan, & Meyers, 1991) that they tend to be ones that are both relatively long and grammatically complex.

The grammatical function of a word

Moments of stuttering during both oral reading and spontaneous speech are more likely to occur on *lexical* words (nouns, verbs, adverbs, and adjectives) than on *function* words (articles, prepositions, conjunctions, and pronouns) when the relative frequencies of occurrence of these two types of words are taken into consideration (Brown, 1945; Williams, et al., 1969b). This is true for both school-age children and adults who stutter (Brown, 1945; Williams, et al., 1969b). It also is true for hesitations (disfluencies) in the spontaneous speech and oral reading of school-age children and adults who do not stutter (Silverman & Williams, 1967; Williams, et al., 1969b). This phenomenon, therefore, appears to be a characteristic of speech disfluency in general rather than of stuttering specifically.

The length of a word

Moments of stuttering during both oral reading and spontaneous speech are more likely to occur on relatively *long* words than on relatively *short* ones, when the relative frequency with which these two types of words occur is taken into consideration (Brown, 1945). This is true for both school-age children and adults (Brown, 1945; Williams, et al., 1969b). It also is true for hesitations (disfluencies) in the spontaneous speech and oral reading of school-age children and adults who do not stutter (Silverman & Williams, 1967; Williams, et al., 1969b). Thus, this phenomenon, like grammatical function, appears to be a characteristic of speech disfluency rather than just of stuttering.

The initial phoneme of a word

Moments of stuttering during both oral reading and spontaneous speech are more likely to occur on words beginning with *consonants* than with *vowels*, when the frequency with which words beginning with consonants and vowels occur is taken into consideration (Brown, 1945). This is true for both school-age children and adults (Brown, 1945; Williams, et al., 1969b). It also is true for hesitations (disfluencies) in the spontaneous speech and oral reading of school-age children who do not stutter (Silverman & Williams, 1967; Williams, et al., 1969b). The cause does not appear to be phonological difficulty, at least for young children who stutter (Throneburg, Yairi, & Paden, 1994). This phenomenon, like grammatical function and word length, appears to be a characteristic of speech disfluency in general rather than of stuttering.

The speaker's degree of familiarity with a word

There is some evidence suggesting that both stutterers and nonstutterers are less likely to be disfluent on words with which they are familiar than on those with which they are not familiar, particularly during oral reading (Hubbard & Prins, 1994). This finding, if replicated, would suggest that difficulties with word retrieval and/or phonological encoding can precipitate moments of stuttering (Hubbard & Prins, 1994).

Syllable stress

Moments of stuttering on polysyllabic words appear more likely to occur on stressed syllables than on unstressed ones (Prins, Hubbard, & Krause, 1991). Perhaps this is why moments of stuttering rarely occur on the final syllable of polysyllabic English words.

The consistency effect

Moments of stuttering, during both oral reading and spontaneous speech, occur on words on which they occurred previously more often than would be expected by chance (Johnson & Knott, 1937b). This phenomenon, which is referred to as the consistency effect, is present in the speech of both school-age children and adults (Johnson & Knott, 1937b; Williams, Silverman, & Kools, 1969a). This also appears to be true for hesitations (disfluencies) in the spontaneous speech and oral reading of persons who do not stutter (Williams, et al., 1969a). Consequently, this phenomenon—like grammatical function, word length, and initial phoneme—appears to be a characteristic of speech disfluency in general rather than just of stuttering.

The location within a word

Moments of stuttering during both oral reading and spontaneous speech are more likely to occur on the *initial syllables* of multisyllable words than on any of their other syllables (Starkweather, 1987). They almost never occur on final syllables (Lebrun & Van Borsel, 1990).

Distance from previously stuttered words

For some stutterers, moments of stuttering tend to occur in clusters more often than would be expected by chance. This phenomenon has been observed in the speech of children as well as that of adults (Hubbard & Yairi, 1988).

The Expectancy (Anticipation) Phenomenon

The tendency for moments of stuttering not to be distributed randomly may be at least partially due to the *expectancy (anticipation) phenomenon*. This is the ability exhibited by some stutterers to predict *with greater than chance accuracy* the words on which they are going to stutter (Johnson & Sinn, 1937; Johnson & Solomon, 1937; Knott, Johnson, & Webster, 1937; Van Riper, 1936). The words "greater than chance accuracy" are italicized above because few, if any, stutterers appear able to predict *all* of their moments of stuttering (Johnson & Sinn, 1937; Johnson & Solomon, 1937; Knott, et al., 1937; Van Riper, 1936). This ability is not observed as frequently in children as in adults (Silverman & Williams, 1972a). Anticipatory physiological changes prior to stuttering that are correlated with such predictions have been observed in some stutterers (Baumgartner & Brutten, 1983). Some authorities believe that this phenomenon contributes to the precipitation of stuttering (see chapter 5).

When stutterers anticipate stuttering on a word, they may substitute another for it to avoid stuttering. This technique is of limited usefulness. As several STUTT-L participants commented:

> I was really good at word substitution. That trick no doubt helped me build a massive vocabulary. My tenth-grade English teacher wrote in my yearbook "Bob—the biggest vocabulary I've seen in 30 years of teaching."

> I became a walking thesaurus. Indeed, I could not have existed without word substitution. My world fell apart when, as a young police officer, I was required to give evidence in court. The experience was horrendous, as I stood for several minutes (it seemed liked hours) attempting to say the second word of the oath. ("I sssssssssssssswear"). It also contained many other words that I would, generally, have avoided like the plague, but I had no alternative. My day of reckoning had finally arrived. One cannot substitute the name of the defendant; the date and time of the offence; the location of the illegal occurrence; the make and registration of the motor vehicle; the defendant's oral responses, etc.

> I hated the way I looked when I stuttered—the closing of eyes, the looking up at the ceiling to force a word out, the tongue doing crazy things, the way my lips formed different shapes trying to say my troubled words, the stamping of my foot, my hand pounding on the desk in school to try and force a word out, etc.—not to mention the

way I sounded. I felt ugly and embarrassed. I felt inferior to others. I thought others would think I was stupid, or something was wrong with me. It was seeing the awkwardness in my listener's eyes that drove me to be covert. Their looks of surprise and wonderment made me think stuttering was a bad thing. What were they thinking? Do they think I am stupid? Are they embarrassed to be around me? So if I couldn't control the way my words came out, I would change the words and carefully select which words to say. I would often "lie" about my name, where I have been, where I was going, what I had for lunch, etc. . . . just to avoid feeling like an idiot and feel accepted. Heck, I still do that. I am a living Thesaurus!

Conditions under Which Stuttering Severity Decreases

Stutterers tend to stutter more severely under some conditions than under others (Andrews et al., 1983). While there are individual variations with respect to how specific conditions influence stuttering severity, there are some conditions that appear to affect the majority of stutterers similarly—that is, to increase or reduce their stuttering severity.

Why is it important that stuttering severity varies in a predictable manner under certain conditions? One reason is that such phenomena (like those associated with the distribution of moments of stuttering) tend to make some explanations (theories) for the etiology of stuttering more plausible than others. Another is that they have been incorporated into intervention strategies to reduce stuttering severity. These phenomena, therefore, have clinical as well as theoretical implications.

A number of conditions under which stuttering severity tends to decrease are described below.

Speaking in a nonhabitual (novel) manner

If stutterers modify their speaking behavior in any way, the result is likely to be a temporary reduction in stuttering severity (Bloodstein, 1987). Such a reduction can last as long as several years (see Silverman, 1976b).

In what ways have stutterers modified their habitual speaking behavior that have resulted in increased fluency? They have changed their speaking rate, in most cases reducing it; changed their pitch; whispered; simulated accents; changed the intonational pattern of their speech—as in speaking in a monotone or in a "sing-song" manner; and prolonged vowel sounds. They have also interjected sounds, syllables, words, and/or phrases before words on which they expected to stutter and have accompanied speech with movements such as arm swinging.

Reading in chorus

Few, if any, stutterers will stutter while reading aloud in chorus (unison) with someone (Barber, 1939; Johnson & Rosen, 1937). The person with whom they read can be a normal speaker or another stutterer.

Even if the other person is a stutterer, neither person is likely to stutter when reading in unison. When the second person stops reading with the stutterer, he or she will usually begin stuttering again almost immediately. Choral reading differs from most of the other conditions described in this section because its ability to facilitate fluency does not seem to wear off.

"Shadowing"

Some stutterers become more fluent while "shadowing" or concurrently repeating, another person's speech (Andrews et al., 1983). Shadowing is the spontaneous speech equivalent of reading in chorus. A variation of shadowing is speaking in chorus with one's echo: This phenomenon, incidentally, has been widely used in Poland as a component of treatment programs for stuttering (Adamczyk, 1994).

Singing

Few stutterers, if any, stutter while singing (Andrews et al., 1983). I have worked with two extremely severe stutterers who sang semiprofessionally and neither stuttered while doing so. Mel Tillis, a contemporary country-western singer who is a moderately severe stutterer, apparently never stutters while singing.

Some clinicians who treated stuttering during the first half of the twentieth century utilized this phenomenon in their therapy programs. They encouraged stutterers to speak in a "singsong" manner (Eldridge, 1968; Van Riper, 1973). While this strategy may have reduced stuttering severity (at least temporarily), it probably caused more adverse attention to be called to these people than did their stuttering.

Using a metronome

Many stutterers stutter less frequently (at least initially) when they pace their speech with a metronome—one word or syllable per beat (Andrews et al., 1983; Johnson & Rosen, 1937). The metronome beat can be delivered auditorily, visually, tactilely, or by some combination of these senses. The effect for some stutterers, however, wears off after a period of time (Silverman, 1976b). Some normal speakers also tend to be disfluent less frequently while speaking under this condition (Silverman, 1971b).

Since the early part of the nineteenth century stutterers periodically have been encouraged to pace their speech with the beats of a miniature metronome (Wingate, 1976). There was considerable interest in this approach during the late 1960s and early 1970s (Brady, 1971; Silverman & Trotter, 1973a, 1973b, 1974, 1975). Miniature electronic metronomes intended for this purpose were built into hearing-aid housings (see figure 2-1).

Figure 2-1   Behind-the-ear hearing-aid housing containing a metronome
intended for stutterers.

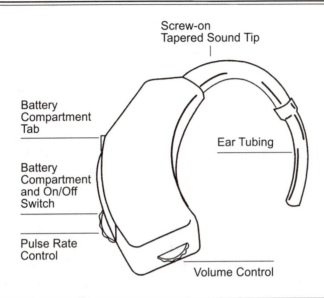

Screw-on
Tapered Sound Tip

Battery
Compartment
Tab

Ear Tubing

Battery
Compartment
and On/Off
Switch

Pulse Rate
Control

Volume Control

Speaking in the presence of loud masking noise

Many stutterers tend to stutter less severely (at least temporarily)
while speaking in the presence of masking ("white") noise that presumably is loud enough to keep them from hearing their own speech
(Cherry & Sayers, 1956). The masking noise may be generated by
either an audiometer or a device specifically designed for this purpose.
It is presented to the stutterer binaurally, using either standard-size
headphones or the miniature type used with hearing aids. Some normal speakers also tend to be disfluent less frequently while speaking
under this condition (Silverman & Goodban, 1972).

There have been attempts to utilize this phenomenon in stuttering
therapy (Moore & Adams, 1985; Silverman & Trotter, 1973a, 1973b,
1974, 1975; Walle, 1980). Beginning in the mid-1960s, miniature
masking-noise generators built into body-type hearing-aid housings
were made available to stutterers. Some used manual switches to turn
the sound on and off (Trotter & Lesch, 1967) and others used voice-
actuated units (Ingham, Southwood, & Horsburgh, 1981). With the
latter, a small disk-shaped microphone is attached to the neck (usually
using tape disks that are sticky on both sides) over the thyroid cartilage of the larynx. When the stutterer begins to phonate, the microphone detects the vibration and turns on the masking noise, and when
he or she stops phonating, the noise is turned off. Some stutterers feel
that they have benefited from using such a device (see Carlisle, 1985).

Experiencing delayed auditory feedback

Some stutterers stutter less severely when they experience delayed auditory feedback while they speak (Andrews et al., 1983; Goldiamond, 1965). Ordinarily, we hear what we say almost immediately after we say it. With delayed auditory feedback we hear what we say a short period of time (usually 0.2 seconds) after we say it. The experience is somewhat similar to that of speaking in an environment in which there is an echo. The electronic device used for creating delayed auditory feedback functions like an audiotape recorder in all but one significant way: It can "record" and "play back" at the same time. The stutterer talks into a microphone and his or her speech is recorded and played back through headphones a fraction of a second later. The recording may be stored on magnetic tape or in a computer's memory. These devices have been made small enough to be used by stutterers outside of the therapy room (Craven & Ryan, 1984; Kalinowski, 2003; Muellerleile, 1981).

Reducing speaking rate

Some stutterers stutter less severely than usual if they speak slowly (Andrews et al., 1983; Johnson & Rosen, 1937). It has been hypothesized that some of the conditions mentioned in this section (such as pacing speech with a metronome) reduce stuttering severity because they cause stutterers to speak more slowly than usual (Bloodstein, 1987).

Speaking while alone and to animals and young children

Stutterers tend to stutter less severely when they speak or read aloud in an environment where no one can hear them (Porter, 1939). They also have been reported to do so when they speak to animals and very young children (Andrews et al., 1983).

Articulating without phonating (lipped speech)

Some stutterers stutter less severely if they do not phonate while producing the articulatory gestures required for speech (Commodore & Cooper, 1978).

Speaking in a monotone

Some stutterers stutter less severely if they speak or read in a monotone—a type of speech pattern in which each syllable is produced at approximately the same pitch and loudness level (Adams, Sears, & Ramig, 1982).

Speaking a language in which the person tends to be relatively fluent

Many stutterers who are bilingual report that they stutter less severely in one language than the other. This has been confirmed in some cases (e.g., Bernstein-Ratner & Benitez, 1985).

Response-contingent stimulation of stuttering

The operant model of B. F. Skinner indicates that behavior that is learned in a particular way—that which is an operant response—can be manipulated in frequency through response-contingent punishment and reinforcement. Shames and Sherrick published a theoretical paper in 1963 in which they suggested that both normal disfluency and moments of stuttering may be operant responses. Their hypothesis was based in part on a study by Flanagan, Goldiamond, and Azrin (1958) in which the frequency of moments of stuttering was temporarily reduced by contingent presentations of a 105-dB tone.

Following publication of the Shames and Sherrick (1963) paper, there was a great deal of research dealing with the effect of response-contingent presentation of stimuli assumed to be "punishing" on the frequency of various behaviors that occurred during moments of stuttering. A number of types of stimuli were used in this research, including electric shock (Martin & Siegel, 1966a; 1966b), blue light (Martin & Siegel, 1966a, 1966b); verbal punishment, such as saying the word "wrong" (Martin & Siegel, 1966b); loud noise (Flanagan, et al., 1958); intervals of delayed auditory feedback (Goldiamond, 1965); and removal of money (Halvorson, 1971). There also was research in which stimuli assumed to be neutral (e.g., the word "tree") or positive (the word "right") were presented in the same response-contingent manner (Cooper, Cady, & Robbins, 1970).

The findings of these and other studies indicate that response-contingent stimulation of behaviors associated with moments of stuttering, *regardless of the nature of the stimulation,* tends to reduce the frequency at which they occur (Andrews et al., 1983; Shames & Sherrick Jr., 1963; Siegel, 1970). Authorities do not agree about the reason (Bloodstein, 1987). Identical noncontingent stimulation in experimentally naive subjects produces no such effect (Andrews et al., 1983).

Utilizing electromyographic (EMG) biofeedback from speech muscles

Some stutterers stutter less severely while monitoring the degree of tension in parts of their speech musculature utilizing electromyography (EMG) biofeedback instrumentation (Guitar, 1975). EMG biofeedback, as it is used with stutterers, is a procedure for monitoring muscle tension to produce relaxation. Electrodes are attached to the skin over the muscle being monitored and the amount of tension in the muscle is communicated to the client in some concrete manner, such as by the pitch of a tone (for example, the more tense the muscle, the higher the pitch). The client is told to change the feedback stimulus in some way. If it were a tone, he or she would be told to lower its frequency. Doing so would result in the muscle becoming more relaxed.

Not desiring to conceal (avoid) stuttering

For many stutterers, the less important they feel it is to conceal or avoid stuttering, the less severely they tend to stutter (Van Riper, 1982). In fact, when they want to stutter, they may not be able to do so. I once offered a severe stutterer money for each time he stuttered "for real" during a specified time period. He did not stutter even once during the allotted time period but began doing so again immediately after it ended. The following case report (Frankl, 1985) also illustrates this phenomenon:

> A similar case . . . was related to me by a colleague. . . . It was the most severe case of stuttering he had met in his many years of practice. Never in his life, as far as the stutterer could remember, had he been free from his speech trouble, even for a moment, except once. This happened when he was twelve years old and had hooked a ride on a streetcar. When caught by the conductor, he thought that the only way to escape would be to elicit his sympathy, and so he tried to demonstrate that he was just a poor stuttering boy. At that moment, in which he tried to stutter, he was unable to do so. (p. 127)

Perhaps one reason why some stutterers tend to be more fluent while speaking to animals and young children and while alone is that they do not attempt to conceal their stuttering.

Not thinking about or attending to speech

Anecdotal reports from stutterers indicate that there is a decrease in stuttering severity when they are not thinking about or attending to speech (Bloodstein, 1987; Kamhi & McOsker, 1982). There is some evidence that stutterers tend to devote more attention to speech than do nonstutterers—for example, they perform more poorly than the latter on attention-demanding tasks that accompany speech (Kamhi & McOsker, 1982).

Playing a "role"

Stutterers who function as actors or actresses may not stutter while doing so. Among the actors and actresses who had a stuttering problem are Marilyn Monroe and Peter Bonerz (the actor who played Pete the dentist on the Bob Newhart television show in the 1970s). Stutterers who attempt to project an image that they feel is not really their own may stutter less severely while doing so. This is particularly likely to be true if the image they are trying to project is more forceful than their usual one (Fransella, 1972).

Suggestion

If stutterers believe that they will stutter less severely than usual under certain conditions, there is likely to be a *temporary* reduction in their stuttering severity under these conditions (Hulit & Haasler, 1989). The message that causes them to develop this belief could be self-generated or communicated to them while they were in a "waking" or "hypnotic" state (Bloodstein, 1987). Some therapies, incidentally, that use relaxation techniques (see Jacobson, 1938; Wolpe, 1958) tend to produce a state that is similar to, or perhaps identical to, a hypnotic one.

Performing an adaptation task

Most stutterers become progressively more fluent if they repeat a speaking task a number of times, one after the other. An example of such a task would be reading the same passage aloud five times without pausing more than a few seconds between readings (Johnson & Knott, 1937b). Most stutterers would have fewer moments of stuttering during their second reading than during their first and still fewer during their third, fourth, and fifth readings than during either their first or second (see figure 2-2). This phenomenon, which is referred to as the *adaptation effect,* also has been studied using repetitions of a spontaneous speech task (Bloom & Silverman, 1973). The tasks that have been used for this purpose include consecutive repetitions of a single word on which stuttering initially occurs (Silverman & Williams, 1972b) and repeated descriptions (one after the other) of an object or event (Bloom & Silverman, 1973). The latter task differs from the others described in this paragraph in that the word(s) said each time is (are) not exactly the same. Most stutterers do not become as fluent while performing spontaneous speech adaptation tasks as they do while performing oral reading. Some normal speakers also tend to exhibit the adaptation effect (Silverman, 1970a, 1970c, 1970d; Williams, et al., 1968).

Conditions under which Stuttering Severity Increases

A number of conditions that reduce stuttering severity were discussed in the preceding section. There also are conditions that increase the severity of stuttering in many cases, at least temporarily (Young, 1985). Some of them are described in this section.

Speaking on the telephone

Many stutterers tend to stutter more severely than usual while talking on the telephone (James, Brumfitt, & Cudd, 1999). In fact, some stutter so severely that they avoid using the telephone whenever possible. To cope with this problem they have someone (such as their spouse) make calls for them, or they talk to people face-to-face when it would be more sensible to speak with them on the phone. For example, they may travel to stores rather than phone to find out if certain items are available.

Figure 2-2   Performance of a typical stutterer on an oral reading adaptation task.

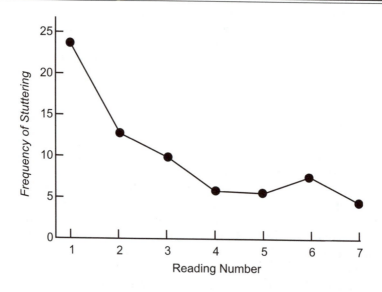

One explanation that has been offered for this phenomenon is that it is due at least in part to the desire to make a good impression (Van Riper, 1982). When stutterers talk to people face-to-face, the listeners' impressions of them are based on both visual and auditory information. Although their speech may not communicate that they are mature, intelligent persons, their visual appearance (such as the way they are dressed) may do so. The impressions people form over the telephone are based solely on auditory data. Hence, stutterers probably have a stronger desire to avoid stuttering while talking on the telephone than they would in other situations. This would tend to increase their stuttering severity on the telephone.

Another explanation offered for this phenomenon is that stutterers fear that people will hang up the telephone if they are unable to initiate speech (Van Riper, 1982). They may have difficulty saying "hello" when they answer the telephone, or they may have difficulty beginning to speak after a person whom they are calling answers. The person being phoned may assume that it is a "crank" call (particularly if he or she hears sounds associated with heavy breathing) and hang up. Obviously, a stutterer who had such a fear would not want to stutter on the telephone, particularly at the beginning of a call, which would tend to increase his or her stuttering severity.

A third possible explanation for this phenomenon is that stutterers feel under pressure to communicate quickly while speaking on the telephone. Consequently, they wouldn't want to stutter because doing so makes it take longer to communicate. This desire to avoid stuttering tends to increase their stuttering severity.

Saying one's name
Many stutterers stutter relatively severely when they say their name (Bloodstein, 1987). This occurs both when they are asked their name and when they voluntarily say it (as when introducing themselves). They also may do so when they say their address and telephone number. A strong desire to avoid stuttering and knowing that they cannot do so by substituting or circumlocuting may be the reasons for stuttering in this instance.

Telling jokes
Some stutterers stutter relatively severely when they tell jokes (Van Riper, 1982). They are particularly likely to do so on the punch lines. Since stuttering on a punch line can ruin a joke, the reason for increased stuttering under this condition is probably a strong desire to avoid doing so.

Repeating a misunderstood message
When asked to repeat a message some stutterers tend to stutter more severely than when they say it the first time (Bloodstein, 1987). They may even stutter when repeating a message that they originally said fluently. Perhaps this increased stuttering results from their desire to transmit the message successfully when they repeat it and a belief that stuttering could keep them from doing so.

Waiting to respond
For some stutterers, the longer they have to wait to say something, the more severely they are likely to stutter while doing so (Young, 1985). If they are a member of a group in which people are taking turns introducing themselves, they are more likely to stutter more severely if they are one of the last persons to do so than if they are one of the first. Some stutterers experience an increase in their anxiety level as the time when they will have to introduce themselves gets closer and closer. The increase in stuttering severity that occurs under this condition probably is a function of both the desire not to stutter when introducing oneself and the longer time available to anticipate and fear stuttering while waiting to speak. An increase in anxiety while waiting to respond may not be unique to stutterers. There is some evidence that nonstutterers also experience it (Miller & Watson, 1992).

Speaking to authority figures
Many stutterers tend to stutter more severely when they speak to people whom they regard as authority figures (Bloodstein, 1987). Such per-

sons could include their parents, employers, and teachers. Actually, it could include anyone on whom they want to make a good impression.

Speaking to a relatively large audience

Some stutterers tend to stutter more severely while speaking to a relatively large audience than to a relatively small one (Porter, 1939; Young, 1985). Perhaps this is true, in part, because they have a stronger desire than usual to be fluent while speaking to a such an audience. Others, at times, tend to be relatively fluent while speaking to large audiences. This seems particularly likely to occur if they believe that they are viewed by their listeners as an authority figure and they are willing to bring their stuttering out into the open (Johnson, 1946, 1961).

Failing to bring one's stuttering out into the open

Not acknowledging to their listeners verbally or otherwise—as through a message printed on a T-shirt (Silverman, 1988a; Silverman, Gazzolo, & Peterson, 1990)—that they have a stuttering problem tends to cause many stutterers to stutter more severely (Johnson, 1946, 1961). For this reason, clinicians usually encourage stutterers to bring their stuttering out into the open.

Desiring to avoid stuttering

Stutterers tend to stutter most when they want to stutter least (Williams, 1982). This may partially explain why some of the other conditions mentioned in this section result in increased stuttering.

Spontaneous recovery

The tendency for stutterers to become progressively more fluent during a series of readings of a passage (the adaptation effect) in which the pause between readings lasts no longer than a few seconds has been described in this chapter. If a stutterer pauses for a period of time after reading a passage repeatedly in this manner and then begins to read the passage yet again, he or she probably will stutter more severely during the first reading of the second series than during the final reading of the first series (see figure 2-3). This phenomenon, which is referred to as *spontaneous recovery* (Johnson & Knott, 1937), does not appear to be exhibited by nonstutterers (Silverman & Bloom, 1973). Hence, it seems to be one that does differentiate stuttering from normal speech disfluency (Silverman & Bloom, 1973).

Experiencing positive emotional arousal (excitement)

The conditions discussed in this section thus far are associated with negative emotional arousal (e.g., anxiety). In some cases children's stuttering has reportedly increased in severity under conditions that

Figure 2-3   Spontaneous recovery following adaptation on an oral reading adaptation task. Note that the frequency of stuttering is higher on the sixth reading than on the fifth.

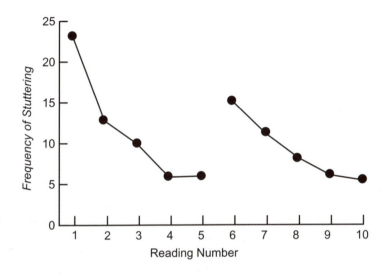

are thought by their parents to generate positive emotional arousal—for example, being excited about their birthday. Whether such an increase in severity results from positive emotional arousal or from the conditions actually producing a negative emotional state is uncertain (Adams, 1992).

Secondary Behaviors (Symptoms) that Accompany Moments of Stuttering

Some behaviors other than disfluencies may occur during moments of stuttering. These behaviors—which are referred to in the stuttering literature as *secondary symptoms* or *secondaries*—more commonly occur in the speech of adult stutterers than in that of preschool-age and primary-school-age children (Van Riper, 1982). Some investigators have questioned whether the difference between children and adults with regard to the presence of secondaries is as large as has been previously assumed (see Yairi, Ambrose, & Niermann, 1993). Observations concerning the presence or absence of secondaries can be helpful when deciding whether a young child is beginning to stutter. Their presence in the disfluent speech of a preschooler would suggest that he or she is doing so (see Conture & Kelly, 1991).

What types of behaviors have been classified as secondaries? Among those that tend to occur most often are:

- looking away from the listener while stuttering; that is, maintaining poor eye contact with the listener (Atkins, 1988)

- jerking or other movements of the head

- blinking (closing) the eyes and/or wrinkling the forehead

- distortions of the mouth (such as pressing the lips tightly together)

- quivering of the nostrils

- interjections of sounds, syllables, words, and phrases that are being used as "starters" and do not contribute to communicating the person's message

- abnormal variations in the loudness and/or pitch of the voice

- abnormal variations in speaking rate

Such behaviors may occur by themselves or in various combinations (Prins & Lohr, 1972).

Why do these behaviors accompany moments of stuttering? The most widely accepted explanation is that they began as devices for avoiding these moments or at least reducing their severity (Bloodstein, 1987). If a stutterer anticipates stuttering on a word, he or she may attempt to avoid it by doing something prior to saying the word, or if the person begins to stutter on a word, he or she may attempt to do something to reduce the duration of the block. A stutterer is likely to continue using the device until he or she no longer believes that doing so will reduce the duration of blocks. By this time, the behavior has become an habitual (learned) component of the blocks. Thus, as mentioned in the previous section, such behaviors may accompany moments of stuttering either because they are being used as devices for coping with moments of stuttering, or because they were used for this purpose in the past but no longer work and have merely become habitual.

Assuming that these devices represent current or past attempts to cope with stuttering, why do they work initially, and why do they subsequently stop working? There are several reasons. First, they cause stutterers to speak in a nonhabitual manner, which causes many stutterers to become more fluent. However, once such a device becomes a habitual part of a stutterer's speaking behavior, it no longer facilitates fluency. A second reason why such devices may eventually stop working has to do with the stutterers' beliefs regarding their efficacy. So long as they believe that a device will in some "magical" way facilitate fluency, it is likely to do so. According to Barbara (1982):

> The various bodily movements and contortions used by a person when he stutters . . . carry with them a sense of implied magic ritual. The pressing of both hands against the sides of the body, the

pinching of himself to get started, the blinking of his eyelids, the placing of the palm of his hand over his mouth, etc., are just some of the many bodily magic gestures used in a particular difficult speaking situation. (p. 50)

However, if a stutterer loses confidence in a device's ability to facilitate fluency, it is likely to cease doing so. *Anticipation of fluency tends to lead to fluency in the same manner that anticipation of stuttering tends to lead to stuttering.*

A third reason why such devices may only work temporarily is a combination of the previous two reasons. Devices initially work because they cause stutterers to speak in a nonhabitual manner. The fluency that they experience while using them causes stutterers to anticipate further fluency. The initial fluency-enhancing effect, therefore, is a function of *both* speaking in a nonhabitual manner and anticipating fluency. Once the nonhabitual manner of speaking begins to become habitual, such devices tend to become less effective. This tends to result in a loss of confidence in stutterers' ability to facilitate fluency, which, in turn, tends to make them less effective at doing so.

A stutterer may continue consciously to use a device beyond the point that it is effective in reducing his or her stuttering severity. This person may believe that using the device tends to make his or her blocks shorter. Obviously, there is no objective way of determining how long a block would have lasted if a device had not been used. He or she may also believe that using the device sometimes prevents stuttering on a particular word. Of course, this person might have been fluent while saying that word without the device. We know that the ability of stutterers to predict their moments of stuttering is far from perfect (Johnson & Sinn, 1937; Johnson & Solomon, 1937; Knott, et al., 1937; Van Riper, 1936). The belief that a device sometimes "works" reinforces its use on a *partial reinforcement schedule* (Brutten & Shoemaker, 1967). The findings of a large number of studies conducted by experimental psychologists suggests that behaviors learned on such a schedule are extremely difficult to extinguish (Brutten & Shoemaker, 1967).

Physiological Events Accompanying Moments of Stuttering

Thus far, we have considered moments of stuttering from the perspective of their observable, or rather acoustic and visual, characteristics. There are several other perspectives from which they can be viewed, one of which is physiological. Moments of stuttering are accompanied by abnormal physiological events that intermittently influence the processes of respiration, phonation, and/or articulation.

Because abnormal physiological events occur during moments of stuttering, it does not necessarily follow that they are at least partially responsible for them. Physiological *consequences* of a psychological process may be the cause of their occurrence. If, for example, moments of stuttering were at least partially caused by anxiety, there would be an increase in the level of activity of the sympathetic division of the autonomic nervous system (Brutten & Shoemaker, 1967). A number of abnormal physiological events tend to occur whenever there is such an increase (Brutten & Shoemaker, 1967).

Some abnormal physiological events associated with respiration, phonation, and articulation that reportedly occur during moments of stuttering are described in this section. Other aspects of physiological functioning that differentiate persons who stutter from their peers are described in chapter 3.

Respiration

Abnormalities in respiratory functioning sometimes occur during moments of stuttering. There were efforts during the first half of this century to partially explain stuttering on this basis. Types of abnormalities include

> . . . antagonisms between abdominal and thoracic breathing, irregularities of consecutive respiratory cycles, prolonged expirations or inspirations, complete cessation of breathing, interruptions of expiration by inspiration, and attempts to speak on intake of air. (Bloodstein, 1987, p. 11)

Most stutterers tend not to exhibit these abnormalities when they are silent or speaking fluently (Bloodstein, 1987).

Phonation

A number of abnormalities in the functioning of the laryngeal mechanism during moments of stuttering have been reported. In fact, there were a number of attempts during the 1970s and 1980s to explain stuttering on the basis of such abnormalities. Among those that are commonly observed clinically are breath-holding and glottal fry. Many stutterers have reported to their clinicians that their "throat closes tightly" during moments of stuttering.

A number of studies on laryngeal functioning during moments of stuttering have utilized instrumentation-based measurement approaches such as electroglottography and electromyography (Borden, Baer, & Kenney, 1985). Among the reported abnormalities in laryngeal functioning during moments of stuttering are:

- breaks in the rhythm of vocal fold vibration and a clonic fluttering of the folds (Borden, et al., 1985)

- vocal folds fixed in either an open or closed position (Conture, McCall, & Brewer, 1977)

- a more gradual buildup in voicing than in fluent utterances (Borden, et al., 1985)
- excessive muscular activity (Freeman & Ushijima, 1978)
- simultaneous contractions of antagonistic (abductor and adductor) laryngeal muscles (Freeman & Ushijima, 1978)

Articulation

The functioning of the articulators during moments of stuttering has been studied extensively using such techniques as electromyography, x-ray motion pictures, and measures of intraoral air pressure and rate of airflow. Among the abnormalities that have been reported are:

- defective synchronization of the action potentials of the paired musculature, such as the masseter muscles (Williams, 1955)
- a buildup of muscular tension, reaching a peak near the termination of a block (Sheehan & Voas, 1954)
- excessive muscular activity (Van Riper, 1982)
- tremors (Van Riper, 1982)
- prolonged articulatory postures on stop consonants (Van Riper, 1982)
- lack of coordination between articulatory movements and onset of phonation (Hutchinson & Watkin, 1976)
- abnormally rapid articulatory movements at the moment of release from a block (Hutchinson & Watkin, 1976)

Psychological (Introspective) Concomitants of Moments of Stuttering

Thus far, we have examined the moment of stuttering from the perspective of listeners and physiologists. One important perspective we have not yet considered is that of persons who stutter. What they experience prior to and during moments of stuttering and how they react to it can influence not only their attitude toward their stuttering, but also their stuttering behavior itself.

Stutterers ordinarily experience their moments of stuttering auditorily and through feelings they report to be associated with muscle tension and anxiety (Brutten & Shoemaker, 1967). These feelings may occur prior to as well as during moments of stuttering. In fact, they may partially explain the ability of many stutterers to predict their moments of stuttering with greater-than-chance accuracy (Johnson & Sinn, 1937; Johnson & Solomon, 1937; Knott, et al., 1937; Van Riper, 1936).

Stutterers' auditory perception of their moments of stuttering

Stutterers probably do not experience their moments of stuttering auditorily in exactly the same manner as do their listeners. Some seem surprised when they hear audiotape recordings of their speech. There could be several reasons for this difference. One is that while they are speaking stutterers are attempting to do things to cope with, or reduce, the severity of their stuttering, which would tend to divert their attention from monitoring their speech auditorily (Van Riper, 1982). Another is that during at least some of their moments of stuttering they experience "a kind of momentary loss of contact" (Bloodstein, 1987, p. 24).

Stutterers' tactile-kinesthetic perception of their moments of stuttering

Stutterers experience their moments of stuttering tactile-kinesthetically as well as auditorily. They experience them as feelings of abnormal muscle tensing (Snidecor, 1955) and as feelings resulting from the articulators touching (contacting) each other with excessive force. If, for example, stutterers were blocking on /f/, they probably would be aware of their upper teeth pressing against their lower lip. If a block is a particularly "hard" one, the stutterer may experience pain. This is particularly likely if a stutterer blocks and bites his or her tongue while producing a voiced or voiceless *th*.

Stutterers may judge the severity of their stuttering in a particular situation as much, if not more, on the basis of how it "feels" than how it "sounds." If they don't perceive much abnormal muscle tension or many "hard contacts" while they speak, stutterers may conclude that their stuttering is not very severe. On the other hand, if they are aware of a great deal of abnormal muscle tensing or a number of hard contacts (particularly those accompanied by pain) while they speak, they are likely to conclude that their stuttering is relatively severe.

We have considered elsewhere in this chapter how a stutterer's desire to avoid stuttering can result in increased stuttering. One reason why a stutterer may desire to avoid stuttering is to avoid the discomfort, the abnormal muscle tensing and hard contacts associated with it. Few people enjoy biting their tongue or lip!

Listeners may not be aware of all a stutterer's stuttering and for this reason will experience it differently than the stutterer does. Some moments of stuttering that are unlikely to be detected by a listener visually or auditorily can be detected by a stutterer who experiences them as abnormal feelings of muscle tensing and/or hard contacts between articulators. People for whom this type of stuttering is predominant are referred to as *internal stutterers* (Freund, 1966).

Stutterers' perceptions of anxiety before moments of stuttering

The preceding section addressed feelings associated with the muscle tensing that occurs *during* moments of stuttering. Similar feelings can also occur *before* moments of stuttering. Such feelings appear to be associated with increases in anxiety level. According to Bloodstein (1987):

> Prior to the block there is often an apprehension of impending difficulty, varying in severity from mild uneasiness to extreme panic. . . . (p. 24)

Whether such apprehension *causes* stutterers to anticipate stuttering or whether it *results* from their doing so has not been established unequivocally.

SYMPTOMATOLOGY AND PHENOMENOLOGY OF CLUTTERING

A number of symptoms and phenomena (speech, language, and behavioral) are evinced by persons who have this disorder. St. Louis and Hinzman (1986) compiled the list in table 2-1 from six publications dealing with the symptomatology and etiology of cluttering. Few persons who clutter are likely to exhibit all of them. However, judging by the data presented in this table and other literature on cluttering (including the study by St. Louis, Hinzman, & Hull, 1985), there are certain symptoms that tend to be manifested by most persons who have the disorder. These include a rapid speaking rate, speech disfluencies (particularly repetitions), a lack of awareness of the disorder (including the disfluencies and the rapid speaking rate), and articulation and language problems. St. Louis and Hinzman (1986) synthesized the following description of persons who have this disorder from the data they distilled from the literature (see table 2-1):

> Their speech is noticeable because it usually sounds "cluttered" as though they are talking without a clear idea of what they want to say. Their conversation is hard to follow because they seem to talk too fast, in a jerky fashion, and seem to run words and sentences together. Clutterers may also repeat sounds, syllables, or phrases excessively. Despite these characteristics, they are typically unaware of any difficulty and may be talkative and outgoing.
>
> Clutterers may also have academic problems in various subjects, yet they may not be severe enough to require specialized educational placement. In fact, some clutterers may excel in certain areas, such as mathematics.
>
> Overall, clutterers seem disorganized, always in a hurry, and unable to concentrate, perhaps due to a poorly developed attention span. In many things a clutterer does—speaking, writing, reading or working at specific activities—there is a curious tendency to function in constant disarray. (pp. 134–135)

The speech disfluency of clutterers differs from that of stutterers in several ways (see table 2-2). The first concerns their level of aware-

Table 2-1.   A Sampling of Symptoms and Other Characteristics that the Literature Associates with Cluttering

Fast speech rate	Interjection overuse
Run-on sentences	Motor coordination problems
Disorganized thinking	Language delay
Irregular speech rate	Learning disabilities
Unawareness of the problem	Struggle during speech
Word repetitions	Neurological impairment
Sound/syllable repetitions	Tension during speech
Phrase repetitions	Prolongations
Inability to get to the point	Handwriting difficulties
Reduced attention span	Family history of cluttering
Revisions	Monotone speech
Academic achievement difficulties	Social maladjustment
Misarticulations	Secondary behaviors
Poor syntax	Poor music abilities
Circumlocutions	

Source: Reprinted from *Journal of Fluency Disorders*, Vol. II, St. Louis, K. O., and Hinzman, A. R., "Studies of Cluttering: Perceptions of Cluttering by Speech-Language Pathologists and Educators," 1986, with permission from Elsevier.

ness of their disfluency: stutterers tend to be aware of their disfluencies, but clutterers do not.

Clutterers, like stutterers, tend to be more fluent in some situations than in others. However, the impact of some situations on their fluency levels is quite different (see table 2-2). While stutterers tend to be *less* fluent when they feel it is important to be fluent, clutterers tend to be *more* fluent in this circumstance. Thus, stutterers tend to be less fluent with authority figures than with young children, and clutterers tend to be less fluent with young children than with authority figures.

Asking clutterers to pay attention to their speech usually results in less disfluency—at least for a few minutes after they are told to do so (see table 2-2). Asking stutterers to attend more to their speech usually results in increased disfluency.

Some children are at higher risk than others to develop cluttering. Like stuttering, more males than females develop the disorder (Myers & St. Louis, 1992); and, also like stuttering, it is more likely to occur in families in which there is a history of the disorder than in those in which there is no such history (Myers & St. Louis, 1992).

As Weiss (1964) and others have noted, clutterers appear to have a language disorder in addition to a fluency disorder. Children who have this disorder are more likely to be delayed in language development than are their peers (Daly, 1992).

Table 2-2 Differences between Stuttering and Cluttering

	Cluttering	Stuttering
Awareness of disorder	Absent	Present
Speaking under stress	Better	Worse
Speaking in relaxed situation	Worse	Better
Calling attention to speech	Better	Worse
Speaking after interruption	Better	Worse
Short answers	Better	Worse
Foreign language	Better	Worse
Reading a well-known text	Worse	Better
Reading an unknown text	Better	Worse
Handwriting	Hasty, repetitious, uninhibited	Contracted, forced, inhibited
Attitude toward own speech	Careless	Fearful
Psychological attitude	Outgoing	Rather withdrawn
Aptitude (academic)	Underachiever	Good to superior
EEG	Often diffuse dysrhythmia	Usually normal
Goal of therapy	Directing attention to speech details	Diverting attention from speech details

Source: From Weiss, 1967.

While stuttering and cluttering are separate disorders, a person can have both. Based on a review of the literature, Daly (1993b) has estimated that between one-third and two-thirds of stutterers exhibit some symptoms associated with cluttering. According to Freund (1966):

> In a typical case of cluttering-stuttering, the expectancy of difficult speech sounds, tonic efforts, postponements and avoidance devices, etc., are much less marked than in typical cases of common . . . stuttering. In the former, the stutter symptoms, consisting usually of quick reiterations often of vowels within or between syllables with not too much effort combined, vary in direct proportion to the severity of the underlying "cluttering." The latter can be clinically defined as an overly hasty and poorly organized speech. (pp. 140–141)

SYMPTOMATOLOGY AND PHENOMENOLOGY OF NEUROGENIC ACQUIRED STUTTERING

The types of abnormal disfluency behaviors observed in the speech of persons who have this disorder include repetitions and/or dysrhythmic phonations. The specific symptomatology is determined, in part, by the neurological condition (site of lesion) with which the disorder is associated. The following three descriptions from published case reports are representative:

1. *A 62-year-old man who had a stroke.* Conversational speech was characterized chiefly by repetitions of syllables and short words and by sound prolongations, for example, "be-be-because," "until-til," and "I was, I was, I was. . . ." Repetitions were dysrhythmic and both clonic and tonic in nature. He frequently attempted to avoid disfluencies by pausing and restarting phrases. (Helm-Estabrooks, 1986, p. 196)

2. *A 22-year-old woman who had an episode diagnosed as viral meningitis.* She stuttered on 95 percent of the words she spoke, repeating initial consonants four to six times and medial consonants three to four times. The stuttering was not specific to any phoneme or group of phonemes. There was no adaptation effect. Whispering made no difference. She demonstrated marked effort in the production of speech but not poor eye contact, distracting sounds, or excessive body movement. (Nowack & Stone, 1987, 142–143)

3. *A 62-year-old man with right cerebral damage.* Disfluency was characterized by sound, syllable, word, and phrase reiterations. Word and phrase repetitions were more frequent than sound and part-word repetitions. The latter occurred primarily in initial position, while word and phrase iterations could occur anywhere in the sentence, including at the end. . . . On one occasion, the target sentence *I can't walk* was actualized as "can't-can't-can't-can't walk-can't-can't-can't walk-can't-can't-walk." Having been asked what a robin was, the patient answered, "A bird-a bird-a-a-a bird-bird-bird-bird, a robin-robin is a bird b-b-b-b-b-bird." Disfluencies were more numerous in spontaneous speech than in repetition and in oral reading. Few iterations occurred in recitation and none could be observed in singing. (Lebrun & Leleux, 1985, p. 138)

While the symptomatology of this disorder appears to vary, in part depending on the neurological condition with which it is associated, are there characteristics other than time and nature of onset that tend to differentiate it from stuttering? Canter (1971) has suggested seven such characteristics, all of which he cautions are *unlikely* to apply to any one client:

1. Repetitions and prolongations are not restricted to initial syllables.

2. The phonemic foci of the disfluency may differ from developmental stuttering, that is, the /r/, /l/, /h/ sounds may be targets for disfluency.

3. There is no particular relationship between disfluency and the grammatical function of words, so that small function words may be as troublesome as substantives.

4. Disfluency is not necessarily in direct relationship to propositionality, so that self-formulated speech may be easier than more automatic speech tasks such as the Lord's Prayer.

5. There is no observed adaptation effect, that is, improved fluency with repeated readings of a passage.

6. The speaker may be annoyed, but not necessarily anxious about his stuttering.

7. There may be no secondary symptomatology such as facial grimacing or fist clenching.

While Lebrun, Leleux, Rousseau, and Devreux (1983) have raised questions concerning whether these are characteristics of the speech of most adults with the disorder, Market, Montague Jr., Buffalo, and Drummond (1990) have reported data supporting this conclusion, particularly for the first, second, sixth, and seventh characteristics.

SYMPTOMATOLOGY AND PHENOMENOLOGY OF PSYCHOGENIC ACQUIRED STUTTERING

Less is known about the symptomatology and phenomenology of psychogenic acquired stuttering than of stuttering, cluttering, and neurogenic acquired stuttering. The following list of symptoms and onset characteristics that *may* at least partially define this disorder was adapted from Deal (1982, p. 304):

1. The onset is sudden.

2. The onset is related to a significant event that could have resulted in extreme psychological stress.

3. The abnormal disfluency behavior consists primarily of repetition of initial or stressed syllables.

4. This disfluency behavior is affected little by choral reading, white noise, delayed auditory feedback, singing, or other conditions that have been reported to influence the disfluency behavior of "ordinary" stutterers.

5. There may be no conditions under which a person who has this disorder is completely fluent.

6. The person may appear to have an indifferent attitude toward the disorder. "He seems to feel no responsibility for what he does. He is relatively detached from the symptom" (Freund, 1966, p. 139). This phenomenon has been referred to in the psychiatric literature as *la belle indifférence* (Roth et al., 1989).

7. The person does not exhibit secondary symptoms. He or she does not appear to avoid sounds, words, or speaking situations.

8. The person maintains normal eye contact (Deal & Doro, 1987).

9. The person may evidence the same pattern of repetitions during mimed reading aloud. This phenomenon also was reported by Deal & Doro (1987). According to Deal (1982):

> The continuation of stuttering-like behaviors during miming may be analogous to Hoover's sign, which is observed in some hysterias. When a supine patient is asked to lift one leg, the other leg also tends to lift; however, this action is absent in patients presenting hysterical paralysis of one leg. It is as if the patient's mind is unaware of body mechanics. By analogy [the patient with this disorder may be unaware] that stuttering-like movements rarely occur when miming words. (p. 304)

Consequently, a typical patient who has this disorder is an adult, with no previous history of stuttering, who suddenly begins to stutter after (or while) experiencing a great deal of psychological stress and who has no neurological condition that could account for the behavior. Furthermore, the patient's disfluency may not vary on a situational basis, and he or she may not exhibit any behavior that indicates a desire to avoid it.

ASSIGNMENTS

Stuttering Checklist

From a videotape of a stutterer reading a passage or doing a spontaneous speech task, select six words on which moments of stuttering occur. Use the Checklist of Stuttering Behaviors (see Appendix C) to catalogue the behaviors that occur during each of these moments. The behaviors you will be cataloging have been described in this chapter. Have a fellow student (or some other person) also do the checklist for these words. How well do your judgments agree? Why are there disagreements? Is your use of the checklist reliable enough for clinical purposes?

Stuttering Severity Rating

Watch a videotape of a stutterer reading a passage or doing a spontaneous speaking task and rate the severity of the stuttering on the Iowa Scale of Severity of Stuttering (see Appendix C). Have a fellow student (or some other person) also perform this task. How well do your severity ratings agree? If they are different, how do you explain the difference? Is your use of this scale reliable enough for clinical purposes?

Cluttering Simulation

One of the main symptoms of cluttering is tachyphemia—a very rapid speaking rate. Speak to a friend or read a passage at a very rapid rate and record yourself doing so. Listen to the recording. What effect did speaking very rapidly have on your speech fluency? Did you repeat syllables and words more frequently than usual? If your rate of repetition increased, how aware were you of it happening while you were speaking?

Delayed Auditory Feedback

Persons who have neurogenic acquired stuttering are disfluent because certain parts of the brain are functioning abnormally. One way that you can temporarily simulate such abnormal brain functioning, thereby enabling you to gain a little insight into what it's like to be unable to speak fluently for this reason, is to speak in the presence of delayed auditory feedback. (A delay in auditory feedback, of course, is not the reason why persons who have this disorder are disfluent.) In addition to speaking with delayed auditory feedback yourself, have a few other nonstutterers do it and describe their reactions to being unable to speak fluently.

3

The Person Who Has a Fluency Disorder

INSTRUCTIONAL OBJECTIVES

By the end of this chapter, you should be able to:

▸ Describe some aspects of the cardiovascular functioning of persons who stutter and compare them to their nonstuttering peers.

▸ Describe some aspects of the biochemical functioning of persons who stutter and compare them to their nonstuttering peers.

▸ Describe some aspects of the central nervous-system functioning of persons who stutter and compare them to their nonstuttering peers.

▸ Describe some aspects of the autonomic nervous-system functioning of persons who stutter and compare them to their nonstuttering peers.

▸ Describe some aspects of the auditory-system functioning of persons who stutter and compare them to their nonstuttering peers.

▸ Describe some aspects of the tactile-kinesthetic functioning of persons who stutter and compare them to their nonstuttering peers.

▸ Describe some aspects of the visual functioning of persons who stutter and compare them to their nonstuttering peers.

> ▸ Describe some aspects of the intelligence of persons who stutter and compare them to their nonstuttering peers.
>
> ▸ Describe some aspects of the emotional adjustment of persons who stutter and compare them to their nonstuttering peers.
>
> ▸ Describe some personality traits of persons who stutter and compare them to their nonstuttering peers.
>
> ▸ Describe the self-concepts of persons who stutter and compare them to those of their nonstuttering peers.
>
> ▸ Describe some speech and language skills of persons who stutter and compare them to their nonstuttering peers.
>
> ▸ Describe essential aspects of the physiological and psychological characteristics of persons who manifest cluttering.
>
> ▸ Descrbe essential aspects of the physiological and psychological characteristics of persons who manifest neurogenic acquired stuttering.
>
> ▸ Describe essential aspects of the physiological and psychological characteristics of persons who manifest psychogenic acquired stuttering.

Do persons who have a particular fluency disorder share anything other than the symptomatology and phenomenology of their abnormal disfluency? That is, do they share any other attributes? This chapter focuses on the literature that addresses these questions.

While there is some overlap between the literature reviewed in this and the preceding chapter, the orientation is different. In this chapter the focus is on the person who has the disorder rather than on his or her hesitation phenomena. Characteristics of persons who have a fluency disorder were discussed in chapter 2 to help explain the symptomatology and phenomenology of their disorder. Relevant data are used in this chapter to help explain how persons who have a particular fluency disorder function physiologically, how they feel about and react to themselves and others, and how they communicate aside from evincing abnormal disfluency.

Because there is more information in the fluency disorder literature about persons who stutter than about those who have one of the other disorders, considerably more information about stutterers appears in this chapter than about those whose disorder is cluttering, neurogenic acquired stuttering, or psychogenic acquired stuttering.

Caution is necessary when interpreting the information presented in this chapter. Even if the majority of persons who have a particular fluency disorder appear to differ in some way from their normal-speaking peers, it is not safe to assume that the difference is related somehow to the etiology of their disorder. It may be the result, for example, of living with the disorder rather than its cause.

A second reason why caution should be exercised is that "mind" and "body" are not independent entities. Physiological differences between groups can result from psychological differences between them and vice versa (Kent, 1983). A difference in anxiety level between groups, for example, can produce a difference between them in physiological events that occur when there is an increase in the level of activity of the sympathetic division of the autonomic nervous system—for example, an increase in the amount of perspiration on the skin (Brutten & Shoemaker, 1967).

It is important for clinicians to be aware of how persons who have a fluency disorder differ from their normal-speaking peers in ways other than speech fluency. There are several reasons. First, it provides them with information they need to formulate hypotheses about the etiology of behaviors they want to modify. Before an intervention strategy for modifying a behavior can be formulated, it is necessary to make an assumption, or formulate a hypothesis, about why it occurs. If the strategies clinicians develop are consistent with their hypotheses and their hypotheses are valid, they are more likely to be successful in modifying the behavior (Williams, 1979).

Second, this awareness can help them understand their clients' attitudes, feelings, and reactions. If they do not, they will tend to be less effective regardless of the therapy approaches they are using (Van Riper, 1979).

Third, it provides clinicians with information they need to identify the *set of behaviors* that defines a client's stuttering problem. This set is likely to include behaviors other than those directly related to the moment of stuttering (Silverman, 1980a, 1980b). While no client is likely to exhibit all the behaviors referred to in this chapter, those mentioned occur often enough that they are worth checking for during an evaluation.

Fourth, the awareness can influence the prognosis for improvement. The presence or absence of certain attitudes, feelings, and reactions can influence (reduce or increase) the likelihood that a client will benefit from therapy (Van Riper, 1979).

THE PERSON WHO STUTTERS

Thousands of studies have been published, during the past and current centuries, in which physiological and psychological attributes of persons who stutter were compared to those of peers who did not stutter. Following is an overview of this literature as well as of the literature on stutterers' speech and language attributes (other than their moments of stuttering).

Physiological Characteristics

While no differences in physiological functioning, other than those that occur during the moment of stuttering, have been demonstrated unequivocally to differentiate persons who stutter from their normal-speaking peers, some investigators believe that there may be such differences. This belief, in part, is based on the findings of a number of studies that report such differences. Also, some believe that investigators may have failed to find them because they searched in the wrong place and/or used methodologies that were not sufficiently sensitive.

If there are physiological differences between persons who stutter and those who don't other than those occurring during moments of stuttering, where would they most likely be found? Since such differences probably would be found where previous research suggests they exist, following is a summary of the findings of studies where such physiological differences have been reported.

Respiration

Because of the obvious anomalies in breathing movements that occur during moments of stuttering, it is not particularly surprising that this was one of the first areas in which investigators searched for a physiological cause for stuttering. Systematic research on the breathing movements of persons who stutter started at the beginning of the twentieth century (Beech & Fransella, 1968). Most research findings support the following conclusions:

- Various kinds of abnormalities in breathing movements may occur during moments of stuttering.

- Breathing patterns of stutterers during fluent speech may be abnormal.

- The same types of breathing abnormalities tend to occur during both moments of stuttering and expectancy of stuttering.

- Patterns of chest wall posturing for phonation exhibited by stutterers are qualitatively identical to those exhibited by nonstutterers.

- Abnormalities observed in the breathing movements of persons who stutter during moments of stuttering usually are not present during silence.

- During silence, the breathing movements of persons who stutter do not differ from those of their normal-speaking peers.

Cardiovascular functioning

Systematic research on the cardiovascular functioning of persons who stutter has been ongoing for more than 75 years. The impetus for much of this research was the finding that the pulse rate of persons who stutter tends to increase (accelerate) before and during moments of stuttering (Fletcher, 1914). Those phenomena investigated that are associated with cardiovascular functioning include pulse rate, heart rate, sinus arrhythmia, blood pressure, and basal metabolic rate. Research findings on cardiovascular functioning while stutterers are silent (and presumably not contemplating speaking) are mixed. While some studies indicate that these cardiovascular-related phenomena differ in some way(s) between stutterers and their normal-speaking peers, others do not.

Biochemical functioning

Research on the chemical makeup of persons who stutter has been ongoing for more than 60 years. Among the biochemical phenomena that have been studied directly or indirectly are alveolar carbon dioxide level, salivary pH, chemical composition of the blood, and plasma levels of adrenergic neurotransmitters and primary amino acids. While some of these studies report differences between stutterers and nonstutterers, others do not.

Central nervous-system functioning

Research on the central nervous-system (CNS) functioning of persons who stutter has been going on for more than 60 years. There were times during this period when differences between stutterers and nonstutterers appeared to have been found. During the 1930s, for example, a number of studies suggested that persons who stutter are less likely than normal speakers to have established unilateral cerebral dominance.

Much of the recent physiological research on stuttering has dealt with central nervous-system functioning (see, Ingham, 2001). Several investigators have reported finding differences between persons who stutter and their nonstuttering peers, some of which are considered in the following paragraphs.

A number of studies of the *cortical potentials* (brain waves) of persons who stutter suggest they may differ from those of their normal-speaking peers during silence, auditory presentation of words, visual presentation of words, anticipation of speaking, and speaking (see table 9 in Bloodstein, 1987, pp. 136–140). However, in most studies there were stutterers whose brain waves (cortical potentials) did not differ from those of normal speakers. Also, the areas of the cerebral cortex in which irregularities were detected were not the same in all studies.

The prevalence of stuttering among persons with known brain damage has been reported to be higher than in the general population (approximately 1.0 percent). This conclusion is based on the findings of a number of studies. The populations surveyed included persons with epilepsy, cerebral palsy, and/or mental deficiency. The prevalence of stuttering in these studies ranged from 1.5 to more than 20 percent.

An aspect of central nervous-system functioning in stutterers on which there has been considerable research is *cerebral lateralization of function* (Penfield & Roberts, 1959). Investigators have used several strategies for determining (directly or indirectly) whether stutterers differ from their normal-speaking peers in the lateralization of certain functions within their cerebral cortex. Aspects of their sensory, motor, and language functioning that are thought to be mediated by either the right or left side of this structure have been studied. These strategies will now be discussed along with the major findings obtained when using them.

One of the first strategies used to investigate cerebral lateralization of function in persons who stutter was to assess their handedness and other manifestations of cerebral sidedness, such as eyedness and footedness. The subjects were required to complete questionnaires and do tasks (such as writing or catching a ball) designed to assess whether they consistently performed them with the hand, foot, and eye on the same side of the body (right or left) or whether they were ambidextrous and lacked a dominant foot and eye. Since the cerebral cortex is responsible, in part, for the performance of such tasks, inferences can be made about the roles of the right and left halves of the cerebral cortex in carrying them out by observing how they are executed. Consistent use of the left side of the body for doing the tasks would indicate that the right side of the cerebral cortex is dominant for hand, foot, and eye functions and vice versa. However, use of both the right and left extremities and eyes for doing tasks would indicate lack of dominance of one side of the cerebral cortex over the other for mediating hand, foot, and eye functions.

Many of the early studies of peripheral sidedness (such as Van Riper, 1935) suggested that persons who stutter, as a group, are less likely than their normal-speaking peers to have established unilateral cerebral dominance; they are more likely to be ambidextrous. This lack of unilateral cerebral dominance was thought to be a cause of stuttering (see chapter 5). It was hypothesized, for example, that left-handed persons who are forced to write with their right hand begin to stutter because becoming skillful with their right hand causes them to become ambidextrous, and as a consequence they lose unilateral cerebral dominance. After 1940, interest in the peripheral sidedness of persons who stutter lessened because of research suggesting that the methodology used in these studies was faulty (Williams, 1955). When these studies were replicated using methodologies regarded as appropriate, stutterers no longer seemed more likely than their peers to lack unilateral cerebral dominance.

Interest in the cerebral lateralization of persons who stutter lay dormant for several decades. There was renewed interest in this topic during the 1960s, in part because of research indicating that cerebral lateralization for speech and language does not necessarily correspond to that for handedness and other aspects of peripheral sidedness (Penfield & Roberts, 1959). Earlier investigators of cerebral lateralization in persons who stutter appeared to have implicitly or explicitly assumed that they could infer lateralization for speech and language from that for handedness, footedness, and eyedness.

The *Wada Test* was one of the first methodologies used during this period to study stutterers' cerebral lateralization for speech and language. This test is used by neurosurgeons preoperatively to determine which half of the cerebral cortex is dominant for these functions (Penfield & Roberts, 1959). Sodium amytal is injected into the right and left carotid arteries, one at a time. The right carotid artery provides the blood supply to the right half of the cerebral cortex, and the left carotid artery provides it to the left half. If a person temporarily loses the ability to speak when sodium amytal is injected into a carotid artery, it is assumed that a center for mediating speech and language is located in the hemisphere of the cerebral cortex to which the artery supplies blood. By injecting sodium amytal into the carotid arteries one at a time it can be determined whether control for speech and language functions is located in the right half of the cerebral cortex, the left half of the cerebral cortex, or both. For most persons it appears to be located in one half of the cerebral cortex, almost always the left (Penfield & Roberts, 1959).

A report was published by a neurosurgeon on four of his patients who stuttered in which he indicated that Wada tests administered before surgery demonstrated a lack of lateralization—that is, all four appeared to have a center for language processing in both hemispheres (Jones, 1966). Investigators who attempted to replicate this finding (such as Rosenfield, Jones, & Liljestrand, 1981) did not detect such a lack of lateralization in any of their stuttering subjects.

A second methodology that was used during this period to study cerebral lateralization in persons who stutter was *dichotic listening*. This task, like the Wada test, was used to infer cerebral lateralization for speech and language processing. It is administered by having the subject listen simultaneously to pairs of different words, one with the right and one with the left ear. Most persons report the words they hear through their right ear more accurately than those they hear through their left ear. Since words heard with the right ear are sent to the left half of the cerebral cortex for processing, the fact that most persons understand more of what they hear with their right than with their left ear provides additional support for the hypothesis that the left hemisphere of the cerebral cortex is usually dominant for speech and language processing.

If, on dichotic listening tasks, persons who stutter do not do as well with their right ear as do normal speakers, this would suggest that the left hemisphere of their cerebral cortex was less dominant than is normal for language processing. In other words, it might indicate that their right hemisphere had a greater-than-normal role in mediating language functioning. It is not surprising, therefore, that a number of investigators have used dichotic listening to test the hypothesis that at least some persons who stutter lack unilateral cerebral dominance for speech and language processing. While the findings of some studies are consistent with this hypothesis, those of others are not. In studies that could be interpreted as supporting the hypothesis, persons who stuttered, as a group, did less well than normal speakers in comprehending words heard through their right ear.

A third methodology that has been used to study cerebral lateralization for speech and language in persons who stutter is electroencephalography. Changes in brain waves (usually alpha waves) that occur in the right hemisphere are compared to those that occur in the left during tasks requiring linguistic processing. Normal speakers tend to evince a larger change in the left than in the right hemisphere while performing such tasks. Some persons who stutter, on the other hand, have been reported to evince a larger change in the right hemisphere than in the left while doing so (Moore, 1986).

One reason why some stutterers may differ from normal speakers in level of right-hemisphere activity is that the tasks may produce more stress (anxiety) in those who stutter than in those who don't. There is some evidence that stress results in greater activation of the right hemisphere (Boberg, Yeudall, Schopflocher, & Bo-Lassen, 1983). Hence, the increase in right-hemisphere brain wave activity evinced by some persons who stutter may have resulted from conditioned anxiety to the receptive/expressive aspects of the speech act rather than from the use of the right hemisphere for language processing (Boberg, et al., 1983).

Several other methodologies have been used to study cerebral lateralization for speech and language in persons who stutter. These include auditory tracking, the presentation of words in different halves of the visual field using a tachistoscopic viewing procedure, and finger tapping with right and left hands while performing speech tasks. The findings of studies that used these methodologies are mixed. Some findings suggest that at least some persons who stutter use their right hemisphere more than normal speakers do to process speech and language. However, those of others did not indicate any differences between groups in this regard. The findings of studies using these methodologies, therefore, are the same as those using the others discussed in this section—that is, although some persons who stutter seem to evince higher levels of right-hemisphere activity on some tasks involving language processing than their normal-speaking peers, the available evidence does not indicate that this is true for all persons who stutter.

The motor capabilities of the speech mechanism are determined, in large part, by the functioning of the central nervous system. Since the musculature of this mechanism functions abnormally during moments of stuttering, it is not particularly surprising that investigators have researched the possibility that persons who stutter have less than normal ability to control the movements of at least some parts of this musculature. Most of the early studies on the motor capabilities of persons who stutter dealt with general bodily coordination. Investigators reasoned that if persons who stutter had a neuromuscular disorder or apraxia that affected their speech mechanism, it would be likely also to affect other parts of their musculature, including that of the upper extremities. While differences were reported in some of these studies between persons who stutter and their nonstuttering peers, they were not reported in others. The findings of these studies, therefore, suggest that the general motor capabilities of some persons who stutter tend to be inferior to those of their normal-speaking peers but do not establish this unequivocally for the majority of them.

During the past 30 years, much of the research on the motor performance of persons who stutter has focused on the musculature of the speech mechanism. Subtle oral-motor coordination differences between them and their normal-speaking peers have been reported, particularly involving the functioning of the larynx (Perkins, Rudas, Johnson, & Bell, 1976; Riley & Riley, 1986). The phrase "oral-motor discoordination" has been used to refer to these differences (Perkins et al., 1976; Riley & Riley, 1986). Many stutterers have been reported to exhibit such abnormalities in laryngeal functioning during moments of stuttering. From time to time hypotheses have been advanced suggesting that stuttering results from some disturbance in the functioning of the laryngeal mechanism. A relatively large number of studies have been published during the past 30 years that were designed, at least in part, to determine whether stutterers differ from nonstutterers with regard to phonatory reaction time—the time it takes a person to initiate or terminate phonation after being given a signal to do so. While the findings of most of these studies indicate that the typical (mean or median) stutterer tends to be slower than the typical normal speaker, they also indicate that some overlap exists between groups. That is, some stutterers have faster phonatory reaction times than some normal speakers. There is also some evidence, incidentally, that stutterers who tend to have relatively slow phonatory reaction times also tend to have relatively slow reaction times for nonspeech movements (Cross & Luper, 1983).

Autonomic nervous-system functioning

For more than 50 years investigators have been interested in the possibility that abnormalities in the functioning of the autonomic nervous
system contribute to the etiology of stuttering. Interest in this possibility is not particularly surprising, considering that the level of activity of its sympathetic division is positively related to anxiety (Brutten
& Shoemaker, 1967) and that some explanations for the moment of
stuttering attribute it, at least in part, to anxiety (see chapter 5).

Seeman (1934) was one of the first to look into the possibility that
an abnormality in the functioning of the autonomic nervous system
could contribute to the etiology of stuttering. He believed that such an
abnormality could do so by causing the sympathetic division to become
hyperactive, or more irritable than normal. His hypothesis received
some support from the findings of several studies of stutterers' sympathetic reactivity during silence. Unfortunately, the numbers of stutterers evincing particular abnormalities in these studies were not
compared to those in matched control groups of normal speakers.
While there is a paucity of studies designed to determine whether
stutterers differ from nonstutterers in sympathetic division reactivity,
it is possible that some stutterers have a tendency toward higher-
than-normal levels of such reactivity, resulting in lower thresholds for
autonomic response to stress.

Auditory functioning

Even though the prevalence of stuttering in the hearing-impaired
population appears to be lower than that in the general population
(Andrews et al., 1983), a number of investigators have looked into
the possibility that persons who stutter have an anomaly in their
auditory system that somehow contributes to the etiology of their
disorder. Aspects of auditory functioning that have been investigated include: threshold for pure tones; relative phase angle of air-
and bone-conducted sounds; and right-ear versus left-ear presentation of stimuli—as in dichotic listening, effect of delayed auditory
feedback on oral activity not involving speech, central auditory functioning at the level of the brainstem, and reflex response of the middle ear muscles to sound. The findings of these studies, like those for
all aspects of the physiological functioning of persons who stutter,
are mixed. While some investigators who have researched a particular aspect of auditory functioning report differences between persons
who stutter and their peers, others do not. Incidentally, in many of
the studies in which a group difference was reported, the author(s)
concluded that the subjects who stuttered behaved more like their
normal-speaking peers then they did like persons who were known
to have auditory-system lesions. Perhaps, as some investigators
have speculated, the reported differences in auditory functioning

between persons who stutter and those who do not result, in part, from differences in anxiety levels.

Tactile-kinesthetic functioning

A disturbance in tactile-kinesthetic feedback can have a detrimental effect on the performance of motor acts. While such acts are occurring, information is continuously being sent to the brain from receptors in the muscles and the skin about the state of contraction of the various muscles and the location in space of the various structures involved in performing the acts. Could a disturbance in tactile-kinesthetic feedback disrupt movements of the articulators and vocal folds in a way that would cause a breakdown in speech fluency? A few investigators have attempted to answer this question. The aspects of tactile-kinesthetic functioning that they studied included threshold for vibratory sensation, intra-oral two-point discrimination, and oral recognition of forms. The findings of their studies (like those of the other aspects of physiological functioning discussed in this chapter) are mixed. While the available evidence does not rule out the possibility that a disturbance in tactile-kinesthetic feedback contributes to the etiology of stuttering, neither does it provide strong support for the existence of such an etiologic factor.

Visual functioning

A number of investigators have studied the visual performance of persons who stutter. While the functioning of the eyes and central visual nervous system is only indirectly related to that of the speech mechanism, differences between persons who stutter and those who do not during the performance of visual tasks could point to differences between them in central nervous system functioning for speech.

The aspects of visual functioning that have been studied in persons who stutter include: visual acuity, phoria, binocular perception, color vision, visual perseveration, and perception of visual symbols. In addition, there has been research on the prevalence of stuttering among persons who are blind and partially sighted. The findings of these studies suggest that the prevalence of stuttering among blind and partially sighted persons is the same as that in the general population and that the visual acuity, phoria, binocular perception, and color vision of persons who stutter are within normal limits. It is uncertain, however, whether the performance of persons who stutter is within normal limits on visual perseveration and visual symbol perception tasks. While the findings of some studies suggest that they perform differently than normal speakers on the tasks, those of others do not. Consequently these findings are, as for most other aspects of physiological functioning discussed in this chapter, mixed.

Psychological Characteristics

There are few, if any, psychological attributes that have not been discussed somewhere in the stuttering literature. Many are discussed in autobiographies of persons who stutter (see Carlisle, 1985; Johnson, 1930; Murray & Edwards, 1980; Wedberg, 1956). Many are also discussed in the writings of clinicians who have treated persons who stutter, including those of psychiatrists, psychologists, and speech pathologists. In addition, a great deal of information about such attributes has been published in research journals, particularly those in the fields of speech pathology, psychology, and psychiatry. This section makes use of information from all these sources.

Intelligence

While most estimates of the average I.Q. of stutterers that have been reported fall in the general region of 100 (the theoretical average for the population at large), in studies in which they have been compared to nonstutterers their I.Q.s tended to be slightly lower, approximately half a standard deviation. This deficit is evident in both verbal and nonverbal intelligence tests.

The prevalence of stuttering among the mentally retarded (i.e., cognitively impaired) that has been reported in some studies (see Bloodstein, 1987, table 20) is approximately three percent. This exceeds the rate in the general population, which is approximately one percent.

Emotional adjustment

While the available data (both clinical and research) do not provide strong support for the conclusion that stuttering is usually a symptom of a neurosis or other type of emotional disorder, they do not rule out the possibility. These data come from two sources. The first is from studies in which persons who stutter were evaluated for the presence of psychopathology by means of psychological tests. The second is from studies and case reports in which the impact of psychotherapy on stuttering was reported.

There have been many studies in which psychological tests were administered to persons who stutter by investigators who wanted to determine whether they have a type of psychopathology of which stuttering could be a symptom. The findings of many of these studies indicate that persons who stutter, as a group, tend to be a little less well adjusted than their normal-speaking peers, but they are more similar to nonstutterers than to persons who are known to be emotionally disturbed.

Several factors could have contributed to stutterers appearing less well adjusted than their peers on some of these tests. One was the inclusion of items that relate to attitudes toward speaking (such as "Do you find it difficult to speak in public?"). Most older children and adults who stutter are aware that, in at least some situations, they tend to have poorer speech skills than nonstutterers (Watson, 1988). Therefore, they are likely to respond "inappropriately" to such items for different reasons than do normal speakers who are emotionally disturbed. A second factor was their being less well adjusted than nonstutterers as a consequence of living with stuttering. Living with almost any disability can adversely affect a person's emotional adjustment.

Another type of evidence that supports the conclusion that stuttering usually is not a symptom of some type of emotional disorder are reports addressing the impact of psychotherapy on stuttering. If stuttering were a symptom of an emotional disorder, we would expect it to be reduced considerably in severity or eliminated by "successful" psychotherapy, particularly successful psychoanalysis. Reports in the literature about the impact of psychoanalysis and other forms of psychotherapy on stuttering do not indicate that it is often successful by itself in eliminating the disorder or dramatically reducing its severity. *This should not be interpreted to mean that persons who stutter are unlikely to benefit from psychotherapy*; many have benefited from it. However, the ways in which they do so are unlikely to include the amelioration of their stuttering.

While the available evidence does not support the conclusion that stuttering is a symptom of psychopathology for the majority of persons who stutter, it does not disprove that it may be such for some persons. There are case reports suggesting that it can be such a symptom (see Van Riper, 1979). Also, the available evidence does not disprove that there are stutterers who are severely emotionally disturbed. The prevalence of severe emotional disturbance in the stuttering population is at least as great as that in the general population. Finally, the available evidence does not disprove that the emotional adjustment of persons who stutter influences the severity of their stuttering. It undoubtedly does do so for at least some persons who stutter.

Personality traits

While there has been considerable speculation (particularly in the psychiatric literature) about personality traits common to persons who stutter, their presence has not been established empirically. There is no personality trait that almost all persons who stutter have been shown unequivocally to possess (Bloodstein, 1987). However, there are some traits that many of them appear to possess. The reason may be, in part, that they have been reacted to negatively in a similar manner by their normal-speaking peers—for example, they have often been teased, mocked, laughed at, patronized, and treated as intellectually inferior.

Many persons who stutter are *not as outgoing* as they probably would be if they did not have the disorder. This is not particularly surprising, considering how they are perceived and consequently reacted to by some people with whom they interact. They tend to avoid social situations in which they expect people to react negatively to them because they stutter; and when they do enter such situations, they tend to talk less than they would if they did not stutter. They are particularly likely to avoid social interactions that involve talking on the telephone—a situation in which most stutterers tend to stutter relatively severely (see chapter 2). There is a little evidence, however, that at least some tend to become less concerned about their stuttering—and, consequently, less likely to avoid talking because of it—after they are 50 years old (Manning, Dailey, & Wallace, 1984).

Is it an abnormal tendency on the part of many stutterers to avoid situations in which they would have to do a lot of talking? While it increases the extent to which they are handicapped by their stuttering problem, it does not appear, in most cases, to indicate the presence of psychopathology. It is normal to try to avoid pain—both physical and psychological! Since persons who stutter are likely to experience negative reactions to their stuttering as pain, and since most of them probably are not masochists, their attempts to reduce the pain in their lives by avoiding talking (and, hence, stuttering) whenever possible are understandable. The problem is that the price they pay for avoiding this source of pain may be too high. It can, for example, cause them to choose an occupation in which they will not have to do much talking, particularly on the telephone. Since most relatively high-paying jobs in our society do entail a great deal of talking (including on the telephone), their choice of a job that does not require much talking can adversely affect them economically.

A second way that persons who stutter may pay too high a price for avoiding this source of pain is restricting their social relationships—including romantic relationships. Many teenage (and older) males who stutter, for example, avoid dating because of concern about how their date will react to their stuttering, particularly if they would have to make the date by telephone (Carlisle, 1985). One way that a speech-language pathologist can be helpful to such persons is to increase their awareness of the price they are paying for avoiding this source of pain.

While many persons who stutter are not very outgoing, there are some who are so in spite of reactions to their stuttering. They sometimes choose occupations in which the ability to communicate well is important, including teaching, law, medicine, sales, speech pathology, psychology, social work, entertainment, accounting, politics, and the ministry. They may also choose avocations that cause them to be actively involved with various groups in their community.

A second personality trait shared by many persons who stutter is *unwillingness to express anger openly when doing so would be appro-*

priate (Barbara, 1982). This trait, which appears to result from living with stuttering, can influence its severity. The more anger they feel and the less willing they are to express it openly, the more severely they are likely to stutter. The effect of openly expressing anger on fluency can be dramatic—very few people tend to stutter while they are swearing! Why might many persons who stutter sometimes be unwilling to express anger openly? One reason may be that they believe people will not like them as well if they do so. That is, they believe that openly expressing anger will cause them to be rejected (Rubin, 1969).

A third personality trait that is shared by many stutterers is depression related to coping with stuttering. The depression they evince, of course, is not solely from this source. Stutterers can be depressed for the same reasons as their normal-speaking peers—both psychological and biochemical. Why might stuttering cause clients to be depressed? There are several possible reasons. First, they may be depressed as a consequence of the grieving process (Tanner, 1980). This is a normal, predictable, healing process that people go through when they experience a loss. The first stage is denial, the second is anger, the third is bargaining, the fourth is depression, and the fifth is acceptance. The loss that the stutterer has sustained is the ability to speak normally and all that this implies for interpersonal relationships. While the length of time people normally spend at each stage of this process can vary considerably, depending on the nature of the loss and their ability to cope, some persons remain at a particular stage so long that it is likely that they have become _fixated_ (Tanner, 1980). Some persons who stutter appear to have become fixated at the depression stage (Johnson, 1946). They have not reached the acceptance stage at which they would accept the fact that they stutter, then do what they can to reduce its severity, and get on with their lives.

A second reason why stuttering may cause clients (particularly adults) to become depressed is that they believe their failure to overcome stuttering is their fault. That is, they believe it is possible to overcome stuttering, and their failure to do so means that they have not tried hard enough or are too weak-willed. The belief that it should be possible to cure their stuttering could have been based on information from any of several sources, including books about the disorder (such as Schwartz, 1976; Schwartz & Carter, 1986) and statements made to them by speech-language pathologists and other clinicians. Their belief may not be accurate (Cooper, 1987).

A third reason why clients may experience depression because of stuttering is that they are overreacting to their disfluency, possibly because they are perfectionists—that is, they are reacting more negatively to it than others are likely to. Some persons who have become quite fluent as a result of therapy experience depression from this very source. Rather than comparing their present fluency level to what it was before therapy and feeling good about what they have accomplished, these persons compare their present fluency level to an idealized level of perfect fluency. As a result, they perceive themselves as having failed and become depressed. Such persons have what Johnson (1946) referred to as the "IFD disease," going from idealism to frustration to demoralization. Their internal standard for acceptable fluency is vague and/or unrealistically high. Either would result in their judging their fluency as unacceptable, which, in turn, would lead to frustration and finally demoralization (depression). Even a few mild moments of stuttering a month could cause a person with this orientation to become depressed. Some extremely mild stutterers may become depressed for this reason.

The following comment by a middle-aged STUTT-L participant illustrates the tendency evinced by some persons who stutter to focus more on their stuttering as self-defining, in contrast to the way that others view them:

> I have recently had the experience of finding out that the kids I knew in high school don't remember me as "the kid who stuttered" at all. They might remember that I stuttered, but that's not their definition of me as they remember me. For me, or course, it was. My "speech problem" was the focus of my daily existence.

A fourth personality trait shared by many persons who stutter is guilt about stuttering. This guilt could have arisen from several sources. One is the belief that they are somehow responsible for beginning to stutter because they did not do what was necessary to talk correctly. This belief could have had its origin in advice they received as children from their parents and others to talk more slowly, or to take a deep breath before beginning to talk, or to think of what they are going to say before they say it, and it may have been reinforced by one or more of the following reactions:

- being rejected, punished, or mocked because of their stuttering;

- having people (particularly their parents) look away or sometimes have a pained expression on their face while their stuttering occurred; or

- having people, particularly their parents, participate in a conspiracy of silence about their stuttering. This may communicate to stutterers that what they are doing is so bad that it cannot even be mentioned.

All of these reactions could be interpreted to imply that someone stutters because he or she did not try hard enough to stop.

This belief could also have been reinforced by speech-language pathologists. They may, for example, have made comments to their clients suggesting that they stutter "because they do things that interfere with talking." While this may be true, and it may be necessary to make such comments to motivate clients to work on their speech, it is important to recognize that these remarks can reinforce their guilt.

A second source of guilt for many stutterers is that they believe they are somehow responsible for their continuing to stutter. This belief can be reinforced by information they receive from the media and from professionals (including speech-language pathologists), which suggests that it is possible for them to be cured or learn to speak with considerably less abnormality. This may not be true for some persons who stutter (Cooper, 1987). Their guilt can also be reinforced by their certainty that they should be able to change any aspect of their behavior.

A third source of guilt is that people who have improved their fluency through therapy may believe they are somehow responsible if they relapse following termination of the therapy—that is, if they fail to maintain the fluency they gained while in therapy. This belief may result, in part, from comments made by their clinician suggesting that if they had been doing what they should have been doing to maintain their fluency, they would not have relapsed. This may or may not be true.

A fourth belief that may contribute to guilt is that when people stutter, they may feel they take too much of other people's time. Having this belief is likely to put them under time pressure to speak fluently, which tends to increase stuttering severity, and motivate them to avoid words on which they expect to stutter. Stutterers, for example, may order something in a restaurant they do not want, believing that if they order what they really do want, they will stutter and take too much of the server's time.

Experiencing guilt about stuttering can lead to feelings of shame or embarrassment. This accounts, at least in part, for the poor eye contact that many stutterers evince during moments of stuttering. Psychologists have found that looking away is one of the main behavioral changes associated with feeling ashamed about something (Atkins, 1988). Hence, one strategy that could be used for improving the eye contact of persons who stutter would be to reduce their feelings of shame or embarrassment about stuttering. It can be argued, incidentally, that having feelings of shame about stuttering is irrational. As one STUTT-L participant commented:

> Why feel shame? One does not typically feel shame if one is not too athletic. Would you feel shame that you cannot pitch a ball perfectly or play good basketball? No. But that need not stop you from playing and practicing to do the best you can. But when stuttering comes into the picture, we suddenly feel a need to attain perfect fluency. Why feel we should not talk unless we are perfectly fluent? And believe me, fluency is the last thing that will help you be an effective communicator. I've seen some boring, very fluent speakers and some very engaging, stuttering speakers.

A fifth personality trait that is shared by many persons who stutter is anxiety about speaking. Such anxiety can result from anticipating stuttering in a speaking situation and desiring to avoid it. Some authorities have speculated that it contributes to precipitating moments of stuttering (see chapter 5). Persons whose stuttering is relatively mild often tend to experience a higher level of such anxiety than those whose stuttering is relatively severe, particularly if they try to conceal the fact that they stutter. They can be successful in concealing their stuttering by using such strategies as word substitution and reduced verbal output. Anticipating stuttering while with persons from whom they have tried to conceal the disorder can cause them to experience anxiety because they are afraid that if these persons find out, they will no longer accept them. The longer stutterers try to conceal their stuttering and the more they value a personal relationship, the more intense this anxiety is likely to be. Persons who stutter relatively severely may experience less anxiety about the effect of stuttering on their relationships. Because they are unable to conceal it completely, they usually find out fairly quickly whether they will be accepted.

A sixth personality trait shared by many persons who stutter is an external locus-of-control orientation for speech (McDonough & Quesal, 1988). The construct of *locus of control* implies a continuum, the ends of which represent two different general expectancies about reinforcement: internal and external. According to McDonough and Quesal (1988):

> An individual with an internal locus of control believes that his/her own behaviors, abilities, or attributes determine "reinforcements." Those individuals with an external locus of control believe that reinforcements are under the control of "luck," "chance," "good days," "bad days," "powerful others," etc., rather than under their personal control. (p. 98)

While stutterers do not appear to differ from nonstutterers in their expectancies on *overall* locus of control, there is a little evidence that they tend to differ in their expectancies concerning *speech-specific* locus of control—they are more likely than nonstutterers to believe that their disorder is controlled by external factors (McDonough & Quesal, 1988). Since the presence of such a belief would be likely to interfere with many approaches to therapy, clinicians should be alert for such a tendency. Strategies addressing this situation are described in chapters 7 and 8.

Self-concept

Considerable data exist to indicate that the self-concepts of many persons who stutter are adversely affected by their stuttering. Aspects of their self-perception that have been studied include how they perceive their body, personality, and social status and how they believe others perceive them. Some of the ways in which these aspects of self-concept are likely to be affected by stuttering are described in this section.

Persons who stutter are likely to have a conflicting body image—normal one moment and deviant the next. A conflicting body image can be more difficult to cope with than one by which you are always likely to be regarded by yourself and others as being abnormal in some way. One young woman who stutters stated:

> I'd rather be blind or deaf, or have a huge birthmark on my face, or be bald than stutter. Then I would always have the trouble and could get used to it. I'll never be able to accept a face that only sometimes suddenly jumps around and makes horrible sounds. How can you learn to bear something that comes and goes so erratically? (Van Riper, 1982, p. 227)

Hence, stress from living with a conflicting body image can add to the severity of a client's stuttering problem.

There are several strategies that persons who stutter may use alone or in combination to lessen the stress that results from living with a conflicting body image. The first (which has already been discussed in several contexts) is avoiding or concealing stuttering. The less frequently a person stutters, the less often he or she experiences stress from it.

A second strategy stutterers may use for this purpose is to secure therapy. However, even if it is successful and they become much more fluent than they were previously, stutterers may continue to experience stress from their stuttering. Some of them are so highly aware of their stuttering that even occasionally having a few mild blocks (ones of which most listeners probably would not be aware) can adversely affect their body image. Consequently, reducing the severity of their stuttering, by itself, may not "normalize" their body image. Their *reaction* to their stuttering (or the meaning it has for them) must also change (Johnson, 1946).

A third strategy they may use is *denial*—not abstracting (not paying attention to) at least some of the abnormality that occurs during their moments of stuttering. The less attention they pay to their stuttering, the less they tend to react to it and, consequently, the less likely they are to experience this source of anxiety. The use of this strategy, however, can interfere with some approaches to therapy (intervention), particularly those that attempt to teach clients to modify or control their moments of stuttering in some way. If they are unaware of what they are doing while they are stuttering, they probably will find it difficult to learn to modify their disorder (Van Riper, 1973).

Thus far, our discussion of aspects of self-concept that may be adversely affected by stuttering has focused on body image. Another aspect that may be affected is how persons who stutter view their social status. Social status in our culture is determined primarily by one's occupation, education, and evidence of success as measured by wealth and possessions and by the number of people on whom one has claims. You acquire claims on people by putting them in your debt (such as by doing favors for them) and/or by viewing them as inferior (e.g., having the ability to hire or fire them). Persons who stutter tend to be more comfortable and, consequently, more fluent when they speak to persons on whom they have claims. In this regard, a successful businessman said:

> If I know that I can hire or buy them, I don't mind stuttering so much and I don't stutter so hard. I'm on top and they're down under. I don't give a damn what they think. It's my equals who bother me. (Van Riper, 1982, p. 231)

Some stutterers who regard themselves as having relatively high status tend to stutter more severely when talking to persons whom they believe are not aware of their status. A university professor who stutters, for example, may find that his stuttering increases when ordering food from a waiter or waitress who is not aware of "who he is." This increase may result, at least in part, from the stutterer's belief that people who don't know them are likely to regard those who stutter as "inferior" unless they have information to the contrary. Hence, stutterers would want to be fluent while speaking to such persons, which would tend to increase the severity of their stuttering. As mentioned earlier, stutterers tend to stutter most when they want to stutter least!

Some persons who stutter blame the disorder for causing them to have a lower social status than they would have had otherwise. They tend to view themselves as being "a giant in chains" ("If only I hadn't stuttered, I would have achieved. . . ."). There is evidence, incidentally, that some stutterers perceive high levels of discrimination against them in the area of employment. However, others do not view themselves as having a lower social status because of stuttering (see Tillis & Wager, 1984).

Persons who stutter, of course, are not the only ones who view themselves as being "a giant in chains." Many persons in our society feel that they have been kept from achieving a higher social status by some sort of chain (as in not having been able to go to college). Viewing yourself in this manner can have both positive and negative consequences. Positively, it can keep your perceived lack of achievement from adversely affecting your self-concept ("I'm good, but circumstances beyond my control kept me from achieving."). Negatively, it can keep you from trying to achieve until the chains are removed. Some persons who stutter tend to assume, for this reason, that they can't achieve their goals until their stuttering is cured. Though it certainly is desirable for them to reduce the severity of their stuttering through therapy, it may not be necessary for them to wait until they have done so to get on with their lives!

In addition to the ways in which stutterers view themselves, another aspect of self-concept that is likely to be affected is how they feel *others* view them. How we believe others view us affects how we view ourselves. According to Van Riper (1992):

> We construct our personal identities by internalizing the reactions
> and evaluations of the people who play important parts in our lives—
> parents, siblings, mates, friends, employers, and fellow workers.
> What we think we see in the eyes of others often determines what
> and whom we think we are. (pp. 229–230)

The impact on self-concept of how persons who stutter believe others
view them is likely to be felt early in the development of the disorder.
Parents tend to look upon stuttering as undesirable behavior and
respond negatively to it (Johnson & Associates, 1959). Also, teasing,
mockery, and rejection from peers are common experiences for children of all ages who stutter.

In adulthood, persons who stutter may feel the force of negative
evaluation from peers of both sexes. This can adversely affect their
self-concept and, thereby, their behavior in a number of ways. For
example, it can affect their choice of a lover or spouse (Boberg &
Boberg, 1990; Carlisle, 1985). According to Van Riper (1982, p. 233), a
man who stutters may seek a person who evaluates his speech with
unusual tolerance and is willing to protect him against communicative
trauma and stress. Such a companion probably would be willing to
make some phone calls for him. He may also seek one whom he feels
others would not regard as very desirable. The reason is that he
believes a person whom others would regard as desirable probably
would not find him attractive because of his stuttering.

How persons who stutter *expect* others to view them can influence
their perception of how others actually *do* view them. People "filter"
the reactions of others to support their expectations (Johnson, 1946).
According to Fransella (1972):

> It cannot be reiterated too often that how we construe an act, person,
> place, or thing determines how we behave in relation to that act, per-
> son, place, or thing. No situation is intrinsically dangerous, anxiety-
> provoking or beautiful, it is only so if we construe in that way. (p. 69)

This impact of expectation on perception has several clinical implications. First, it has to be taken into consideration when evaluating clients' reports of how people react to their stuttering. The reactions they
report may or may not be accurate. And second, knowledge about it
can be used as a "tool" (in combination with others) for desensitizing
clients to their stuttering. Their perceptions of people's reactions to
their stuttering can be distorted by how they *expect* others to react.
The more aware they are of this possibility, the less certain they
should be (in at least some situations) that people really are reacting
negatively to their stuttering and, hence, the weaker should be their
desire to avoid it. Also, the less certain they are that listeners really do
react negatively to them because they stutter, the less likely they
should be to signal to them that they are embarrassed or ashamed

because they stutter and, consequently, the less likely their listeners should be uncomfortable while talking to them. When listeners react negatively to them while they are stuttering, the listeners may be reacting more to the "discomfort" they evince than to their stuttering per se (Hugh-Jones & Smith, 1999; Murphy & Quesal, 2002).

How persons who stutter believe others view them also affects their stuttering severity. The more certain they are that listeners react negatively when they stutter, the more likely they are to try to conceal their stuttering and, as a consequence, they stutter relatively severely while talking with others (see chapter 2). There is some evidence, incidentally, that nonstutterers tend to perceive the intelligence and personality of persons who stutter more positively if the stutterers acknowledge their stuttering rather than attempt to conceal it (Collins & Blood, 1990).

It should be evident from the information presented in this section that many persons who stutter tend to have relatively poor self-concepts. This, of course, contributes to the severity of their stuttering problem and the extent to which they are handicapped by it. It may also contribute to the likelihood that they will recover from stuttering. Perkins (1993, p. 11) has hypothesized that "prevention of a self-image of stutterer [in children] would be equivalent to prevention of stuttering as a chronic clinical problem."

The fact that some stutterers do not have relatively poor self-concepts is important. *It indicates that it is possible for persons to stutter and still have a relatively good self-concept.* It may be possible, therefore, to improve your clients' self-concepts at least a little without first improving their fluency. In fact, doing so may help to improve their fluency because the better they feel about themselves, the less severely they are likely to stutter (see chapter 2).

Language Skills

Thus far, we have considered persons who stutter from the perspectives of physiological and psychological functioning. One perspective we have not yet considered is speech-language functioning other than stuttering. Do persons who stutter, as a group tend to differ from their nonstuttering peers in this aspect? The majority of investigators who have compared attributes of speech-language functioning have found differences. There is some evidence that children who stutter are late in passing their speech milestones: The extent of delay has been reported to be about six months (Andrews et al., 1983). Also, they appear to make more articulation/phonological errors than their peers do (Andrews et al., 1983). Furthermore, their expressive language skills do not appear to be as highly developed as those of their peers (Andrews et al., 1983). However, their receptive language skills, their narrative ability, and their reading ability appear to differ little, if at all, from those of their nonstuttering peers.

Is there any reason to believe that a linguistic performance deficit can contribute to the onset and development of stuttering? Some speech-language pathologists believe that the demands language places on the speech motor planning and execution capacities of persons who have such a deficit can contribute to the disorder's etiology. See Watson, Freeman, Chapman, Miller, Finitzo, Pool, and Devous (1991) for a review of the literature supporting this point of view.

THE PERSON WHO MANIFESTS CLUTTERING

Practically no systematic research has been published on the physiological and psychological characteristics and language skills of persons who clutter (www.mankato.msus.edu/dept/comdis/kuster/cluttering/clutterbib.html, accessed 5/16/03). What has been published is mainly observations made while treating persons who have this disorder. Most of these observations pertain to how persons who clutter differ from persons who stutter.

Physiological Characteristics

Unfortunately, the available data provide little information about the physiological characteristics of such persons. About all that it seems relatively safe to conclude about their physiological characteristics is that they probably have some type of cerebral dysfunction that interferes with their ability to monitor their speech rate, fluency, and possibly also their articulation and language functioning. The conclusion that their disorder results from a deficit in cerebral functioning is based on a number of reports (largely from clinical case studies) which indicate that persons with this disorder evince behaviors that are thought to be symptoms of such a deficit, including auditory perceptual difficulties, distractibility, hyperactivity, and/or a limited attention span (see the Web site cited above for a bibliography of such reports).

Psychological Characteristics

Perhaps the most frequently mentioned psychological characteristic of persons who have this disorder is their lack of awareness of their speech being abnormal (e.g., too rapid and excessively disfluent). This sharply differentiates them from persons who stutter, who, once they're beyond preschool age, are usually highly aware of their disfluency.

What we know about the personalities of persons who clutter is based largely on observations by clinicians who have treated a relatively large number of persons who have this disorder. The personality characteristics mentioned below are similar to those reported by other such clinicians.

Klencke characterizes clutterers as carefree, careless, and lacking in persistence and sense of responsibility. The majority, indeed, seem to have some of these characteristics in common. They are generally of pleasant temperament and do not take life's problems very seriously, including, alas, their treatment. They have a short attention span, which precludes their carrying a grudge, persisting in a given task, or keeping a promise for long (although their promises are sincere and their transgressions sincerely regretted). They tend to be overactive, but change pace occasionally and change their mind frequently. For instance, a young clutterer may change toys frequently, or request food urgently but leave it untouched and then wonder because his lack of direction is questioned. In more mature clutterers we are apt to find personal untidiness, disorder of possessions, and lack of punctuality. Clutterers often sit restlessly, squirming or assuming unusual positions—each for a short time. Impatience is their basic characteristic. (Weiss, 1964, p. 53)

Since this description of the clutterer's personality is based on informal clinical observation rather than systematic research, its generality is uncertain.

If persons who have this disorder are unaware of the effect that it has on their speech, it would seem reasonable to assume that it shouldn't adversely affect their self-concept. This, unfortunately, isn't a safe assumption to make. We recently saw a woman in our clinic who developed a poor self-concept, at least in part as a result of having this disorder. While she wasn't aware of the abnormality in her speech, she had been told repeatedly since childhood that she spoke poorly and her acceptance of this opinion had adversely affected her self-concept.

Language Skills

There appears to be general agreement among authorities on cluttering that some of the language skills of persons who clutter tend to be less highly developed than those of their peers. Language skills that have been reported to be affected include receptive oral language, expressive oral language, reading, and writing. Some of the specific deficits that are mentioned in the literature are indicated in this section. The percentage of clutterers who evince each of them is uncertain.

Receptive language impairments

Clutterers are reported to have difficulty listening and following instructions. Furthermore, clutterers are reported to be more likely to have a reading disorder than their normal-speaking peers. These impairments are probably due, at least in part, to difficulty concentrating and/or a relatively short attention span.

Expressive language impairments

Language errors tend to occur more often in the speech of clutterers than in that of their normal-speaking peers. The types of errors that clutterers have been reported to evince while speaking include (Daly & Burnett, 1999, pp. 230–231):

- narrative discourse with inappropriate syntax or word order, or poor sequencing of ideas

- frequent interjections, repetitions, and revisions

- syllabic or verbal transpositions

- improper pronoun referents or overuse of pronouns

- excessive use of empty words or filler words

- inappropriate language use, including inappropriate turn-taking and inappropriate topic introduction, maintenance, and/or termination

- frequent "slips of the tongue"

- immature and imprecise articulation and sound or syllable transpositions or omissions

Language errors also tend to occur more often in the writing of clutterers than in that of their peers. According to Roman (1959):

> Disintegrated writing is the hallmark of the clutterer, who spills out the written word in headlong haste, clipping letters, omitting syllables, slurring substitutes, transposing words, hence producing in his almost illegible hand the counterpoint of his inarticulate speech. (p. 29)

Consequently, the language deficit that clutterers evince would appear to affect both their writing and speech similarly.

THE PERSON WHO MANIFESTS NEUROGENIC ACQUIRED STUTTERING

What little information we have about the impact of neurogenic acquired stuttering on those who have it is from clinical case studies. Unfortunately, these studies focused almost exclusively on the etiology of the disorder, on the symptomatology of the resulting disfluency, and/or on ameliorating the disfluency, rather than on the person who had it. Consequently, we know very little about this person, aside from the symptomatology, etiology, and treatment of his or her disfluency behavior.

Physiological Characteristics

A person who has this disorder is more likely to be an adult than a child. He or she will have developed a temporary, progressive, or non-progressive neurological disorder prior to the onset of stuttering. The disorder is likely to affect aspects of the person's functioning other than speech fluency. Those effected will be determined by the part of the brain that is impaired (see chapter 5).

Psychological Characteristics

One characteristic that all older children and adults who develop this disorder will share is the need to go through the grieving process. The grieving process begins with shock and denial, progresses to depression and anger, and, hopefully, ends with acceptance. This process is triggered whenever somebody experiences a loss. Persons who develop this disorder sustain a substantial loss—the loss of the ability to speak fluently, and probably more.

Persons who develop this disorder are usually aware of it and are likely to seek help. Thus, it seems reasonable to assume that its presence probably adversely affects their self-concept, at least a little. Consequently, the resulting impairment in their ability to speak fluently may also be both a significant disability and a handicap.

Language Skills

If there is damage to the cerebral cortex and/or to the pyramidal or extrapyramidal tracts, the person's ability to communicate may also be impaired, at least minimally, by aphasia and/or dysarthria. He or she may, for example, have word-finding difficulties and/or multiple articulation errors. Furthermore, the person may develop an overlay of stuttering (see chapter 8).

THE PERSON WHO MANIFESTS PSYCHOGENIC ACQUIRED STUTTERING

The available information about persons who evince psychogenic acquired stuttering is obtained largely from clinical case studies. These case studies (like those about persons who evince neurogenic stuttering) have focused almost exclusively on the etiology of the disorder, on the symptomatology of the resulting disfluency, and/or on ameliorating the disfluency, rather than on the person who had the disorder. Consequently, we know very little about this person, aside from the symptomatology, etiology, and treatment of his or her disfluency behavior.

Physiological Characteristics

Persons with this disorder share one negative physiological characteristic—they do not appear to have a neurological condition that can explain (or explain completely) the onset of their abnormal disfluency. In fact, the possibility of neurological origins for sudden-onset stuttering must be ruled out before it can be considered psychological, because neurogenic acquired stuttering appears to be far more common than psychogenic acquired stuttering (Baumgartner, 1999).

Psychological Characteristics

About the only psychological characteristic shared by persons who have this disorder is a short- or long-term unpleasant (possibly traumatic) experience prior to the onset of the disorder that stressed the person sufficiently to precipitate it.

Some of those who develop this disorder have a prior history of psychopathology. However, according to Baumgartner (1999):

> Psychopathology need not always be present for stuttering to be psychogenic. Reports of distress or of stress as a normal reaction to life events, or anticipation of them, may precipitate stuttering just as they are commonly said to precipitate dysphonia or aphonia. (p. 278)

Language Skills

The only speech or language deficit that is universal (or close to it) among persons with this disorder is abnormal disfluency. Some of those who have this disorder may also evince the

> . . . presence of unusual grammatical constructions, e.g., "Me get sick," and bizarre speech such as multiple repetitions of nearly all phonemes with simultaneous head bobbing, facial grimacing, and tremor-like arm movements. (Helm-Estabrooks, 1999)

ASSIGNMENTS

Eye Contact

Many adults who stutter do not maintain normal eye contact, particularly while they are stuttering. Talk to three persons and, at times, stare at the ceiling or the floor while doing so. How did you feel while your eye contact was abnormal? Were your listeners aware when you failed to maintain eye contact, and if they were, did they react differently to you when you did so? If you are uncertain, ask them.

Impact of Mind-Set on Perception of Self

Some adults who stutter expect people to react negatively to them because of their impairment. Consequently, they often enter speaking situations with a mind-set that causes them to perceive such reactions when they aren't there. ("Seek and ye shall find.") For a period of several hours, assume that the people whom you engage in conversation are going to react negatively to you. While doing so, keep the following questions in mind: Is there anything in their behavior that could be interpreted as supporting your expectation (your "certainty")? If there is, do you think you would have interpreted it in this way if you hadn't had this mind-set? (See chapter 7 for a detailed discussion about certainties.)

4

Onset and Development

INSTRUCTIONAL OBJECTIVES

By the end of this chapter, you should be able to:

▸ Describe eight aspects of the symptomatology and phenomenology of stuttering at or near onset.

▸ Describe the reactions of parents and others to a child's "stuttering," at or near onset.

▸ Describe the onset of stuttering in adults.

▸ Describe Bluemel's, Bloodstein's, and Van Riper's stages through which stuttering evolves into its fully developed adult form.

▸ Specify why some older adults may recover from stuttering.

▸ Describe essentials of the onset and development of cluttering.

▸ Describe essentials of the onset and development of neurogenic acquired stuttering.

▸ Describe essentials of the onset and development of psychogenic acquired stuttering.

Our focus in this chapter is on the onset and development of stuttering, cluttering, neurogenic acquired stuttering, and psychogenic acquired stuttering. All fluency disorders have a beginning (onset), and their symptomatology tends to change in predictable ways as they develop. Because much more is known about the onset and development of stuttering than about the onset and development of any of the other fluency disorders, considerably more space is devoted to stuttering than to the others.

ONSET OF STUTTERING

Although stuttering can begin at any age, its onset, in most cases, is reported to be between the ages of two and five years (Johnson & Associates, 1959). The mean ages of onset that have been reported range from 32 (Yairi & Ambrose, 1992c) to 46 months (Darley, 1955). Age of onset here refers to the age at which an informant (usually a parent) reports that he or she first concluded that a child's repetitions and/or other hesitations probably were abnormal. Unfortunately, very few children have been evaluated by speech-language pathologists within days or even weeks of the time the disorder was reported to have begun. Consequently, almost all the information we have about stuttering at onset is from reports by informants who are not speech-language pathologists made months (or even years) after the disorder probably began. However, the fact that data from thousands of such reports from many different countries tend to agree fairly well makes it probable that at least some of the information we have is reliable.

Our information about the onset of stuttering also is incomplete because much of it is based on what can readily be observed by a layperson through vision and hearing. There are undoubtedly associated physiological and psychological events that either cannot be observed without instrumentation or that a layperson observing would be unlikely to regard as being related to the onset of the disorder. This has one, or possibly two, implications. First, it means that the onset of stuttering as described here is incomplete, possibly in some important ways. And second, it could mean that the onset of stuttering occurs at an earlier age than a layperson's reports would suggest. That is, it could mean that the presence of relatively high levels of syllable and word repetition and/or other hesitation phenomena is not the first stage in the development of the disorder—it is just the first one about which laypersons are likely to become concerned.

Symptomatology and Phenomenology of Stuttering at or Near Onset

The following questions are discussed in this section:

1. Does the onset of stuttering tend to be sudden or gradual?

2. What are the speech characteristics of early (primary) stuttering?

3. How similar is early stuttering to normal childhood disfluency?

4. How aware of and concerned about their stuttering do young children tend to be?

5. To what extent do children at the initial stage in the disorder's development do things to avoid stuttering?

6. How well are children at the beginning stage of the disorder able to predict their moments of stuttering?

7. To what extent does stuttering at (or near) onset tend to vary on a situational basis?

8. How representative does stuttering observed in the "therapy room" tend to be of stuttering observed in other situations?

9. During its initial stage, what impact is stuttering likely to have on a child's self-concept? How are reactions to the child's stuttering likely to influence this impact?

1. *Does the onset of stuttering tend to be sudden or gradual?* This question is difficult to answer because most of the relevant data (such as Johnson & Associates, 1959) are from reports by parents and other laypersons months (or even years) after the disorder is thought to have begun. Such reports may be inaccurate because the persons making them classified at least some of the child's normal repetitions and other hesitations as the beginning of stuttering. This would tend to make the onset of the disorder appear to have been more gradual than it really was. The reports may also be inaccurate because the persons making them either were not aware of the child's earliest moments of stuttering or considered them to be normal hesitations. This would tend to make the onset of the disorder appear more sudden than it really was.

Though the relevant data have to be interpreted with caution for the reasons indicated earlier, they do seem to indicate that the onset can be either sudden or gradual, with a gradual onset being more usual (Van Riper, 1982).

2. *What are the speech characteristics of early (primary) stuttering?* When children begin to stutter, what is the nature of their hesitations? Of what behaviors do their moments of stuttering tend to consist? In other words, what are they doing that causes someone (usually a parent) to first decide that something is wrong with their speech? Almost all reports of their speaking behavior agree that what these children are most likely to be doing is repeating single-syllable words and the first syllables of multisyllable words (particularly the latter). Since a single-syllable word is also a syllable, the repetition of such a word can be classified as a syllable as well as a word repetition. What they are repeating, therefore, is syllables. Their syllable repetitions may call attention to themselves not only because they are judged to occur frequently, but also because the number of units per

instance of repetition is considered to be excessive. For example, they might say "I-I-I-I-I want . . ." rather than "I-I want. . . ."

The repetitions evinced by at least a third of the children diagnosed as beginning to stutter are accompanied by signs of tension at least some of the time (Johnson & Associates, 1959; Yairi, 1993). Whether such signs usually are present from the moment the child begins to stutter or whether they tend to develop after a few days, weeks, or months has not been established empirically.

While the first type of disfluency that usually causes someone to become concerned about a child's speech is sound, syllable, and/or single-syllable word repetition (Yairi, 1993), in some cases it is complete stoppages, or rather, prolonged articulatory postures, which may be silent or accompanied by prolonged sounds (Yairi, 1993). These usually occur on the initial sounds of words. When they occur within words, they may not be at syllable boundaries—for example, "v—ery." When such blockages occur within a word, the word is referred to as *broken*. The blockages almost never occur on the final sounds of words. Some of them are accompanied by behavioral events usually associated with developed stuttering, such as eyelid opening and closing, eyeball movement (lateral or vertical), head movement, limb movement, torso movement, audible inhalation, vocal intensity change, audible exhalation, lip movement, or some combination of these (Schwartz, Zebrowski, & Conture, 1990).

The percentage of children who evince prolonged articulatory postures during the first few weeks after the onset of the disorder is not known for certain. However, Van Riper (1982, pp. 69–70) has shed some light on this. Over a period of years he evaluated 61 children within three weeks of the reported onset of the disorder. Of these children, approximately one-third evinced articulatory postures that lasted at least two seconds.

3. *How similar is early stuttering to normal childhood disfluency?* Some of the data referred to in the previous answer indicate that what young children usually are doing when someone becomes concerned about their speech fluency is repeating single-syllable words and/or the first syllables of multisyllable words in a relatively relaxed manner. To what extent do their normal-speaking peers repeat single-syllable words and/or the first syllables of multisyllable ones? Since most cases of stuttering are reported to begin between the ages of two and five, preschoolers are the age group from which the data used here were obtained for answering this question.

Most normal-speaking preschool children repeat single-syllable words and the first syllables of multisyllable words (Johnson & Associates, 1959; Silverman, 1972a). Hence, the fact that a child does so does not, *by itself*, indicate that he or she is beginning to stutter.

While the presence of syllable repetition does not allow one to differentiate children beginning to stutter from their normal-speaking peers, perhaps the amount and/or the manner in which they do so would allow one to distinguish between them. Do children beginning to stutter tend to repeat syllables more often than their normal-speaking peers? The most comprehensive study of the syllable repetitions of both groups of preschoolers was reported by Johnson and Associates (1959). These data (see table 1.1) show considerable overlap between the groups. While most children who are thought to be beginning to stutter repeat syllables more often than the majority of their normal-speaking peers, not all appear to do so. In fact, there are children about whose fluency no one seems to be concerned who repeat more often than some children who are thought to be beginning to stutter (see table 1.1). The overlap between the groups was confirmed by Yairi and Lewis (1984) and Meyers (1986), though the degree to which it occurred in their subjects was considerably less than reported by Johnson and Associates (1959). Consequently, if a clinician decides whether children are beginning to stutter *solely* on the basis of whether they repeat syllables, he or she is likely to misdiagnose some of them—and according to the diagnosogenic theory (see chapter 5), such a misdiagnosis can precipitate stuttering.

Do children who stutter differ from their normal-speaking peers in the number of times they are likely to repeat the first syllable of a multisyllable word or a single-syllable word? When they repeat, do they tend to have more *units* of repetition per instance of repetition than do their normal-speaking peers? Would an instance of repetition such as "I-I-I-I-I want . . ." ever occur in the speech of a normal-speaking child? The available data (Johnson & Associates, 1959) indicate that there is overlap between groups. While the typical preschool-age child who stutters tends to produce more units of repetition per instance of repetition than his or her normal-speaking peers, there are normal-speaking preschool-age children who produce more of them than some of their peers who have the disorder. In fact, normal-speaking four-year-olds have been observed repeating a syllable as many as seven times (Silverman, 1972a). Hence, it would not be safe to conclude that a child is beginning to stutter solely because he or she *occasionally* repeats a syllable a large number of times.

Some children who are beginning to stutter evince prolonged articulatory postures—which may be silent or accompanied by prolonged sound. Do normal-speaking preschool-age children ever evince such postures? The available evidence (see Johnson & Associates, 1959) indicates that they do. However, the typical child who stutters evinces them more often and for longer periods of time than does his or her typical normal-speaking peer. There appears to be less overlap between groups for prolonged articulatory postures than for syllable

repetitions. Nevertheless, an *occasional* prolonged articulatory pos-
ture—particularly when a child is upset or seems to have a great deal
to say—is not necessarily indicative of early stuttering.

While the data indicate unequivocally that syllable repetitions
and prolonged articulatory postures occur in the speech of normal-
speaking children as well as in the speech of those beginning to stutter, this does not necessarily mean that information about such hesitation phenomena should be ignored when deciding whether a child is
beginning to stutter. There are some children for whom the amount of
repetition, the number of units per instance of repetition, the frequency and duration of prolonged articulatory postures, or some combination of these, is clearly abnormal. To deny this would be playing
the "Emperor's New Clothes" game. If the hesitation phenomena are
abnormal, the child is in need of help.

4. *How aware of and concerned about their stuttering do young
children tend to be?* Most young children who are judged to be beginning to stutter because they are repeating excessively and/or have frequent prolonged articulatory postures do not usually seem to be aware
that there is anything abnormal about their speech fluency. Even if
they are aware of their hesitations, most of the time they tend to
evince much less concern about them than do adults who have the disorder. Van Riper (1982, pp. 95–107) reported that the stuttering of 68
percent of the 300 children he studied developed along Track I or
Track II (see tables 4-1 and 4-2 for descriptions of these tracks). A
characteristic of both is "no awareness" of stuttering during the beginning stage of the disorder. Yairi (1993) reported, based on parental
questionnaire data, that 77 percent of the children in his sample did
not seem to be aware of their stuttering when it first began. Bloodstein (1987, p. 42) concluded, after examining the clinical case histories of 418 children who stutter, that "Most of the time children in the
first phase of stuttering show little evidence of concern about the
interruptions in their speech." However, some children do appear to be
highly aware of and concerned about stuttering almost from the
moment of the onset of the disorder. Twenty-seven (9 percent) of the
300 children Van Riper (1982) studied appeared to evince such awareness and concern, and a few of the 20 preschool-age children studied
by Ambrose and Yairi (1994) did also.

5. *To what extent do children at the initial stage of the disorder's
development do things to avoid stuttering?* Since most children at the
initial stage of the disorder's development usually do not seem to be
concerned about (or even aware of) their moments of stuttering, they
would not be expected do things to avoid them. Those who are aware
of and concerned about them, however, sometimes seem to do things
to avoid stuttering. Van Riper (1982) reported evidence of such avoid-

ance by approximately 9 percent of the 300 children in his sample who were at the initial stage in the development of the disorder. Children who appear to be trying to avoid stuttering definitely are in need of professional help. The presence of avoidance behavior can provide useful information when trying to determine whether children are aware of and concerned about stuttering. If they try to avoid stuttering, this means that they are aware of and concerned about it at least *some* of the time.

6. *How well are children at the beginning stage of the disorder able to predict their moments of stuttering?* Those children who are not aware of their moments of stuttering are unable, of course, to predict them with greater-than-chance accuracy. Those children who are aware of them—like the 9 percent in Van Riper's (1982) sample—*may* be able to do so. However, even by elementary-school age most children's ability to predict them is not nearly as good as that of most adults who have the disorder (Silverman & Williams, 1972a).

7. *To what extent does stuttering at (or near) onset tend to vary on a situational basis?* Many (perhaps most) children in the initial stage do not stutter the same amount in all situations. Bloodstein (1987, p. 41), for example, included the following two among his six characteristics of the beginning of stuttering: that the difficulty has a definite tendency to be episodic; and that the child stutters most when excited or upset, when seeming to have a great deal to say, or when under other conditions of communicative pressure. (See Bloodstein's "Four Phases" later in the chapter.) The tendency for stuttering to vary on a situational basis also is a characteristic of the disorder in adults (see chapter 2).

8. *How representative does stuttering observed in the "therapy room" tend to be of that in other situations?* The stuttering observed in the therapy room *may not* be representative of that in other situations. When it is not representative, in most cases the child is more fluent there than in other situations (Silverman, 1975). The reason may be that children are less likely to be excited, upset, or under communicative pressure in this situation than in some others. Regardless of the reason, it is not safe to assume that a child's speech in the therapy room is representative of that in other situations, particularly if it is quite fluent. Some children who stutter may not do so at all in a therapy room environment! (See Silverman, 1975.)

9. *What impact is stuttering during its initial stage likely to have on a child's self-concept? How are reactions to a child's stuttering likely to influence this impact?* During its initial stage, the disorder is unlikely to affect significantly the self-concepts of children who have it, if those with whom they interact do not express concern about it

(Johnson & Associates, 1959). However, the disorder can, during its initial stage, adversely affect the self-concepts of children who are often aware of and concerned about their stuttering. This is particularly likely to happen if someone whom they respect gives them the message that what they are doing when they hesitate is "bad" and that they could stop doing it if they really wanted to or tried hard enough (Johnson & Associates, 1959). There are several ways such children may communicate they have accepted the judgment that their hesitations are "bad" and, hence, something about which to be embarrassed or ashamed. One is maintaining poor eye-contact during moments of stuttering. (We have already mentioned research that shows how "looking away" expresses feelings of embarrassment or shame [Atkins, 1988]). Another way is by doing things to avoid these moments, such as the avoidance of talking in some situations and use of the devices employed for the purpose by older children and adults—such as word substitution (Van Riper, 1982).

Reactions of Parents and Others to a Child's "Stuttering" at (or Near) Onset

How do people tend to react to young children whom they believe are beginning to stutter? Our primary focus will be on the parents, since they are the ones who usually are the first to become concerned about their children's speech fluency. Most parents will react in some manner if they believe that something about their child is abnormal. However, they differ with respect to what they consider abnormal as well as how they react when they classify something as such. A behavior that will cause one parent concern may not come to the attention of another (may not be abstracted) or, if it does, it does not cause concern (the parent does not classify the behavior as abnormal). Also, while one parent will react to believing a behavior is abnormal by remaining calm and seeking professional help, another will do so by becoming anxious or depressed.

Are parents of children who stutter more likely than those of their nonstuttering peers to be aware of and to classify repetitions and prolonged articulatory postures as abnormal? The answer to this question is not certain (Johnson & Associates, 1959; Zebrowski & Conture, 1989). If they are, perhaps it is because they are more likely to have a mind-set to see and hear them as stuttering. The findings of a number of studies (such as Berlin, 1960; Williams & Kent, 1958) indicate that whether repetitions and other types of speech hesitations are classified as stuttering is a function, in part, of whether the person doing the classifying has a mind-set to hear it. If there is a history of stuttering in their family, for example, parents may be more likely to have a mind-set to hear stuttering in their children's speech than they would otherwise. And, as has been pointed out earlier in this chapter, there is a history of stuttering in the families of persons who stutter more often than in those of their normal-speaking peers.

Once parents have classified their children's hesitations as stuttering, they may react in a number of ways, including the following:

- They may try to ignore the hesitations or not communicate concern about them to the child. There are several reasons why they may do so. First, they may be grieving for the loss of their child's ability to speak normally. The first stage of the grieving process is denial (Tanner, 1980). Second, they may hope that by not communicating concern to the child, the stuttering will just be a phase through which he or she will pass.

- They may react to the hesitations in a way that is likely to increase the child's awareness of and concern about them. Among the ways they may do this are using body language—such as looking away (Atkins, 1988)—when the child hesitates, which communicates that they are embarrassed by it, or by saying things that communicate this feeling.

- They may give the child advice about what to do to be more fluent (Johnson & Associates, 1959). The advice is likely to reflect why they think he or she is stuttering. If they think the reason is speaking too rapidly, they are likely to tell the child to slow down. If they suspect that the child is not adequately formulating the message before beginning to speak, they are likely to tell him to "think of what he is going to say before he says it" or to "stop and start over again." If they think the stuttering is caused by inadequate breath support, they are likely to tell the child to "take a deep breath before speaking."

Since many children are raised in either a single-parent family or one in which both parents work at least part of the time, the persons other than parents who probably spend the most time with preschool children are those who provide them with daycare. These persons can range from family members (such as grandparents or older siblings) to professional daycare workers. Their reactions to the hesitations of children beginning to stutter are likely to influence both how the children view these hesitations and how they view themselves (their self-concept). Therefore, it is important when evaluating a child who is thought to be beginning to stutter to determine how those who take care of the child during the day react to his or her hesitations.

Onset of Stuttering in Adults

Stuttering tends to be regarded as a disorder of childhood because the relevant data indicate that its onset almost always occurs before the age of eighteen, usually before the age of five. However, there are a number of reports in the literature of persons who began to stutter after the age of eighteen (see Van Riper, 1982, pp. 44–46). While some of these may be cases in which the person stuttered for at least a short time during childhood (but doesn't remember doing so), stopped, and then began again as an adult, it seems unlikely that they all are. It seems probable, therefore, that stuttering can have its onset during adulthood.

DEVELOPMENT OF STUTTERING

Thus far in this chapter we have considered how the symptomatology and phenomenology of stuttering at (or near) onset in children differs from that in adults. In this section we will consider how the symptomatology and phenomenology of the disorder at (or near) onset evolve into their adult form—that is, the process through which stuttering *increases* in complexity (severity). In not all cases, however, do the symptomatology and phenomenology of the disorder increase in complexity. In some the opposite seems to occur: The person eventually recovers completely or almost completely. Consequently, in this section we also will consider how the symptomatology and phenomenology of the disorder evolve into normal (or near normal) speech fluency —the process through which persons have been reported to recover from the disorder.

Stages through which the Disorder Evolves into Its Fully Developed Adult Form

There have been several attempts to describe how the symptomatology and phenomenology of stuttering in preschool children evolves into that evinced by most adults. The three that are discussed in this section appear to have had the most impact on how the development of the disorder is currently viewed.

Bluemel's "primary" and "secondary" stages

One of the first attempts to describe the development of the disorder was by Dr. Charles Bluemel (1957). He referred to the stuttering evinced during the first stage as "primary" stuttering and that evinced during the second as "secondary" stuttering. He described primary stuttering as consisting of relatively effortless repetitions and prolonged articulatory postures ("blocks"). This is the type that would be exhibited by most children at (or near) onset. According to Bluemel (1957), secondary stuttering

> . . . is marked by the conscious physical struggle to articulate while the mental process of speech is momentarily halted. The stammerers' [Bluemel used the term *stammerer* instead of *stutterer*.] breathing is

disturbed; likewise his vocalization and articulation. He uses starters and wedges to get the speech going. He becomes conditioned against difficult words and difficult situations, and he develops speech aversion and avoidance. He resorts to synonyms and circumlocutions to avoid his stammering. He remains silent when he should speak. Confusion and phobia enter into the speech situation. (p. 128)

Bluemel's scheme has been criticized for several reasons. One is that much, if not all, of the behavior he indicates as being symptomatic of primary stuttering can be observed in the speech of normal-speaking preschool-age children. A second basis on which Bluemel's scheme has been criticized is that stuttering does not always begin with relatively relaxed hesitations of which the person is unaware. Cases have been reported in which children exhibited behaviors characteristic of secondary stuttering immediately following the onset of the disorder. A third criticism is that Bluemel did not describe in sufficient detail the *transition* between beginning stuttering and the fully developed form of the disorder. A final criticism is that Bluemel's scheme does not adequately describe the symptomatology of the disorder in school-age children, particularly in those of elementary-school age.

Bloodstein's "four phases" in the development of stuttering

Bloodstein (1960) proposed a four-stage scheme that includes aspects of the symptomatology of the disorder in school-age and preschool children and adults. He appropriately points out that there is considerable variation in the age at which a person evinces the symptomatology associated with each phase. However, the "typical" person who stutters will evince symptoms associated with *Phase I* while a preschooler, symptoms associated with *Phase II* while in elementary school, symptoms associated with *Phase III* during late childhood and early adolescence, and symptoms associated with *Phase IV* by late adolescence or adulthood. Not all persons who stutter, incidentally, eventually reach Phase IV: The symptomatology evinced by some adults is that of Phase II or III.

According to Bloodstein (1960), the symptomatology associated with each phase is at follows:

PHASE I

1. *The difficulty has a distinct tendency to be episodic.* One of the best indications that stuttering is still in its most rudimentary form is that it appears for periods of weeks or months between long interludes of normal speech. During this phase there is apparently a high percentage of spontaneous recoveries from stuttering that consist essentially of cases in which episodes of stuttering have failed to recur. How high this percentage is would be very difficult to determine. It is not

improbable that single episodes of stuttering so mild and brief that they are overlooked or soon forgotten are exceedingly common during these years.

2. *The child stutters most when excited or upset, when seeming to have a great deal to say, or under other conditions of communicative pressure.*

3. *The dominant symptom is repetition.* This must be hastily qualified. Practically any of the integral or associated symptoms of stuttering may be seen in some of the youngest stutterers, and in some cases there seems to be little or no repetition. For the most part, however, the more severe symptoms appear briefly and intermittently in these children, and relatively simple repetition is far more common. In some cases repetition is practically the only symptom to be observed. While much of it consists of repetition of initial syllables, as it does in older stutterers, there is also usually a conspicuous tendency to repeat whole words.

4. *There is a marked tendency for stutterings to occur at the beginning of the sentence, clause, or phrase.* In some of the youngest children stuttering seems to be limited almost entirely to the first word of the sentence.

5. *In contrast to more advanced stuttering, the interruptions occur not only on content words, but also on the function words of speech—the pronouns, conjunctions, articles, and prepositions.* Stuttering on such words often tends to consist of whole-word repetitions. In short, there is frequent repetition of such words as "like," "but," "and," "so," "he," "I," and "with."

6. *Most of the time children in the first phase of stuttering show little evidence of concern about the interruptions in their speech.* This is not to say that they are completely unconscious of them. It is commonplace for children as young as two or three to show acute frustration when they stutter by refusing to speak, crying, beating the wall with their hands, or saying, "Why can't I talk?" Such reactions are usually brief and sporadic, however, in contrast to the chronic fear and embarrassment of many older stutterers. Furthermore, the characteristic reaction of the Phase I stutterer may be epitomized by saying that when there is any reaction at all it is apparently in response to the immediate experience of being thwarted in efforts to communicate rather than to the ramified implications of the knowledge on the part of the child that he or she "is a stutterer."

PHASE II

1. *The disorder is essentially chronic.* There are few, if any, intervals of normal speech.

2. *The child has a self-concept of a stutterer.*

3. *The stutterings occur chiefly on the major parts of speech—nouns, verbs, adjectives, and adverbs.* There is much less tendency to stutter only on the initial words of sentences and phrases, and whole-word repetitions are no longer quite as common.

4. *Despite a self-concept as a stutterer, the child usually evinces little or no concern about the speech difficulty.* There is an absence of such features of more advanced stuttering as conscious anticipations of stuttering; substitution; circumlocution; avoidance of speaking; and word, sound, and situation fears.

5. *The stuttering is said to increase chiefly under conditions of excitement and when the child is speaking rapidly.*

PHASE III

1. *The stuttering comes and goes largely in response to specific situations.* Among the situations the person often reports to be especially difficult are classroom recitation, speaking to strangers, making purchases in stores, and using the telephone.

2. *Certain words or sounds are regarded as more difficult than others.*

3. *In varying degrees, use is made of word substitutions and circumlocutions.* This tends to be done only occasionally and more often as a reaction to frustration, or its imminence, than to actual fear of stuttering.

4. *There is essentially no avoidance of speech situations and little or no evidence of fear or embarrassment.*

PHASE IV

1. *Vivid, fearful, anticipations of stuttering.*

2. *Feared words, sound, and situations.*

3. *Very frequent word substitutions and circumlocution.*

4. *Avoidance of speech situations, or other evidence of fear and embarrassment.*

While Bloodstein's scheme provides a more complete description of the development of the disorder than that of Bluemel, it does have one of the same limitations. Five of the six "symptoms" characteristic of Phase I stuttering also are exhibited by many normal-speaking preschool-age children. That is, the amount they repeat (or otherwise hesitate) tends to vary considerably from day to day (Yairi, 1981, 1982); they tend to hesitate most "when excited or upset, when seeming to have a great deal to say, or under other conditions of communicative pressure"; they frequently repeat syllables and whole words (Johnson & Associates, 1959; Yairi, 1981, 1982); they tend to hesitate frequently at the beginnings of sentences, clauses, and phrases; their hesitations occur on both content and function words; and most of the time they ". . . show little evidence of concern about the interruptions in their speech." The only symptom that may differentiate the groups is the tendency to hesitate most when excited or upset, when seeming to have a great deal to say, or under conditions of communicative pressure. There is some evidence that normal-speaking preschool-age children, as a group, do not tend to hesitate more frequently in "stress" than in "neutral" situations (Wexler, 1982).

Van Riper's four tracks along which stuttering can develop

Van Riper (1982) agreed with Bloodstein that the process through which the symptomatology of the disorder in preschool children evolves into the adult form is not dichotomous. However, he concluded that the continuum (track) along which it developed was not the same for all persons. He indicated that there are at least four continua, or tracks, along which it can develop (see tables 4-1 and 4-2). Their existence has been verified by two other investigators (Daly, 1981; Preus, 1981). Track I, which his data suggest more than 50 percent of cases follow, is quite similar to the continuum defined by Bloodstein's four phases. As such, it has the same limitation as the scheme proposed by Bloodstein—the symptoms that define the beginning of this track also are exhibited by some normal-speaking preschool-age children.

Is the disorder that develops along tracks II, III, and IV the same as that which develops along track I? Though all are labeled "stuttering," they may not be the same disorder. The symptomatology evinced by the children on track II (see tables 4-1 and 4-2), for example, seems to be that of cluttering.

Development of stuttering during middle age and beyond

In the schemes that have been reviewed thus far there is an implicit assumption that once stuttering has reached its most severe form—usually during adolescence or early adulthood—it ceases to develop in a predictable manner. Research pertaining to this assumption began during the 1980s (Manning et al., 1984). Does the severity and symptomatology of the disorder tend to change during middle age and beyond? There is some evidence that personality and attitudes tend to change in predictable ways during the adult life cycle (Sheehy, 1976). Since personality attributes and attitudes influence stuttering severity (see chapter 2), it would not be particularly surprising if stuttering did change during middle age and beyond. There is a little evidence that this does, in fact, happen. According to Peters and Starkweather (1989), the following changes tend to occur after the age of 30:

> During this period, a gradual decline in the severity of stuttering usually is seen. New behaviors are no longer acquired, and although the tendency for a reduction of abnormality has largely stopped, the increased self-confidence and maturity seem to reduce the frequency with which all stuttering behaviors occur. Occasionally, there is complete remission. (pp. 316–317)

Table 4.1.   Onset Characteristics

Track I	Track II
Begins 2½ to 4 years.	Often late; at time of first sentences.
Previously fluent.	Never very fluent.
Gradual onset.	Gradual onset.
Cyclic.	Steady.
Long remissions.	No remission.
Good articulations.	Poor articulations.
Normal rate.	Fast spurts.
Syllabic repetitions.	Gaps, revisions, syllable and word repetitions.
No tension; unforced.	No tension.
No tremors.	No tremors.
Loci: first words, function words.	Loci: first words, long words, scattered throughout sentence, content words.
Variable pattern.	Variable pattern.
Normal speech is well integrated.	Broken speech with hesitation and gaps, even when not disfluent.
No awareness.	No awareness.
No frustration.	No frustration.
No fears; willing to talk.	No fears; willing to talk.

Track III	Track IV
Any age after child has consecutive speech.	Late, usually after 4 years.
Previously fluent.	Previously fluent.
Sudden onset, often after trauma.	Sudden onset.
Steady.	Erratic.
Few short remissions.	No remissions.
Normal articulation.	Normal articulation.
Slow, careful rate.	Normal rate.
Unvoiced prolongations.	Unusual behaviors.
Laryngeal blockings.	
Much tension.	Variable tension.
Tremors.	Few tremors.
Beginning of utterance after pauses primary.	First words; rarely on function words; content words especially.
Consistent pattern.	Consistent pattern.
Normal speech is very fluent.	Normal speech is very fluent.
Highly aware.	Highly aware.
Much frustration.	No frustration.
Fears speaking; situation and word fears.	No evidence of fear; willing to talk.

Source: Reproduced from Van Riper, 1982, p. 106, with permission of the publisher.

In addition, older stutterers tend to perceive their stuttering as less of a handicap than they did when they were young adults (Manning et al., 1984).

Table 4.2 Developmental Characteristics

Track I	Track II
Repetitions of syllables increase in frequency and speed and become irregular.	Behaviors remain the same but the speed increases; their number also increases.

Then:

Repetition of syllables begins to end in prolongations.	Little change in form.

Then:

Prolongations show increased tension, tremors, struggle. Evidence of frustration.	Little change; little awareness; little frustration.

Then:

Overflow of tension; facial contortions; retrials; speech output decreases; signs of concern.	Duration of nonfluencies increases; more syllabic repetitions; little awareness.

Then:

Word fears and avoidance occur. Fears of certain sounds arise. Then situation fears develop. Repetitions and prolongations turn into silent fixations with struggle (blocking). Poor eye contact and tricks to disguise the difficulty are observed. Shows hesitancy, embarrassment.	Occasional fears of situations, not of words or sounds. Long strings of syllabic repetitions at fast speed are added to other behaviors. Some fears of situations. Good eye contact. No disguise. Output of speech increases. Little avoidance. Primarily repetitive. Unorganized.

Track III	Track IV
An increase in the frequency but the behavior at first changes little. Signs of frustration.	The number of instances increases, and they are shown in more situations.

Then:

More retrials are seen; lip protrusions and tongue fixations appear; prolongations of initial sounds.	Little change in form; monosymptomatic and symbolic.

Then:

Tremors; struggling; facial contortions; jaw jerk, gasping; marked frustration.	Little change.

Then:

Interruptor devices become prominent; rate slows; more hesitancy; more refusals to talk.	Little change in type but duration and visibility increase; no interruptions or new forcings; increased output of speech.

Then:

Intense fears of words and sounds; many avoidances; patterns change in form and grow more bizarre; much overflow; output of speech decreases; will cease trying to talk. Poor eye contact; the normal speech becomes hesitant. Nonvocalized blockings are frequent. Primary tonic blocks with multiple closures.	Very few avoidance or release behaviors. Not much evidence of word fears. Few consistent loci. Very aware of stuttering. Stutters very openly. Good eye contact. Little variability in the stuttering behavior. Normal speech very fluent. Talks a lot. Consistent pattern; few silent blockings. Either tonic or clonic.

Source: Reprinted from Van Riper, 1982, p. 107, with permission of publisher.

Recovery from Stuttering

Considered thus far in this chapter is how the symptomatology of the stuttering problem, following onset, evolves into a more severe (complex) form. There is a second way in which the disorder can evolve: The person can recover. A recovery apparently can occur at any age from pre-school to adulthood. According to Ainsworth and Fraser-Gruss (1981):

> It has been estimated that for every person who stutters today, there are three other people who have stuttered at some point in their development. The reasons these people and their parents give for their recovery are extremely varied. . . . (p. 10)

How do we know that some persons recover from stuttering? The evidence comes from several sources. One is anecdotal reports from persons who claim to have stuttered and no longer do so. I have met more than ten people during the past 30 years who claim to have recovered from stuttering whom I am fairly certain really did stutter at one time. Various explanations were offered by them for their recovery. For example, one attributed it to manipulation by a chiropractor; another to learning diaphragmatic breathing; a third to the healing power of a television evangelist; a fourth to learning to talk more slowly; a fifth to having his lingual frenum cut; and a sixth to elocution lessons. All indicated directly or indirectly that they had had confidence in the ability of the technique and/or the person who administered it to cure their stuttering and that they no longer thought of themselves as having a stuttering problem.

Further evidence that some persons recover from stuttering comes from surveys in which participants (mostly high school and college students) were asked whether they had stuttered at any time during their lives (e.g., Culton, 1986). The percentages of persons in these surveys who reported to have stuttered ranged from less than one percent to more than 10 percent, and the percentages of those who reported that they had stuttered but recovered in all of them exceeded 35 percent. While this percentage may be somewhat inflated because it is likely to include some persons who considered their normal repetitions and/or other hesitations to be stuttering, it nevertheless provides strong evidence that some persons do recover from the disorder.

Evidence that some persons recover from stuttering is also found in longitudinal research. Yairi and Ambrose (1992b) have reported data that are consistent with this conclusion on 27 preschool-age children who were followed for a period of from two to twelve years after they began stuttering.

Assuming that recovery from stuttering is possible, at what ages does it tend to occur? The available data suggest that it can do so at any age. Seider, Gladstein, and Kidd (1983), for example, reported ages of recovery that ranged from three to thirty-eight years. However, younger persons appear more likely to recover than older ones

(Seider et al., 1983). From an analysis of the findings of several studies, Andrews et al. (1983) estimated that approximately three times as many who are stuttering by age four than are stuttering by age ten will have recovered by age sixteen. Of course, some of those who were looked upon as stuttering at age four may actually have been normally disfluent. However, it is unlikely that enough were misdiagnosed to account for their probability of recovery declining as a function of age.

If some children recover before reaching adulthood, the prevalence of the disorder in preschool and elementary-school-age children would be expected to be higher than in high-school-age children and adults. While this has not been demonstrated unequivocally to be the case, the available data (see Brady & Hall, 1976) suggest that it is.

Is there any relationship between the severity of a person's stuttering and the likelihood that he or she will recover? There is some evidence that there is a negative relationship between them (Dickson, 1971; Sheehan & Martyn, 1970). That is, the more severe the stuttering, the less the likelihood of recovery.

Another factor that may influence how likely a person is to recover is the degree to which he or she is perfectionistic. According to Amster (1994):

> A young stuttering child who is perfectionistic may react more strongly to disfluency and, in order to control his or her speech, use more effort, tension, struggle, and avoidance, making the disorder more severe and less likely to spontaneously remit. (p. 150)

Once a person has recovered from stuttering, how likely is it that he or she will begin to stutter again? That is, how likely is it that the person will relapse? There is considerable anecdotal evidence that suggests that relapse is very common within the first five years following "recovery." Relapse can occur after this period, but it seems to be less likely. Richter (1982), a German speech pathologist, reported beginning to stutter again after a period of recovery that lasted twenty-eight years. One of my clients began to stutter again after a period of recovery that he reported had lasted 40 years. Unfortunately, there is insufficient data available to estimate the probability of relapse for persons who have been "recovered stutterers" for more than five years.

ONSET AND DEVELOPMENT OF CLUTTERING

Onset

Cluttering usually begins during early childhood (before the age of five). Its initial speech symptoms are a relatively rapid speaking rate, part-word and word repetitions, and multiple articulation errors that reduce speech intelligibility. The child is usually not aware of there being anything abnormal about his or her speech. A reduction in speaking rate results in fewer repetitions and an increase in intelligibility. Most (if not all) aspects of the child's language development are likely to be delayed, at least a little.

The syllable repetitions of beginning clutterers, like those of beginning stutterers, can easily be confused with normal childhood syllable repetitions. Descriptions of young clutterers' repetitions by Weiss (1964) and others are similar to the normal repetitions of young children, and young clutterers' lack of awareness of them is similar to that for both young stutterers and normal speakers. The only speech characteristic that really differentiates young clutterers from young stutterers and normal speakers is a very rapid speaking rate that precipitates syllable repetitions and articulation errors.

Weiss (1964) and others have speculated about a link between beginning cluttering and beginning stuttering. They believe that stuttering can develop from cluttering. Consequently, many persons who are regarded by themselves and others as stutterers may really be clutterer-stutterers. They tend to be regarded as stutterers for two reasons: First, the stuttering component of their symptomatology is more conspicuous than the cluttering one; and second, speech-language pathologists and others, particularly in the United States, knew very little about cluttering until relatively recently and therefore didn't look for it as often as they should have when making diagnoses.

Development

If clutterers continue to speak rapidly (as most do), they will continue to be excessively disfluent. Furthermore, they will continue to have a low level of awareness of their rapid speaking rate and the hesitation phenomena (disfluencies) and articulation/language errors that it precipitates.

One of the main ways that the symptomatology of this disorder appears to change as it develops pertains to language deficits (see chapter 3). Reading and writing deficits, for example, are more likely to be evident in older children and adults than in young children.

ONSET AND DEVELOPMENT OF NEUROGENIC ACQUIRED STUTTERING

Onset

While this disorder can begin at any age, it's more common for it to do so during adulthood than during childhood. The main reason is that the neurological conditions that can precipitate this disorder (see chapter 5) tend to occur in adults more often than in children. The onset of the disorder follows (often almost immediately) the onset of the neurological condition that precipitates it.

Development

Whether the amount of abnormal disfluency changes over time is largely a function of the neurological condition that precipitates it. If, for example, the neurological condition resulted from a side effect of a medication and the person ceased taking that medication, there would probably be at least some reduction in the amount of abnormal disfluency. On the other hand, if the neurological condition that did so was a tumor or a degenerative disease, the amount of abnormal disfluency would be likely to increase.

One way that this disorder may change over time is an overlay of stuttering being acquired. It is particularly likely if a person who has the disorder is highly motivated to avoid speaking disfluently (see chapter 8 for strategies for reducing the likelihood of such an overlay).

The types of disabilities and handicaps that are evinced by some older children and adults who stutter are also evinced by some persons who have this disorder. Consequently, the strategies described in chapter 7 for reducing the disabilities and handicaps of persons who stutter can also be used for persons who have neurogenic stuttering.

ONSET AND DEVELOPMENT OF PSYCHOGENIC ACQUIRED STUTTERING

Onset

While this disorder, like neurogenic stuttering, can begin at any age, it's more common during adulthood than during childhood. The onset of the disorder follows (sometimes almost immediately) the psychological trauma or condition that precipitates it.

Development

Whether the amount of abnormal disfluency changes over time is largely a function of the status of the psychopathology that precipitates it. If the psychopathology is reduced, either spontaneously or through therapy, the amount of abnormal disfluency would be likely to decrease.

Persons who have psychogenic acquired stuttering, like those who have neurogenic acquired stuttering, can develop an overlay of stuttering as well as the types of disabilities and handicaps evinced by stutterers. It isn't necessary, however, for them to develop an overlay of stuttering to have such disabilities and handicaps.

ASSIGNMENTS

Preschoolers' Hesitation Phenomena

Record the spontaneous speech of a three- or four-year-old child who is not regarded as having a fluency disorder. Describe the hesitation phenomena in his or her speech. To what extent are they similar to those of Bloodstein's Phase I stuttering?

Stuttering Mind-Set

Listen to the syllable repetitions of a three- or four-year-old child who is not regarded as having a fluency disorder with the mind-set that his or her repetitions are abnormal. Did you hear beginning stuttering? If you heard it, do you think that you would have if you hadn't had this mind-set?

5

Etiology

INSTRUCTIONAL OBJECTIVES

By the end of this chapter, you should be able to:

▸ Spell out five theories that have been used to explain the cause of stuttering (and possibly other fluency disorders) during the past 5,000 years.

▸ Explain the following scheme for categorizing hypotheses about stuttering: Predisposing cause versus precipitating cause versus maintaining cause.

▸ Explain the following scheme for categorizing hypotheses about stuttering: Etiology of stuttering versus moment of stuttering.

▸ Explain the following scheme for categorizing hypotheses about stuttering: Breakdown versus repressed need versus anticipatory struggle.

▸ Understand the arguments a little better for the etiology of stuttering being physiological, psychological, or some combination of the two.

▸ Specify at least 10 factors that can put a child at higher than normal risk for beginning to stutter.

▸ Explain several breakdown hypotheses, repressed-need hypotheses, and anticipatory-struggle hypotheses for predisposing, precipitating, and/or maintaining stuttering.

▸ Explain the continuity hypothesis for predisposing, precipitating, and/or maintaining stuttering.

▸ Explain shocks and fright, illness, imitation, and conflicts as possible causes for predisposing, precipitating, and/or maintaining stuttering.

▸ Explain "demand for fluency exceeding capacity" as a possible cause for predisposing, precipitating, and/or maintaining stuttering.

▸ Explain "reduced ability to generate temporal patterns" as a possible cause for predisposing, precipitating, and/or maintaining stuttering.

▸ Explain "linguistic and paralinguistic components being dyssynchronous when the speaker is under time pressure" as a possible cause for predisposing, precipitating, and/or maintaining stuttering.

▸ Describe at least three reasons why a person may continue to stutter after the disorder has been precipitated.

▸ Specify aspects of stuttering that may be learned and how they are learned.

▸ Explain how stuttering can be viewed as a member of a class of disorders that's characterized by anticipation of difficulty increasing the likelihood of abnormality occurring.

▸ Briefly describe the etiology of cluttering, neurogenic acquired stuttering, and psychogenic acquired stuttering.

Our focus in this chapter will be on both what has been and what currently is thought to be the cause of stuttering, cluttering, neurogenic acquired stuttering, and psychogenic acquired stuttering. There is considerable agreement about the etiology of cluttering, neurogenic acquired stuttering, and psychogenic acquired stuttering. This, unfortunately, is not true for stuttering. Consequently, because stuttering is the most common fluency disorder and there is a lack of agreement about its etiology, considerably more space was devoted to it in this chapter than to the other fluency disorders.

HOW HAVE FLUENCY DISORDERS BEEN EXPLAINED HISTORICALLY?

Until the middle third of the twentieth century, all fluency disorders were lumped together and referred to as stammering or stuttering. Thus, we can't be certain which fluency disorder(s) were being explained in the literature prior to this time (though they undoubtedly included stuttering). It's probably safest in this section, therefore, to view *stuttering* as a generic term for a fluency disorder.

People have been aware of and have tried to explain and cope with stuttering for thousands of years. The ancient Egyptians are said to have had a hieroglyphic symbol for it (Curlee, 1993, see figure 5-1). Perhaps what this hieroglyph depicts is a tremor—an earthquake—being conducted from the ground to the mouth: If this is so, then the Egyptians used the earthquake as a metaphor for the moment of stuttering.

Stuttering is mentioned several times in the Bible. Moses, who is thought to have stuttered, exhibited a behavior that is frequently a component of the stuttering problem—a desire to avoid talking. Because of his "slow tongue," he wanted God to have his brother Aaron speak to the Pharaoh instead of him:

> And Moses said unto the Lord: "Oh Lord, I am not a man of words, neither heretofore, nor since Thou has spoken unto Thy servant; for I am slow of speech, and of a slow tongue." And the Lord said unto

Figure 5-1   Egyptian hieroglyphic symbol for stuttering.

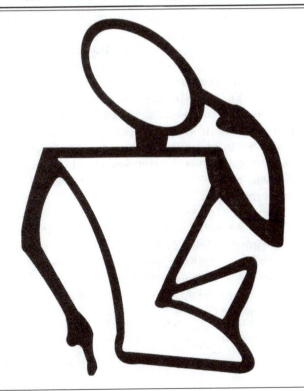

Source: From Curlee, 1993.

him: "Who hath made man's mouth? and who maketh a man dumb, or deaf, or seeing, or blind? Is it not I the Lord? Now therefore go, and I will be with thy mouth, and teach thee what thou shalt speak." (Exodus, 4:10–12)

The cause of Moses' stuttering, according to the Talmud, was physiological—abnormal functioning of his oral speech mechanism (Goldberg, 1989):

> While Moses was still an infant the Pharaoh was advised to kill him, for one day, it was predicted, Moses would rise up against him. The Pharaoh at first shrugged, then decided to put Moses to the test. He placed two bowls before Moses, one filled with gold, the other, with hot coals. If Moses chose the gold, he would be slain. Of course Moses reached for the gleaming gold, but an angel intervened and struck his hand. So he grabbed a hot coal and put it in his mouth. And thereafter stuttered. (p. 71)

The Bible also refers to stuttering in Isaiah (32:4): "And the tongue of the stammerers shall be ready to speak plainly."

During this century, some authorities have expressed the belief that stuttering is caused, at least in part, by an abnormality in the functioning of the peripheral speech mechanism. Some of the abnormalities to which they have attributed it are discussed elsewhere in the chapter.

In this section we will consider how stuttering has been viewed historically, which is important because our present views on both the etiology and management of stuttering are built upon the experience of the past. Clinicians who are unaware of how stuttering has been treated in the past are more likely than are those who have this knowledge to use intervention strategies that have been shown again and again to be of little or no long-term value. These strategies may produce a rapid reduction in stuttering severity, but the vast majority of clients on whom they are used are likely to relapse within five years following termination of therapy (Boberg, 1981; Boberg, Howie, & Woods, 1979).

People have attempted to explain stuttering (and stammering) in various ways during the past 5000 years. Their explanations have usually reflected what physicians, psychologists, psychiatrists, theologians, and philosophers thought at the time to be the cause of misfortune or abnormal behavior. Almost all such explanations (theories) have one of the following themes:

- punishment for sin

- physiological factors other than those directly related to the speech mechanism

- defects in the structure or function of the speech mechanism

- symptom of psychopathology
- learned behavior

Representative explanations having each theme are discussed in the following sections.

Punishment for Sin

Some explanations that have been around for thousands of years imply that stuttering is a punishment for sin—either that of the person who stutters or that of somebody in his or her family. Battus (the son of Polymnestros, a notable Theraean of the fifth century B.C.) went to Delphi to inquire of the prophetess how to cure his stammering. She indicated that his disability resulted from angering Apollo and that he must follow her instructions to placate the god; hopefully, doing so would cause Apollo to be merciful (Herodotus, 1821).

Although punishment for sin, to my knowledge, has not been advocated by any contemporary authorities on stuttering, one occasionally encounters a stutterer or parents of a stutterer who appears to believe it. They may say they believe that this is the cause of their or their child's stuttering, or they may indicate such a belief indirectly by praying for a cure or participating in healing services. There appears to be a fairly generally held belief in our society that "bad things happen to bad people" judging, for example, by the popularity of such books as *Why Bad Things Happen to Good People* (Kushner, 1981).

Physiological Factors Other than Those Directly Related to the Speech Mechanism

Stuttering has been attributed for thousands of years to physiological processes that are not directly related to the mechanisms of respiration, phonation, and/or articulation. Hippocrates, the father of medicine and the author of the Hippocratic oath, stated in the fifth century B.C. that speech disorders, including stuttering, were caused by a disturbance in the harmonious mingling of the four "humours," which are referred to as either heat, cold, moisture, and dryness or blood, bile, phlegm, and a "watery humour" (Hippocrates, 1923a, 1923b, 1923c). Mercurialis, a sixteenth-century physician, felt that the cause of chronic stuttering was a disturbance in the humidity of the brain (Appelt, 1911). Twentieth-century theories of this type have attributed stuttering to abnormalities in (1) the structure and/or function of the hearing mechanism, (2) the bones of the head, (3) the endocrine system, (4) the autonomic nervous system, and (5) the central nervous system.

Defects in the Structure or Function of the Speech Mechanism

These theories attribute stuttering to some abnormality in the structure or function of the mechanisms of respiration, phonation, and/or articulation. Demosthenes, in the fourth century B.C., is reported to have overcome stuttering by practicing speaking with pebbles under his tongue: A generally accepted theory of the time cited the tongue as being responsible for all abnormalities of speech (Cicero, 1942). Aristotle (who had been born in the same year as year as Demosthenes) also blamed the tongue for causing stuttering:

> When people stammer it is due, not to an affection of the veins, but to the movement of the tongue; for they find a difficulty in changing the position of the tongue when they have to utter a second sound. (cited in Eldridge, 1968, pp. 15–16)

The belief that an abnormality in the structure and/or function of the tongue causes stuttering appears to have been the most widely held view between the time of Aristotle and the Renaissance (about A.D. 1500).

Between the Renaissance and the beginning of the twentieth century the tongue continued to be blamed for stuttering. Other abnormalities of the structure or function of the speech mechanism also were regarded as the cause. Several scholars during the seventeenth century blamed the hyoid bone for stuttering. A seventeenth-century Italian anatomist believed that two holes of abnormal size, somewhere in the middle region of the palate, were responsible for causing stuttering. An eighteenth-century scholar attributed stuttering to a weakness of the soft palate, uvula, and root of the tongue.

During the nineteenth century there was considerable speculation about the cause of stuttering, much of which focused on a defect in the structure or function of the speech mechanism. In a book published in 1817, Itard, a French physician, speculated that stuttering was caused by a general debility of the nerves that stimulated the movements of the tongue and larynx (Hunt, 1861). This was one of the first times that the etiology of stuttering was attributed to the larynx, a topic on which there was considerable research during the 1970s and 1980s. Itard recommended exercises for improving tongue strength that involved placing a fork beneath the tongue.

In early nineteenth-century America a physician named Yates developed what became known as the "American Method" for treating stuttering. This method apparently regarded the etiology of stuttering as involving, at least in part, the functioning of the tongue, because it instructed the stutterer to keep the tip of the tongue resting continually on the alveolar ridge (Appelt, 1911). At night a small roll of wet linen was placed under the tongue to help the person maintain this position. Between 1825 and 1830 more than 100 cases were reported to have been cured by this method.

Colombat de l'Isère in 1831 classified moments of stuttering into two groups: (1) those in which the blockings resulted from spasms of the lips and tongue and (2) those in which the spasms occurred in the larynx, pharynx, or respiratory muscles (Eldridge, 1968). He recommended various types of exercises for improving the functioning of the mechanisms of respiration, phonation, and articulation. He also developed a small metronome-type device—known as the *muthonome*—with which stutterers were encouraged to pace their speech (Wingate, 1976, p. 155). More than one hundred years later (in the late 1960s) there was again considerable interest in the use of miniature metronomes for stutterers (see chapter 7).

A German surgeon, Johann Frederick Dieffenbach, believed that stuttering was caused by a spasm of the glottis, and early in 1841 he began treating it by surgery (Lebrun & Bayle, 1973). His operation to cure this spasm consisted of making a horizontal incision at the root of the tongue and excising a triangular wedge across it. More than 250 stutterers in France and Germany were reported to have undergone this operation in 1841 (incidentally, without anesthesia). Though Dieffenbach claimed successful results, some stutterers who underwent the procedure died, and other surgeons who experimented with it did not substantiate his results. Consequently, by the end of 1841 the procedure was apparently abandoned (Hunt, 1861).

Dieffenbach's approach was not the only medical-surgical one to be tried and abandoned during this period. According to Eldridge (1968), others included severing the hypoglossal nerve, piercing the tongue with hot needles, blistering the tongue with embrocations, encouraging smoking as a sedative for the vocal folds, and administering tincture of peppermint oil and chloroform to allay diaphragmatic spasms.

During the second half of the nineteenth century theories continued to be advanced that attributed stuttering to a defect in the structure or function of the speech mechanism, though the primary emphasis during this period appeared to be on psychological mechanisms. A number of devices were introduced, presumably, to help overcome the effect of such defects on speech and, thereby, to cure stuttering. One of these, which was invented by an American named Bates, consisted of a narrow flattened tube of silver, seven-eighths of an inch in length and three-eighths of an inch in diameter, which was held in close proximity to the hard palate by a piece of wire that was fastened to the anterior teeth (Rieber, 1977). The tube was positioned so that the anterior end was lodged just behind the teeth and the posterior opened into the mouth, looking upward and backward toward the fauces. The tube was intended to overcome spasms when producing lingua-palatal sounds by preserving a continuous flow of air. The Committee of Science and Arts of the Franklin Institute in Philadelphia (which was one of the most respected U.S. institutions supporting science and technology during this period) in 1854 presented Bates with one of their most prestigious awards for "his ingenious and useful invention."

Another instrument invented during this period consisted of a collar that was secured around the neck under a "stock or a cravat" (Rieber, 1977). It was fitted with a metal plate designed to rest upon the thyroid cartilage. A screw, resting in a spring, regulated the pressure of the plate on the cartilage. When the pressure was strong enough "to approximate the thyroid and arytenoid cartilages," muscular spasms of the glottis were claimed to be overcome.

There were also attempts during this period to overcome the defect in the structure or function of the speech mechanism by encouraging the stutterer to speak in a nonhabitual manner. One authority recommended that stutterers open the glottis when beginning to block by pronouncing or droning the schwa vowel. He also recommended the substitution of a "soft drawl" for a stutter (Eldridge, 1968). Encouraging stutterers to speak in nonhabitual manners continued throughout the twentieth century, even though it was demonstrated repeatedly through both clinical experience and systematic research that the reduction in stuttering severity resulting from the use of such strategies was almost always temporary.

The use of surgical approaches unfortunately did not cease after the nineteenth century. People underwent operations at the beginning of the twentieth century under the impression that such measures would cure their stuttering. According to Blanton and Blanton (1936):

> The commonest was tonsillectomy and the removal of adenoids. The clipping of the frenum and uvula were quite common. A method popular around 1922 and 1923 was the widening of the dental arch. Occasionally a patient was seen whose tongue has been nicked, and, very rarely, cases were recorded of trepanning, or cutting a hole in the skull. (p. 119)

During the twentieth century many persons who treated stuttering stated a belief (or demonstrated one indirectly by the strategies they used for treating stuttering) that the condition was caused by a defect in the structure or function of some part of the speech mechanism. Breathing exercises and various types of vocal gymnastics were advocated. Persons who treated stuttering in this manner included those both with and without medical training. Those without medical training included speech (elocution) instructors and public school teachers who had little or no formal training in the treatment of speech disorders as well as those who had received significant amounts of such training, persons who had been trained to be speech therapists and persons who had no formal training in speech disorders but felt they had been successful in overcoming their own stuttering and offered to share their "secret" for doing so (for a price) with others. In the early part of the twentieth century, some persons in this latter group began what are known as *commercial stuttering schools* (Wingate, 1976). One of the most infamous of these was the Bogue Institute in Indianapolis. Such schools, most of which used "secret methods" and were residential, offered a "guaranteed cure" for a fairly high tuition that was usually paid in advance. Following is an example of the type of guarantee that was offered by commercial stuttering schools:

> No matter what caused your stammering, no matter how old you are, how long you have stammered, how many times you have tried to be cured—no matter what you think about your case or whether you believe it is curable—if I have diagnosed your trouble and pronounced it curable, then I can cure YOU. . . . I not only claim to be able to do this for you, I back it up with a past record of success in treating hundreds of cases similar to your own. Like cures like. What has cured others like you, will cure YOU. But I don't ask you to risk a single penny upon even that evidence and proof. The moment you enroll in the Bogue Institute, I will issue to you and place in your hands, a written Guarantee Certificate, over my own signature, binding me to cure you of stammering or refund every cent of the money which you have paid me for tuition fee, and asking you only to follow the easy instructions given under the Bogue Unit Method (Bogue, 1926, pp. 236–237)

Some schools, like the one above, offered to refund the tuition if the stutterer was not cured. In most cases, when a stutterer relapsed after leaving the school and asked for a refund, he or she was held at fault for the relapse—that is to say, the stutterer was told that if he or she had followed instructions precisely, the problem would have been cured.

There have been a number of attempts since the end of World War II to attribute stuttering (at least in part) to a defect in the functioning of some aspect of the speech mechanism. Many speech-language pathologists now believe that such a defect does contribute to the etiology of stuttering. Both these theories and the research that supports them are discussed elsewhere in this chapter.

Symptom of Psychopathology

Explanations of this type, which are based on the *medical* model, regard stuttering as a symptom of some type of psychopathology. By classifying it as a symptom, the implication is that it indicates the presence of a psychological pathological process in much the same way as a fever indicates the presence of a physiological pathological process (an infection). Just as a physician usually would not treat a fever (symptom) but the infection causing it, a clinician who believes that stuttering is a symptom of psychopathology usually would not treat the stuttering (symptom) but the psychological pathological process believed to cause it. Theoretically, if the physician were successful in treating the infection, the fever would go down; and if the clinician were successful in treating the psychopathology, the client would stutter less severely. We will consider in this section how a psychological pathological process underlying stuttering has been conceptualized historically—that is, up to the end of World War II.

There appear to have been few attempts prior to the nineteenth century to attribute stuttering to psychopathology. One of the earliest attempts to do so was by the eighteenth-century philosopher Moses Mendelssohn, who attributed stuttering to "a collision between many ideas, flowing simultaneously from the brain" (Eldridge, 1968, p. 36). The belief that persons stutter because "they think faster than they can talk" or because "they do not think of what they are going to say before they say it," incidentally, still is held by many stutterers and nonstutterers alike. As mentioned earlier, it is not unusual for a pre- schooler whom parents believe is beginning to stutter to tell the child to think of what he or she is going to say before saying it. Unfortu- nately, such a suggestion may be more likely to increase stuttering than to reduce it.

During the first half of the nineteenth century there were several attempts to attribute stuttering to psychopathology—specifically, a lack of harmony between thought and speech. Rullier, for example, stated that stuttering ". . .was caused by a disproportion between the rate at which the brain can produce thoughts and that at which it can transfer them to the different stages of innervation," and Blume held that it was caused by "a lack of harmony between thinking and speak- ing" (Appelt, 1911).

Interest in theories that view stuttering as a symptom of psycho- pathology increased considerably during the latter half of the nine- teenth century. Klencke (1860) published an influential book in which he indicated that stammering reflected the stammerer's need of psy- chological help—his whole personality needed treatment; further, Klencke advocated attention to environmental influences and opened a sanatorium as a place of retreat and treatment for stammerers. He was one of the first clinicians to view stuttering as a symptom of an environmentally induced personality disturbance and to stress the importance of treating the whole person—not just the mouth.

During the first two decades of the twentieth century there contin- ued to be considerable interest in theories that viewed stuttering as a symptom of psychopathology. There was a marked tendency during this period to view Freudian psychology and psychoanalysis as a pana- cea for many ills—including stuttering. A paper was published in Ger- many in 1908 entitled "Nervous Disorders and Their Treatment," in which stuttering was discussed as an anxiety neurosis from the psy- choanalytic point of view. Another published in Germany in 1909 was entitled "A New Treatment for Stuttering" and discussed the applica- tion of psychoanalytic techniques. In 1911 Appelt published the book, *Stuttering and Its Permanent Cure*, which strongly advocated the use of psychoanalytic techniques for the treatment of stuttering.

Considerable enthusiasm was generated by such publications and a number of psychoanalytically trained clinicians attempted to use these methods for treating stuttering. Isidor Coriat (1931) held that every stutterer should have psychoanalysis. However, he expressed doubts about whether a complete cure could be expected because he had seen many examples of relapse. Another psychoanalyst, Abraham Brill (1923), after 11 years of treating a total of 69 stutterers through psychoanalysis claimed only five cures, of which one was reported to have relapsed.

Among the persons reported to be skeptical about the value of psychoanalysis in treating stuttering was Sigmund Freud himself. According to a personal communication by Esti Freud (Freund, 1966, p. 174), he was of the opinion that psychoanalysts did not understand the mechanism of stuttering and that psychoanalytic techniques had been valueless in treating it.

Edward Scripture, an American physician who had cooperated with Brill in applying psychoanalysis to stuttering, advocated a modified Freudian approach to the treatment of stuttering. He felt that even after psychoanalytic techniques had resolved the emotional problem causing the stuttering, the stutterer would still be likely to have some bad speech habits that he or she would have to be taught to eliminate (Scripture, 1931). This was one of the first attempts to combine psychotherapy and speech therapy in the treatment of stuttering.

During and immediately following World War I many soldiers on both sides who developed stuttering as a symptom of war neurosis ("shell shock") were treated at military hospitals. Since their condition was assumed to be psychological in origin (a neurosis), psychotherapy often was used. Some of the physicians treating them felt that psychotherapy alone could not eliminate all of the abnormal behaviors that occurred during their moments of stuttering because the behaviors were habits (learned responses), and thus the doctors advocated treating moments of stuttering directly.

There was an awakening of interest during the 1920s in training clinicians who were not physicians to treat communicatively handicapped persons, including stutterers. These persons offered speech correction services in such settings as university speech clinics and public schools. Many of them had been specialists in speech training and belonged to the National Association of Teachers of Speech. In 1925 some members of this organization who were primarily interested in therapeutic aspects of speech training formed the American Academy of Speech Correction—now the American Speech-Language-Hearing Association (Paden, 1970). Since most of the clinicians who viewed stuttering as a symptom of psychopathology were physicians, and since after the 1920s most of the clinicians in the United States who were treating stutterers were not physicians, it is not particularly surprising that there was less interest after this period in treating stuttering through psychotherapy alone.

Learned Behavior

Some theories, which view stuttering as a bad habit or learned behavior, have been around for at least three centuries. Amman (1700) was perhaps the first to state in print that stuttering is a bad habit. He attempted to help stutterers break the habit by, among other things, encouraging them to practice speaking loudly and slowly. Approximately one hundred years later Erasmus Darwin (1800), a stutterer who was the grandfather of Charles Darwin, attributed the disorder to emotionally conditioned interruptions of motoric speech. His recommendations included encouraging stutterers to begin plosive sounds with loose contacts. Madame Leith, who believed that the disorder resulted from an abnormal tongue-thrust habit, in 1825 trained patients to speak with the tongue tip up against the palate (Hunt, 1861). Arnott (1828), who believed that stuttering resulted from a learned "spasm of the glottis," sought to prevent it by teaching stutterers to prefix each word with an "e" vowel. There were others during the first half of the nineteenth century who viewed the etiology of stuttering in this way (Hunt, 1861).

The belief that stuttering was a bad habit (learned response) attained widespread acceptance, particularly in the United States and Britain, during the middle of the nineteenth century (Van Riper, 1982). One of the persons responsible for bringing this about was Alexander Melville Bell, the grandfather of Alexander Graham Bell (inventor of the telephone). Bell wrote several books promoting the view that stuttering was a habit and recommending that it be treated as such. He stated, "The impediment has been shown to be a habit; it is therefore beyond the province either of medical or surgical treatment, and within that, exclusively, of the educator" (Bell, 1853, p. 47). This view was also accepted by many practitioners during the last third of the nineteenth century (Van Riper, 1982).

During the first third of the twentieth century some persons continued to view stuttering as learned behavior, though the prevailing view (due to the influence of Freudian psychoanalysis) was that stuttering was a symptom of psychopathology—a neurosis. One of the most influential persons during this period who viewed it in this way was Knight Dunlap (1932). He believed that the habit of stuttering could be weakened by voluntarily practicing stuttering. Based on this theory (which Dunlap termed the *beta hypotheses*) the stutterer was told that "when the critic [clinician] commands 'again' he is to say the word over (or to say the initial syllable again if stopped on a syllable) in the same way as that in which he said it before, or in a way as near as possible to the erroneous one" (Dunlap, 1932). After the stutterer did so several times the clinician would say "right," and the stutterer would attempt to say it without stuttering.

The number of persons who viewed stuttering as learned behavior increased considerably during the middle third of the twentieth century. This was due, in part, to the fact that many persons who entered the field of speech pathology with strong interests in stuttering during the 1930s, 1940s, and 1950s received at least some of their graduate training in departments of psychology. The University of Iowa was the institution from which many of these persons received their Ph.D. degree (Moeller, 1975). Two of the most influential were Wendell Johnson and Charles Van Riper. During this period, in psychology departments (particularly at Iowa) there was considerable interest in the possibility that at least some abnormal behaviors that were viewed as symptoms of psychopathology were learned. Hence, during this period a number of theories were formulated and intervention strategies were developed that looked on stuttering as being learned behavior (see the section dealing with "The Iowa Development" in Bloodstein, 1987). The impact of this view on stuttering theory and management during the final third of this century is discussed elsewhere in this chapter.

SCHEMES FOR CATEGORIZING HYPOTHESES ABOUT STUTTERING

Many hypotheses have been proposed to explain stuttering. Some deal with a single aspect of the disorder and others more than one. They have been categorized in a number of ways. Several that are of interest to clinicians are described in this section.

Predisposing Cause versus Precipitating Cause versus Maintaining Cause

The word *cause* in the question "What is the cause of stuttering?" can have three meanings. Each of the following questions illustrates one of them:

1. What factors *cause* one person to be at greater risk than another for beginning to stutter?

2. What actually *causes* a person to begin to stutter?

3. What *causes* a person to continue to stutter after the disorder has begun?

Answers to the first question are hypotheses concerning the *predisposing* cause(s) of stuttering; those to the second are hypotheses concerning the *precipitating* cause(s) of the disorder; and those to the third are hypotheses concerning the *maintaining* cause(s). Some explanations attempt to answer only one of them and others two or three.

Etiology of Stuttering versus Moment of Stuttering

This scheme, which was proposed by Bloodstein (1987), has a some-what different focus than the one just outlined. It is based on the aspect of the disorder being explained rather than its etiology. His *etiology of stuttering category* is a combination of the predisposing and precipitating cause categories in the preceding scheme with a little of the maintaining cause category thrown in. Any hypothesis that attempts to explain an aspect of the cause of stuttering can be placed in the etiology of stuttering category.

Bloodstein's *moment of stuttering category* includes a number of hypotheses, some of which can be placed in the maintaining cause category of the preceding scheme. Any that suggest answers to questions such as the following can be placed in this category:

- What abnormal physiological events result in moments of stuttering?

- Why are moments of stuttering more likely to occur on some words than on others?

- Why does stuttering tend to be more severe in some situations than in others?

- What psychological factors can influence the frequency and severity of moments of stuttering?

- Why does reading in chorus cause moments of stuttering to disappear?

- What behaviors (if any) that occur during moments of stuttering are learned? If any are learned, how are they learned?

- What is the role of expectancy in precipitating moments of stuttering?

Breakdown versus Repressed Need versus Anticipatory Struggle

This scheme, which was also proposed by Bloodstein (1987), categorizes hypotheses by *theme* rather than by the aspect of the disorder being explained. Hence, explanations with similar themes are included in a category regardless of whether they attempt to explain the cause of stuttering (predisposing, precipitating, or maintaining) or the symptomatology and phenomenology of the disorder.

There are three general themes that have appeared over and over again in explanations of both the cause of stuttering and the moment of stuttering. The first of these is the *breakdown* theme. Hypotheses having this theme attribute the aspect of the disorder being explained to some sort of *physiological* breakdown, which may or may not be stress related. Explanations that attribute stuttering to abnormal functioning of the central nervous system would fit into this category.

The second of these themes is *repressed need*. Hypotheses based on this theme view the aspect of the disorder being explained as a symptom of an abnormal psychological process, of which the person is probably not aware on a conscious level. One hypothesis that has a theme of this type is the Freudian one, which views the disorder as a symptom of a fixation at the oral or anal stage of infant sexual development (Glauber, 1982).

The third of these themes is *anticipatory struggle*. Hypotheses having this theme view the disorder as either resulting or worsening from the person *anticipating* with dread the occurrence of stuttering and *struggling* to avoid it. Explanations of this type for both the etiology of stuttering and the moment of stuttering have greatly influenced how the disorder has been managed during the past 40 years.

IS THE CAUSE OF STUTTERING PHYSIOLOGICAL OR PSYCHOLOGICAL?

There have been many attempts to answer this question. Some who have attempted to do so believe the evidence indicates that the cause is probably genetic (see Drayna, 1997; Felsenfeld, 2002), and others believe it indicates that the cause is probably psychological (e.g., learned behavior). Still others believe it indicates that the cause is some combination of the two—neuropsychological. The latter view appears to be the most accepted one at present, with the main focus being on the physiological (Smith, 1990a).

Why have persons knowledgeable about stuttering reached such different conclusions? There are several reasons why they may have done so. One is that they have different beliefs about the most likely cause for abnormal behavior. Each of us has such a belief based on the totality of our life experience. That is, we accept a particular cause unless the evidence to the contrary is so strong that we would feel we were being "irrational" to continue doing so. The beliefs of persons who attempted to answer this question, not surprisingly, have been influenced by their professional training. Psychoanalytically trained psychiatrists, for example, have tended to conclude that the cause is psychological (Glauber, 1982).

A second reason why persons knowledgeable about stuttering have reached different conclusions about its "organicity" is that they weigh the evidence bearing on it differently. While the findings of some studies suggest that the physiological functioning of persons who stutter differs in some way(s) from that of their normal-speaking peers, those of others do not (see chapters 2 and 3). Persons who give greater weight to the former studies are more likely to conclude that the cause is physiological than those preferring the latter. A person's beliefs about the cause of abnormal behavior undoubtedly will influence how he or she weighs such evidence.

During the past 60 years, the beliefs held by the majority of speech-language pathologists about the organicity of stuttering have changed several times (Bloodstein, 1987). As this book is being written, most appear to believe that the cause is largely physiological. During the 1940s, 1950s, and 1960s, most seemed to believe that the cause was in large part psychological. Yet during the 1930s, most seemed to believe that the cause was largely physiological. Such opinion shifts also occurred prior to 1930.

Why would persons knowledgeable about stuttering change their belief from the cause being psychological (functional) to it being physiological (or vice versa) and back again? One reason would be the publication of research reports indicating that the physiological functioning of persons who stutter differs in some way from that of their normal-speaking peers. For example, publication of such reports during the 1970s and 1980s (see chapter 3) changed the minds of many of those who previously had believed the cause to be psychological.

The cause of stuttering appears to be both physiological and psychological (Smith, 1990a). Some aspects of its symptomatology and phenomenology appear to result from physiological factors and others from psychological ones (see chapters 2 and 3). Also, a cause that can be viewed as psychological also can be viewed as physiological. If, for example, you believe that the desire to avoid stuttering contributes to precipitating it (a psychological belief), it follows that such a desire causes persons who stutter to function abnormally physiologically. It would be this disturbance in physiological functioning that precipitates moments of stuttering. Hence, based on this belief the cause of moments of stuttering would be *both* physiological and psychological!

WHAT FACTORS CAUSE ONE CHILD TO BE MORE AT RISK FOR STUTTERING THAN ANOTHER?

Some children appear to be at greater risk than others for beginning to stutter (Andrews et al., 1983). That is, they appear to be more vulnerable to the condition, or conditions, that *precipitate* stuttering. A number of factors are discussed in this section that may influence the probability that a child will begin to stutter. Some of these factors have been referred to as *predisposing causes* of stuttering. While the presence of more than one probably increases the likelihood of a child beginning to stutter, the degree to which it does so has not been established. However, even if a number of these factors do apply to a particular child, the odds still appear to be greater that he or she will *not* begin to stutter than that he or she will do so (Andrews et al., 1983).

The Sex of the Child

The likelihood of a boy beginning to stutter is greater than that of a girl doing so. The sex ratio that has been reported by investigators in a number of countries ranges from 3:1 to 5:1 (Andrews & Harris, 1964; Beech & Fransella, 1968; Bloodstein, 1987; Van Riper, 1982). Since the prevalence of stuttering in the population has been reported to be approximately one percent, this means that fewer than one percent of girls stutter and more than one percent of boys do so.

Why are boys more likely than girls to stutter? While the reason has not been established empirically, there has been considerable speculation about it. Some writers (such as Schuell, 1946) have pointed out that boys are more vulnerable than girls for developing a number of disorders, possibly indicating that they are "weaker" than they are in some ways or are less able to tolerate stress. We know, for example, that boys tend to develop (mature) at a somewhat slower rate than girls in a number of ways, including language acquisition.

A second reason suggested for why more boys than girls begin to stutter is that the *environment* in which boys grow up tends to differ from that for girls in ways that make them more vulnerable to developing the disorder. One difference mentioned is in how parents and others tend to perceive, evaluate, and react to boys. According to Ainsworth and Fraser-Gruss (1981):

> Some psychologists feel that part of this difference comes from our cultural expectations for boys. A boy is expected to act like a man too soon. If he cries for reasons not approved of for boys, [a parent] may think that he is not measuring up. (p. 22)

Some of these explanations assume that the manner in which a child's speech hesitations are perceived, evaluated, and reacted to influences the probability that he or she will begin to stutter and that parents and others are more likely to perceive, evaluate, and react to speech hesitations of boys than those of girls in a manner that could precipitate stuttering. Research bearing on such explanations is summarized in this chapter in the section discussing the diagnosogenic theory for the onset of stuttering.

A third reason that has been suggested for this phenomenon is that a specific biologic sex-related difference contributes to making boys more vulnerable. It has been suggested, for example, that the sex ratio in stuttering is due to higher levels of testosterone in the male than in the female fetus, which affects the development of the central nervous system in a way that makes males more vulnerable to developing the disorder (Geschwind & Galaburda, 1985).

A fourth reason that has been suggested is a genetic predisposition for stuttering (some type of sex-modified inheritance) that is more likely to affect males than females (Ambrose, Yairi, & Cox, 1993; Felsenfeld, 2002). While such a predisposition would cause a child to be more likely than otherwise to begin to stutter, it probably would not precipitate the disorder. The actual precipitating cause probably would be "environmental" in nature.

The Age of the Child

While a person can begin to stutter at any age, the likelihood of doing so is greater before the age of five than after the age of five. According to Andrews (1984), "On the basis of the data presently available, half the risk of stuttering is passed by age four, three-quarters by age six, and virtually all by age twelve."

Very few cases of stuttering that began during adulthood have been reported (Van Riper, 1982). Some persons who claim to have begun to stutter as an adult may actually have stuttered occasionally and/or mildly during childhood. However, they either don't remember doing so or they don't consider it to be the same disorder because they remember their hesitations as being much less tense than those they are presently experiencing. Several persons who initially told me they began to stutter as an adult reported episodes of mild stuttering in childhood after I questioned them about their fluency during this period. Some persons who report that they began to stutter as an adult may actually have one of the other fluency disorders (see chapter 1).

While some cases of stuttering reported to have begun during adulthood may not have done so or may not be stuttering, there undoubtedly have been cases that did begin during this period. Actually, there is evidence (see Silverman, 1988b and the discussion of the "monster" study elsewhere in this chapter) that suggests that a person of almost any age can be made to stutter by reacting to his or her fluency in a negative manner.

Whether Any Members of the Family Stutter

The probability that a person will begin to stutter if he or she has relatives who stutter (or who had the disorder and recovered) is greater than it is for one who has no such family history. The fact that stuttering tends to run in families has been established by investigators in many countries, including the United States. The percentages of persons in these studies who had relatives on the maternal or paternal side who stuttered ranged from 30 to 69; the comparable percentages for normal speakers in these studies ranged from 5 to 18 (Bloodstein, 1987, table 7).

While a child who is born into a family in which there is a history of stuttering is at greater risk for acquiring the disorder, this does not necessarily mean that he or she will do so. All that these data really indicate is that the probability of a child beginning to stutter is greater than 1 in 100 if he or she is born into a family in which there is a history of stuttering. It is important to note that stuttering does occur in families in which there is reported to be no previous history of the disorder. The data referred to earlier in this section (ibid.) suggest that the families of at least 25 percent of the persons who stutter do not have such a history.

Why does stuttering tend to run in families? While authorities do not agree on the answer to this question, they have speculated about it a great deal. Reasons suggested include the following:

- A predisposition for stuttering may be inherited. Hence, stuttering (like diabetes and certain types of cancer) would be more likely to occur in families in which there is a history of the disorder.

- Stuttering can be caused by imitation. Young children, according to this explanation, are likely to imitate the speech of persons with whom they spend time. Hence, having someone in the family who stutters increases the odds that a child will spend time with a person who has the disorder. While some authorities during the first half of this century believed that stuttering can be caused by imitation, few (if any) did during the second half of the twentieth century (Bloodstein, 1987; Van Riper, 1982). One reason why this explanation has been rejected is that the symptomatology of beginning stuttering tends to differ from that evinced by older children and adults. Hence, if young children were imitating family members who stutter, they probably would be exhibiting the symptomatology of an advanced stage of the disorder rather than the initial stage.

- Concern about a child stuttering can cause him or her to stutter. If there is a history of stuttering in the family, parents are more likely than otherwise to monitor their children's fluency and communicate to them that they are concerned about their repetitions and other hesitations. Some authorities (see Johnson & Associates, 1959) believe that such expressions of concern can be a precipitating cause of stuttering (see the discussion of the diagnosogenic theory in this chapter).

Socioeconomic Status of the Family

While stuttering occurs in families of all socioeconomic classes, there is a little evidence suggesting that it tends to do so more often in those that are middle or upper-middle class than in those that are lower class (Morgenstern, 1956). The evidence for this, however, is not clear cut (Andrews & Harris, 1964). Assuming that there is a tendency for stuttering to occur more frequently in middle- and upper-middle-class families, what might be the reason? One reason that has been suggested is that there tends to be a greater drive for achieving a higher status in middle- and upper-middle-class families than in those of other classes. (This, of course, does not mean that persons in other socioeconomic classes do not have such a drive; it only means that there tend to be more status-oriented people in middle- and upper-middle-class families.) Such persons usually want their children to achieve at least as high a status as did they themselves, and they are likely to believe that doing so requires excellence in a number of areas, including speaking. These parents, therefore, would be likely to become concerned if their children's speech appeared to be defective and would likely communicate their concern to them. Some writers, as mentioned previously, have suggested that this can precipitate stuttering (see the discussion of the diagnosogenic theory elsewhere in this chapter).

Nationality of the Family

The prevalence of stuttering in some cultures appears to be higher than in others. While prevalence in Western and other "technologically developed" cultures (including the Japanese) has been reported to be approximately one percent, there are cultures in which fewer than one percent have been reported to have the disorder, and in others more than one percent.

Why might the prevalence of stuttering be higher in some cultures than in others? To answer this question, anthropologists and others have attempted to determine what those cultures with a high rate of stuttering have in common that differentiates them from those with a relatively low rate of stuttering. Bloodstein (1987) summarized their findings as follows:

> To say that there are many stutterers in a given society is very possibly to say that it is a rather competitive society that tends to impose high standards of achievement on the individual and to regard status and prestige as unusually desirable goals, that it is sternly intolerant of deviancy, and that, as a by-product of its distinctive set of cultural values, it in all likelihood places a high premium on conformity in speech. (p. 119)

Hence, the reason for cultural variation in stuttering prevalence may be the same as that based on the socioeconomic status of the family. Reread the above quotation from Bloodstein substituting *socioeconomic class* for *society*. He seems to be describing attitudes that are common in middle- and upper-middle-class families.

Whether the Child Is a Twin

A child who is a twin appears more likely to stutter than one who is not (Howie, 1981). Studies of the prevalence of stuttering in the twin population have consistently yielded percentages that are higher than the one percent in the general population.

If one member of a twin pair stutters, is the other likely to do so? The answer appears to depend on whether the pair is identical or fraternal. While the available evidence on identical twin pairs indicates that it is more common for both twins to stutter than only one doing so, that on fraternal twin pairs indicates that it is more common for only one member of a pair to stutter (Howie, 1981). It should be noted, however, that there are a significant number of identical twin pairs in which only one member stutters. In the studies reviewed by Bloodstein (1987, p. 112) this number exceeded 25 percent.

Why are children who are twins more likely to stutter than those who are not? Several explanations have been suggested. One is that a tendency toward twinning and a predisposition to stuttering are genetically linked in some families (Howie, 1981). A second is that an environmental factor (such as the competitive pressures a twin pair often encounters as a result of comparisons made between them) can make them more likely to stutter (Bloodstein, 1987).

Whether the Child Is Brain Injured

The incidence of stuttering that has been reported in most studies among children who are brain injured—particularly among those who have cerebral palsy or epilepsy—in most studies considerably exceeds one percent (Van Riper, 1982). It is uncertain, however, in how many of them the disorder is stuttering. Dysarthrias, apraxias, and word-finding problems (dysnomias), for example, can cause higher than normal levels of speech disfluency.

Whether the Child Is Mentally Retarded

A relatively high incidence of stuttering has been reported among children who are mentally retarded, particularly among those who have Down syndrome. The percentages of such children who have been reported to stutter in almost all studies considerably exceeds one percent (Bloodstein, 1987, table 20; Van Riper, 1982, table 3.1). The question arises (as it does with children who are brain injured) whether the disorder they evince is stuttering or something else. While the abnormal disfluency of some mentally retarded children undoubtedly is cluttering, disfluency associated with neuropathology, and/or developmentally delayed "normal" disfluency, that of others does appear to be beginning stuttering. Some mentally retarded persons, incidentally, have been reported to exhibit symptoms of advanced (secondary) stuttering including word fears, avoidances, and facial grimaces.

Whether the Child Is Bilingual

A child who is bilingual appears to be more likely to stutter than one who is unilingual (Stern, 1948). The reason for this has not been established.

Whether the Child Is Delayed in Language Development

Most studies of the language development of children who stutter indicate that they are more likely than their peers to be delayed in saying their first words, phrases, and sentences and in acquiring speech sounds (see chapter 3). The reason for this relationship between stuttering and delayed speech and language development has not been established. Several interpretations have been suggested:

- Stuttering and delayed speech and language development are caused by the same thing. It has been suggested, for example, that they can be caused by a common genetic predisposition or developmental apraxia.

- Children who are delayed in speech and language development are likely to acquire a sense of failure as speakers and learn to struggle with their speech attempts.

While there undoubtedly is a tendency for stuttering and delayed speech and language development to occur together, most children who stutter do not have a history of delayed speech and language development, and most children who do have such a history do not stutter.

Other Factors

A number of other conditions have been investigated because it was thought that they might influence the probability that a child will stutter. Some of these are:

- abnormalities in physiological functioning (particularly neurophysiological functioning), abnormalities in emotional adjustment, or abnormalities in sensory and perceptual functioning (see chapter 3)

- medical conditions, including diseases and events associated with birth that could cause brain damage. The findings of most studies suggest that stutterers are not more likely than their peers to have abnormal medical histories (Andrews & Harris, 1964)

- abnormalities in physical and social development. Children who stutter appear to compare favorably to their peers with respect to the ages at which they teethe, are weaned, dress and feed themselves, acquire bowel and bladder control, sit, creep, stand, and walk (ibid.)

WHY DO PEOPLE BEGIN TO STUTTER?

A number of factors were mentioned in the preceding section that could cause one person to be more likely to begin to stutter than another. However, the mere presence of one or more of these factors does not appear to cause someone to do so. Something has to *precipitate* the disorder. There has been considerable speculation about what this "something" is; unfortunately, persons knowledgeable about the disorder do not agree on it. We will consider in this section the three major types of explanations (hypotheses, theories) that have been mentioned in the literature for why persons begin to stutter: breakdown, repressed need, and anticipatory struggle. We also will consider several explanations that do not fit neatly into one of these categories.

Breakdown Hypotheses

Breakdown hypotheses are of two types. The first type suggests that stuttering is precipitated solely (directly) by some sort of breakdown in physiological functioning. Hypotheses of the first type attribute the onset of stuttering directly to some abnormality in physiological functioning that may or may not be genetic in origin. The abnormality is said to interfere with the ability of the speech mechanism to produce normally fluent speech. There has been speculation about the nature of this abnormality for thousands of years. For example, you will recall that in the fifth century B.C. Hippocrates explained it as being a disturbance in the harmonious mingling of the four humours: blood, bile, phlegm, and the "watery humour." If Hippocrates were stating this hypothesis today in contemporary language, he probably would indicate that the abnormality is some sort of chemical imbalance.

The second type of breakdown hypothesis suggests that the breakdown precipitating the disorder is a joint product of some sort of abnormality in physiological functioning and an environmental condition (or conditions) producing stress. Some writers (e.g., Bloodstein, 1987) refer to the physiological abnormality as the predisposing cause and the condition (or conditions) producing stress as the precipitating cause. Such hypotheses indicate that both causes have to be present before someone will begin to stutter. The physiological abnormality may or may not be regarded as genetic. Most present-day breakdown hypotheses are of this type.

Hypotheses of both types that have been suggested during this century are discussed in this section. While these are not the only such hypotheses, they include the ones that have been most influential.

A disturbance in cerebral dominance for speech production

One half of the cerebral cortex (usually the left) normally is dominant over the other for various aspects of speech production. If such dominance is not present to a sufficient degree or if the "wrong" hemisphere is dominant for a particular aspect (or aspects) of speech production, it has been suggested that this could result in a *breakdown* in speech production manifested as stuttering. According to these explanations, the person could either have been born with or acquired this anomaly. If the person acquired it, the cause sometimes was attributed to being forced to write with the nondominant hand. During the first half of this century many people believed that forcing left-handed children to write with their right hand could precipitate stuttering. While most authorities now do not believe that switching handedness *by itself* can precipitate stuttering, the evidence on this is inconclusive and conflicting. For example, while Haefner (1929) reported that 24 percent of the 41 children whose handedness he had shifted stuttered, Ojemann (1931) reported that none of the 23 children he had shifted did so.

Because our society does not consider it more desirable to be left-handed than right-handed, few (if any) able bodied right-handed children are likely to have been forced to write with their left hand. Therefore, if switching handedness is a factor in precipitating stuttering, we do not know whether it is so simply because handedness is switched or because switching handedness affects lateral dominance in a specific way. In this regard, Van Riper (1982) has reported three cases of boys who began to stutter after their handedness was purposefully switched from right to left to be more like their fathers (who were left-handed). Also, Oates (1929) reported an experiment in which twelve "subnormal" right-handed children were shifted to the left hand: All were reported to be stuttering after five months of such training. It would appear, then, that the act of shifting probably is more significant in precipitating stuttering than the direction in which the shifting is done.

If switching handedness does contribute to precipitating stuttering, perhaps it does so indirectly. Forcefully switching a child's handedness may cause him or her to become upset and, as a consequence, more disfluent than usual. This increases the probability that someone will become concerned about the child's fluency and communicate this concern to him or her. On the other hand, switching handedness may not make a child more disfluent but instead may cause an adult to become concerned about the child's "normal" disfluency because he or she has heard that switching handedness can cause stuttering. Here, expecting stuttering causes the person to listen to the child's fluency through a different "filter" than he or she would be likely to use otherwise (Johnson, 1946). Based on the diagnosogenic theory, either scenario could precipitate stuttering.

A biochemical imbalance or difference

Some hypotheses suggest that persons can begin to stutter because of a biochemical imbalance or difference that makes their speech mechanism more vulnerable than normal to the fluency-disrupting effects of emotional stress. One explanation of this type views the moment of stuttering as a kind of miniature seizure somewhat similar to that evinced by those who have a childhood form of epilepsy known as pyknolepsy. Such seizures affect mainly the speech mechanism and are precipitated by emotional stress (West, 1958). According to this hypothesis, children who begin to stutter are seizure-prone persons who would evince more severe epileptiform seizures if it were not for the fact that they had a biochemical *imbalance*, such as a relatively high blood sugar level (West, 1958). In other words, these children have epilepsy but are kept from evincing the usual symptomatology of the disorder, possibly by their high blood sugar levels. (While some studies suggest that persons who stutter have relatively high blood sugar levels, others do not.)

Another explanation of this type for why persons begin to stutter—particularly for why more males than females do so—is based on a biochemical *difference* between the sexes—that is, the level of the male sex hormone testosterone to which they were exposed as fetuses (Geschwind & Galaburda, 1985). There is some evidence that the neuronal development of the fetal brain, particularly that of the left cerebral hemisphere, tends to be retarded if the level of testosterone to which it is exposed is relatively high (Geschwind & Golaburda, 1985). Since the male fetus is exposed to higher levels of testosterone than the female, males are more prone to disturbances in left-hemisphere functioning for speech and language than females, which could make them more prone to use their right hemisphere for processing speech. Since the right hemisphere is less adequate than the left for doing this, the result could be an increase in hesitation, particularly in stressful situations.

Stress

Both normal speakers and persons of all ages who stutter tend to be more disfluent when feeling stressed or anxious (see chapter 2). Stress, or anxiety, has been hypothesized to contribute to precipitating stuttering in three ways. The first is *directly* precipitating the disorder *by itself*. Reports of persons beginning to stutter after extremely traumatic experiences support such an explanation. The second is *directly* precipitating the disorder *in conjunction with some type of abnormality* in physiological functioning—for example, a disturbance in cerebral dominance for some aspect of speech production. This explanation differs from the first by suggesting that stress, by itself, cannot precipitate stuttering and that a particular level of stress can precipitate the disorder in some persons (those with a particular physiological anomaly) but not in others.

The third way is *indirectly* precipitating the disorder by causing the person to repeat more often or otherwise be more disfluent. This would make it more likely that someone would become concerned about the person's speech fluency and "diagnose" it as abnormal. Some persons—including myself—believe that such a diagnosis can precipitate stuttering (see the discussion of the diagnosogenic theory in this chapter). This explanation differs from the other two by suggesting that stress does not directly precipitate stuttering, but does so indirectly by increasing the probability that someone will diagnose a person's hesitations as stuttering and react to them accordingly.

For further information about the impact of stress on stuttering, see Blood, Wertz, Blood, Bennett, & Simpson (1997).

Auditory feedback defect

The fluency of people who stutter improves under altered conditions of auditory perception, such as those produced by delayed auditory feedback devices (see chapter 2). Based on this observation, a number of theories have been proposed that attribute stuttering to aberrant auditory feedback during speech production (see Postma & Kolk, 1992, for a review of these theories). A common theme in these theories seems to be that the disturbance in auditory feedback causes the stutterer to detect errors that probably do not exist: The stutterer's attempts to overcome them produce the types of breakdowns in speech fluency that are classified as stuttering-type disfluencies. These theories are not widely accepted at present (Postma & Kolk, 1992).

Repressed-Need Hypothesis

These hypotheses, which view stuttering as a type of neurosis, posit that children begin to stutter because they attempt to cope with some type of repressed (unconscious) "neurotic" need in a way that causes them to be disfluent (Glauber, 1982). These hypotheses look upon stuttering as being both a symptom of an unsatisfied repressed emotional need and a purposeful behavior. Because it is repressed, the child is usually not consciously aware of this need, nor is he or she aware of attempting to cope with it. Such explanations assume that behaviors occurring during moments of stuttering are symbolic of (have meaning with regard to) the repressed need. The meaning of the behaviors is interpreted differently, therefore, depending on what the repressed need is assumed to be. If, for example, it is assumed to be an infantile need for oral erotic gratification, behaviors occurring during the moment of stuttering may be interpreted as symbolizing "the immature sexual pleasures of nursing, biting, and oral incorporation of objects that the person enjoyed as an infant . . ." (Bloodstein, 1987, p. 49). Those who explain stuttering in this manner assume that the person's need for oral erotic gratification was not fully satisfied while he or she was an infant, possibly because of a disturbance in the mother-child relationship.

What repressed needs has stuttering been interpreted as symbolizing? The following have been mentioned frequently in the literature:

- an unconscious mental conflict or disequilibrium. According to Glauber (1982, p. 57), when it "threatens to emerge in consciousness, the stutter worsens and/or becomes a major concern."

- an infantile need for oral erotic or anal erotic gratification (Glauber, 1982).

- an aggressive expression of hostile feelings that the person is afraid to express openly. Stuttering has been equated with aggression in several ways. One is that it allows the person to make those with whom he or she speaks "uncomfortable" without fear of retaliation. The assumption here is that stuttering is "painful" to the listener, particularly if he or she is a parent or other family member. It is well known, incidentally, that the severity of stuttering tends to increase when a speaker who has the disorder is angry at the listener but not openly acknowledging it. For a discussion of other ways in which stuttering has been equated with (interpreted as symbolizing) aggression, see Bloom (1978).

- a conflict between a conscious desire to speak and an unconscious desire to be silent. Several reasons have been suggested for why persons may experience such a conflict. One is that they may be afraid that if they speak, they will reveal certain desires or feelings or use words that their listeners will find unacceptable. Another is that the act of speaking itself means something to them that they feel should be suppressed. For example, they may secure oral gratification (pleasure) from speaking, and because they do not believe they deserve to be happy they may have guilt feelings for doing so. Also, they may view speaking as an act that will cause others to react negatively to them. They may have had people react negatively to them because of how they spoke (e.g., how they pronounced words), what they had to say, or both. For further information about this type of conflict, see Fenichel (1945, chapter 15).

For further information about stuttering viewed as a childhood neurosis satisfying a repressed need, see Bloodstein (1987), Bloom (1978), Coriat (1931), Glauber (1982), and Van Riper (1973, 1982).

Anticipatory-Struggle Hypothesis

The diagnosogenic theory and the continuity hypothesis both view stuttering (at least in part) as *learned behavior*. They are both discussed below.

The diagnosogenic theory

The most influential hypothesis of this type was formulated by Professor Wendell Johnson of the University of Iowa during the 1940s. This hypothesis, which usually is referred to as the *diagnosogenic theory* for the onset of stuttering (Johnson & Associates, 1959), suggests one set of circumstances (not necessarily the only one) that can precipitate the disorder. This hypothesis also has been referred to as the *semanto-genic theory* and the *interactional theory* for the onset of stuttering (Perkins, 1990a).

What does the term *diagnosogenic* refer to in this context? A diag-nosogenic disorder is one that is caused (precipitated) by its diagnosis (Johnson, 1946). A person's normal behavior is labeled abnormal, and as a consequence he or she begins to behave abnormally. The person begins doing so, at least in part, because he or she wants to *avoid* behaving in the way that has been labeled abnormal and/or because of *fear* of doing so. Trying not to behave in a particular way or fearing such behavior can cause you to behave abnormally more often (Frankl, 1985). For example, the desire to avoid perspiring excessively and the fear of doing so can increase the frequency at which it occurs (Frankl, 1985). As the behavior that was labeled "abnormal" increases in fre-quency, both the person(s) who initially labeled it such and the one who is exhibiting the behavior are likely to become more concerned about it. This is likely to strengthen both their desire to avoid the behavior and their fear of it occurring, and as a consequence it is likely to occur even more often. In this manner a *vicious circle* is established: the fear of behaving in a particular way and the desire to avoid doing so causes the behavior to occur even more often, and the more fre-quently it occurs, the stronger becomes both the desire to avoid it and the fear of not being able to do so.

According to the diagnosogenic theory, there are three events that have to occur before a child will begin to stutter (Johnson & Associates, 1959):

1. The child repeats or otherwise hesitates while he or she speaks. The frequency of occurrence of these behaviors does not have to be high: However, the higher it is, the more likely someone is to become concerned about it. Most, if not all, young children occasionally repeat sounds, syllables, and words and hesitate in other ways (see chapter 4). The amount that they do so appears to be related to a number of factors, including their cognitive stage of development (Lindsay, 1989).

2. A person with whom the child interacts "diagnoses" his or her repetitions and/or other hesitations as being abnormal and reacts to them accordingly. The person may be a parent, a grandparent, a teacher, a daycare giver, or anyone who spends time with the child. Most often, it is a parent. He or she does, however, have to be someone whom the child respects and would like to please. The person may make the child aware of

the disfluencies by occasionally saying one or more of the following when they occur:

- "Stop and start over again."
- "Think of what you are going to say before you say it."
- "Take a deep breath before you talk."
- "Talk more slowly."
- "Stop repeating (or stuttering)."

The person may also communicate that the disfluencies are undesirable by doing one of the following when they occur:

- Looking away from (avoiding eye contact with) the child while he or she is being disfluent.
- Having a pained or concerned expression.
- Refusing to acknowledge the presence of disfluencies when the child indicates awareness of them (in other words, playing the "Emperor's New Clothes" game).

3. The child becomes concerned about the disfluencies and tries not to be disfluent. He or she attends more to the disfluencies than previously and tends to become upset when they occur. Any strategy the child uses to keep them from occurring (such as "thinking of what he or she is going to say before saying it") is likely to fail because repeating is not under one's voluntary control. The more he or she tries to avoid them, the more frequently they tend to occur; and the more frequently they occur, the more he or she tries to avoid them. This vicious circle causes an increase both in the frequency at which the child repeats (or otherwise hesitates) and in his or her desire to avoid doing so. As the child's repetitions increase, expressions of concern about them from listeners also tend to increase. This, in turn, reinforces the child's desire to avoid them. It is in this manner, according to the diagnosogenic theory, that stuttering begins.

When the diagnosogenic theory was originally formulated, one of the main pieces of evidence used to support it was the finding that in several tribes of American Indians (e.g., the Bannock-Shoshoni) in which there appeared to be no word for stuttering, there appeared to be no stutterers (Snidecor, 1947; Stewart, 1960, 1985). However, evidence has been reported relatively recently suggesting both that these tribes do have a word for stuttering and stutterers (Zimmermann, Liljeblad, Frank, & Cleeland, 1983). While the presence in a culture of both a word for stuttering and stuttering itself is consistent with the diagnosogenic theory, it also could be consistent with other theories. Consequently, such data can no longer be interpreted as providing strong support for the theory.

What evidence is there that a child can begin to stutter in the manner specified by the diagnosogenic theory? There are a number of research findings that directly or indirectly support aspects of this theory:

- Some normal-speaking preschool-age children, particularly those between the ages of two and four, tend to repeat sounds, syllables, and single-syllable words a great deal (see Johnson & Associates, 1959; Silverman, 1972b; Yairi, 1981, 1982).

- The repetitions that initially caused the parents of some young stutterers to become concerned about their speech do not appear to have been abnormal (Johnson & Associates, 1959). Hence, it seems quite likely that normal repetitions sometimes are diagnosed as stuttering. It should be noted, however, that for some such children the amount of repetition they were exhibiting at the time someone first became concerned about their speech fluency probably exceeded that exhibited by most of their normal-speaking peers (Yairi & Lewis, 1984).

- After parents diagnose their child's repetitions as being abnormal, they say things or react in a manner that would tend to increase their child's awareness of and concern about the repetitions (Johnson & Associates, 1959). There are data which suggest that parent-child interactions can influence children's disfluencies (see Guitar, Schaefer, Donahue-Kilburg, & Bond, 1992, for a review of the literature in which they are reported).

- Some children appear to accept their parents' "diagnosis" that their hesitations are abnormal and react to them in ways suggesting that they are both concerned about them and attempting to avoid them (Johnson & Associates, 1959).

- There is some evidence (Johnson & Associates, 1959) that if parents who recently have diagnosed their preschool-age children as beginning to stutter are counseled not to perceive their children's hesitations as abnormal and therefore not to react to them as such can reduce the probability that the child will continue to be regarded as having a stuttering problem.

While these findings are consistent with major assumptions of this theory, none provide a direct test of it. To do such a test, it would be necessary to take some children who are normally fluent, cause them to become concerned about their hesitations, and see if they begin to stutter. Even better, children would be selected who are at low risk for beginning to stutter—those over the age of ten who are exceptionally fluent speakers. While their beginning to stutter certainly would not prove that all children begin doing so in this manner, it would certainly provide strong evidence that a child can begin to stutter in the manner specified by this theory. (You would be correct in concluding that this would be a highly objectionable way of obtaining data! However, such a method was actually employed, as the following paragraphs relate.)

The results of an unpublished master's thesis (Tudor, 1939), completed more than 60 years ago, can serve as a direct test of the diagnosogenic theory. This investigation, which is reported to have resulted in normal-speaking children being turned into stutterers, was referred to by those who knew of its existence as the "monster" study (Silverman, 1988b). Because of embarrassment about the outcome (and possibly also because of fear of litigation), the study was not reported in print until almost 50 years after it was completed (Silverman, 1988b).

This study was conducted *before* the diagnosogenic theory was formulated, at a time when the prevailing belief was that stuttering resulted from a lack of unilateral cerebral dominance. Hence, the results of the study probably could not have been predicted. The study was *not* a part of a stuttering research program. It was one of a series of at least five master's theses intended to assess the validity of certain general semantics formulations (Johnson, 1946, pp. 517–518). One of these formulations was *evaluative labeling*: the tendency "to evaluate individuals and situations according to the names we apply to them" (Johnson, 1946, p. 261). None of the other theses addressed stuttering.

One of the primary objectives of Tudor's study was to determine whether labeling a person, previously regarded as a normal speaker, as a stutterer would have any effect on his or her speech fluency. Tudor screened the children in an orphanage and selected six who were regarded as normal speakers to serve as subjects. Their respective chronological ages were 5, 9, 11, 12, 12, and 15. She made the following statement to each child at the beginning of the experiment:

> The staff has come to the conclusion that you have a great deal of trouble with your speech. The types of interruptions which you have are very undesirable. These interruptions indicate stuttering. You have many of the symptoms of a child who is beginning to stutter. You must try to stop yourself immediately. Use your will power. Make up your mind that you are going to speak without a single interruption. It's absolutely necessary that you do this. Do anything to keep from stuttering. Try harder to speak fluently and evenly. If you have any interruptions, stop and begin again. Take a deep breath whenever you feel you are going to stutter. Don't ever speak unless you can do it right. You can see how [the name of a child in the institution who stuttered rather severely] stutters, don't you! Well, he undoubtedly started the same way you are starting. Watch your speech every minute and try to do something to improve it. Whatever you do, speak fluently and avoid any interruptions whatsoever in your speech. (Tudor, 1939, pp. 10–11)

In addition, she made the following statements to the teachers and matrons who interacted with these children:

> The staff has come to the conclusion that these children show definite symptoms of stuttering. The types of interruptions they are having very frequently turn into stuttering. We have handled a number of cases very similar to these children. You should impress upon them the value of good speech, and that in order to have good speech one has to speak fluently. Watch their speech all the time very carefully and stop them when they have interruptions; stop them and have them say it over. Don't allow them to speak unless they can say it right. They should be made very conscious of their speech, and also they should be given opportunities to talk so that their mistakes can be pointed out to them. It is very important to watch for any changes in the child's personality, in his attitude toward his school work, in his attitude toward his playmates, etc. (Tudor, 1939, pp. 12–13)

Tudor spoke to the children and their teachers and matrons at least once a month for a semester to attempt to reinforce the label "stutterer." She reported the following description of the children's speech at the end of the semester:

> All of the subjects . . . showed similar types of speech behavior during the experimental period. A decrease in verbal output of all six subjects; that is they were reluctant to speak and spoke only when they were urged to. Second, their rate of speaking was decreased. They spoke more slowly and with greater exactness. They had a tendency to weigh each word before they said it. Third, the length of response was shorter. The two younger subjects responded with one word whenever possible. Fourth, they were more self-conscious. They appeared shy and embarrassed in many situations. Fifth, they accepted the fact that there was something definitely wrong with their speech. Sixth, every subject reacted to his speech interruptions in some manner. Some hung their heads; others gasped and covered their mouths with their hands; others laughed with embarrassment. In every case the children's behavior changed noticeably. (Tudor, 1939, pp. 147–148)

She concluded that her findings supported the hypothesis that evaluative labeling can influence behavior.

Information came from four persons who were knowledgeable about the outcome of the study (including the late Dean E. Williams of the University of Iowa); from Tudor herself (Halvorson, 1999, pp. 189–206); and from Jim Dyer, an investigative reporter for the *San Jose Mercury News* (June 10 and 11, 2001) who located and interviewed Tudor and several of the orphans who served as subjects. Some time following its completion Tudor's advisor (Wendell Johnson) was notified by the orphanage that not only had the changes in the children's communicative behavior persisted, but there also was concern that at least some of them had become stutterers. Tudor, of course, was concerned about the children and visited them periodically for at least several years. Letters she wrote her advisor about her visits with the children suggest that at least some of them continued to stutter. Interviews of several of them when they were in their 70s, conducted by Dyer in 2001, indicated that their stuttering had persisted throughout their lives. (In June, 2001, both the University of Iowa and the American Speech-Language-Hearing Association issued formal apologies to the orphans and their families that were published in many newspapers in the United States and elsewhere.) For additional evidence that at least some of the children continued to stutter, see Silverman (1988b), Halvorson (1999), and the aforementioned articles by Jim Dyer.

The findings of the Tudor study provide strong evidence that diagnosing normal disfluency as stuttering can cause stuttering. What is particularly impressive about the findings is that fact that five of the six children were considerably beyond the age at which stuttering ordinarily begins. They had experienced being normal speakers for a number of years. The implications of the findings seem clear—asking a child to monitor his or her speech fluency and attempt to be more fluent may lead to increased disfluency and possibly stuttering!

While, to the best of my knowledge, nobody has attempted to do a direct replication of the Tudor study, an experiment has been reported by Newman (1987) providing further evidence that reacting negatively to normal speech repetitions can result in the development of stutter-like behaviors. She had ten normal-speaking adult males speak spontaneously for 15 minutes. While repetitions decreased when the stimulus "you repeated" was said immediately after each occurrence of repetition, several behaviors surfaced that were judged by her to be stutter-like in nature. According to Newman (1987):

> Every subject responded to the situation with behavioral changes that included both speech behaviors. . . as well as other behaviors (facial expressions, posture changes, etc.). In general, speech movements seemed to become overcontrolled and speech was uttered with restrained and precise movements that resulted in a halting, hesitant performance.

> A wide variety of behavioral alterations were noted as each subject tried to speak without repeating. At the start of conditioning, most subjects responded to the instructions by changing their posture in the chair from a relaxed to a more formal position. The subjects sat upright immediately and began to fidget. They started to laugh or smile nervously when reminded of their repetitions. They also began to use their hands more frequently, doing things such as playing with the table edge, the topic cards, or the microphone cord. Other behavior changes noted among the subjects included looking down or away while speaking, closing their eyes after delivery of the adverse stim-

ulus, increasing their depth of inhalation, increasing their vocal intensity, and using a rising vocal inflection at the ends of sentences. These behaviors appeared to be . . . [almost] superstitious . . . in that the subjects behaved as though these behaviors would help them talk without repeating. . . . It may be assumed that the responses just described are not unlike those of the stutterer as he or she attempts to speak without being disfluent. (pp. 60–61)

Newman did not report whether any of these behaviors persisted after the experiment ended. However, regardless of whether they did so, the findings of this study provide further evidence that reacting negatively to normal speech repetition can result in the development of stutter-like behavior.

While it seems likely that the conditions specified by the diagnosogenic theory contribute to precipitating some cases of stuttering, *the evidence reviewed here does not prove that they contribute to precipitating all such cases or that they will always do so.* A number of writers (such as Van Riper, 1982) have argued quite cogently that stuttering may have more than one cause.

The continuity hypothesis

This theory, proposed by Oliver Bloodstein (1961, 1987), also states that stuttering develops from the disfluency exhibited by most young children. However, it does not assume that the reason is someone's misdiagnosis of normal disfluency. According to Bloodstein:

. . . stuttering develops when speech tensions and fragmentations become magnified by communicative pressure. In this view, stuttering develops along a continuum as the child struggles increasingly in the face of a mounting conviction that speaking is difficult. It does not occur . . . as the child's effort to avoid the normal disfluency that was being mislabeled as stuttering. . . . It originates from the child's effort to speak. (Perkins, 1990a, p. 373)

When the speech tensions and fragmentations are magnified to the point that they are severe and chronic, they tend to be identified as episodes of stuttering (Bloodstein, 1961).

One of the main differences between this hypothesis and the diagnosogenic one is in how they explain the similarities between normal childhood disfluency and that exhibited by children thought to be beginning to stutter. According to the diagnosogenic theory:

. . . if one child's speech repetitions are normal there is little justification for calling another child's speech repetitions anything else just because there are more of them. By contrast, the continuity hypothesis says that if one child's speech repetitions are stuttering there is little reason to call another child's repetitions anything else merely because there is a relatively normal amount of them. While these two statements appear to represent only differences in definition of stuttering there is a vast distinction between them in their ultimate implications for theory and therapy. In the first instance we must look for the source of the child's problem largely in the perceptual distortions of a listener by reason of which the child comes to regard disfluencies as a matter of concern and to struggle to avoid them. In the second case we must look for the causes of the problem largely in the nature of the stutterings that are latent in almost all children's speech and in the variety of possible factors that might tend to increase them. (Bloodstein, 1987, pp. 352–353)

While these hypotheses disagree about whether childhood disfluency is normal or abnormal and what initially causes the "tension and fragmentation" in a child's speech to increase, they are not necessarily incompatible. Sooner or later both will result in a child becoming aware of the behavior and desiring to avoid it. Whether a child does so because of the negative reactions of listeners to his or her disfluency (diagnosogenic theory), or the child's own awareness and dislike of it (continuity hypothesis), or both of these, the consequences will be the same.

Other Hypotheses

A number of "old" and "new" hypotheses pertaining to the etiology of stuttering that do not fit neatly into one of the other three categories are discussed in this section.

Shocks and fright

Some persons relate the onset of their stuttering to a particular event—usually a traumatic one. They either remember beginning to stutter after it occurred or were told that they did so by someone. It is necessary to exercise caution when interpreting such reports. In some cases, for example, the onset of the disorder actually preceded the event. We do not know how often this happens because it usually is extremely difficult to document that the person was stuttering before the event occurred. Van Riper (1982) has reported a case in which he was able to do so:

A sixteen-year-old stutterer was brought to us by his mother with a clear history of onset at the age of eight years. Both the mother and the boy remembered the event vividly. The boy was on his way home in the early darkness of a winter evening and stumbled across the body of a dead man on the sidewalk in front of the boy's home. (They had the newspaper clipping to prove it.) The boy rushed into the house, opened his mouth to speak, and was unable to do so for some minutes despite repeated attempts. His stuttering dated from this time, so they said, and it was interesting that his major stuttering behavior was this same wide gaping mouth. The mother was absolutely convinced that the boy had been completely fluent previously. Nevertheless, we were able to find school records, and to get the testimony of his first grade teacher who remembered the boy because of his speech difficulty. It was clearly established that he had been stuttering fairly frequently and severely, though repetitively, before the incident. (p. 72)

While such events may not cause children to stutter, they may contribute indirectly to the onset of their stuttering—that is, they may cause children to repeat more often or to be more disfluent than they were previously (Irwin & Duffy, 1955). This increases the probability that others will become concerned about their speech fluency. Persons with whom they interact who believe that stuttering can be caused by a traumatic incident are particularly likely to do so. ("Seek and ye shall find.") As I have indicated previously, some writers have suggested that communicating to children that their hesitations are abnormal is an event that can precipitate the disorder.

The early twentieth-century literature on stuttering contains many reports of children beginning to stutter after a shock or frightening experience. For example, Makuen in 1914 reported that 28 percent of the stutterers in his sample and Gutzmann in 1900 reported that 14 percent of his stutterers (Luchinger & Arnold, 1965) had suffered shocks or fright prior to onset. The event causing the shock or fright, however, usually was not as "dramatic" as the one reported by Van Riper—finding a dead body. According to Luchinger and Arnold (1965, p. 745), "In most cases minor physical or emotional mishaps are incriminated: a dog barked suddenly; a rooster flew onto the child's shoulder; or the child stumbled over a carpet in a department store."

The evidence that a shock or frightening experience can cause stuttering is both anecdotal and circumstantial. It is based on reports that a shock or frightening event preceded the moment when someone first concluded that the child was stuttering. Even if the disorder really began after such an event, this does not necessarily mean that the event precipitated the disorder.

Illness

There are a number of reports in the literature of children beginning to stutter following an illness. Gutzmann (1939) reported that in almost 10 percent of his cases the onset of stuttering followed severe attacks of infectious diseases and other illnesses. West, Nelson, and Berry (1939) reported that between 16 and 20 percent of their stutterers began to stutter after an illness such as a severe respiratory infection, rheumatic fever, whooping cough, bronchitis, pneumonia, epilepsy, and encephalitis. Goda (1961) reported a case of a seven-year-old boy who began to stutter following an attack of spinal meningitis.

Do children who stutter tend to be ill more often during early childhood than their peers? Perhaps, if illness can be a factor in precipitating stuttering, the likelihood of it being so is a function of the amount of time a child is ill rather than the specific illness that he or she has. This does not seem to be the case. The available data indicate that children who stutter do not tend to have more illnesses during early childhood than their peers (Andrews & Harris, 1964; Johnson & Associates, 1959).

Assuming that some children do begin to stutter after an illness, why do they do so? There are several possible explanations. The first is coincidence. With the number of illnesses that many young children tend to have, it would not be particularly surprising if one occurred before the presumed onset of the disorder.

A second possible explanation is that the illnesses resulted in physiological changes that precipitated neurogenic acquired stuttering. However, the phenomenology of the stutter-like disfluencies that result from such changes differs in several significant ways from that of stuttering. Such disfluencies do not, for example, become less frequent when reading in chorus.

A third possible explanation is that the stress resulting from such illnesses causes children to be more disfluent than usual. In this regard, Luchinger and Arnold (1965) state:

> The causative influence of infections . . . should not be construed to represent a specific neurological damage. What is important is the general debilitation and the reduction of physical and mental resistance. Following such a breakdown of psychophysical well-being, stuttering may develop as a psychic reaction. (p. 745)

If, because of "general debilitation," children become more disfluent following an illness, the concern about it of persons in their environment may be communicated to them. Some authorities believe that this can precipitate the disorder (see the previous discussion of diagnosogenic theory).

Imitation

The onset of stuttering has been attributed to imitation of another person's stuttering. Mygind (1898), for example, reported that imitation was the important precipitating cause in 13 percent of his cases: In most of them there were other family members who stuttered. Otsuki (1958), in Japan, reported it to be a significant causal factor in 70 percent of his cases.

How likely is it that a child's stuttering could be caused by imitation? The available data are insufficient for answering this question with a high degree of confidence. With regard to this, Van Riper (1982) reported:

> For many years we have sought evidence for imitation as a precipitant of the onset of stuttering in every case we examined. Though we never counted up the cases we saw in those years, they constitute a substantial number. We tried to trace every account of imitation as a source of stuttering and only in one single stuttering child did we feel confident that the disorder was triggered in this way. (p. 75)

Perhaps the most compelling argument against imitation, by itself, causing stuttering is that the symptomatology of the disorder at onset almost always differs from that in its developed form. Consequently, if a young child's stuttering resulted from imitating that of an older child or adult, his or her symptomatology would be expected to be that of the developed form of the disorder, including facial grimaces and associated movements.

Conflicts (emotional and communicative)

Conflicts probably have been regarded as precipitating causes of stuttering more often than any of the other factors mentioned in this section. The following four excerpts from case reports illustrate what is meant by a conflict in this context. The conflict in the first three cases is emotional, and in the fourth it is communicative.

> The boy, in constant fear lest one of his obscene terms may slip out in the wrong company, and having experienced this dangerous tendency of words to go astray, soon begins to hesitate over every word which begins in the same way as do those dangerous words; and as the hesitations become a more and more fixed and noticeable habit, it extends to other types of words also. (Dunlap, 1917, p. 46)

> Patty was referred to the clinic at the age of three and a half by her mother who was concerned about the child's stuttering. This symptom had started three months earlier following a spanking administered by the mother after the child had run into the street and narrowly missed being run over by a car. Shortly afterward the stuttering had cleared up but a few weeks later, after a second spanking for running into the street, she again began to stutter. (Harle, 1946, p. 156)

> The onset of Nana's stuttering occurred at a time when her mother, because of an acute illness, had become inaccessible to the child. Nana consequently experienced a break in a previously well-established speech chain. This disruption coincided with a critical period in Nana's language development. (Wyatt, 1969, p. 93)

> When I was four years old my mother took a job and put me in a day nursery. . . . We moved to an apartment at about that time which was located on the top floor and we were required to run up five flights of stairs to get up to it. One of my habits was to run up the five flights and upon getting into the house I would try to speak while out of breath. This is the first time I can remember "stumbling" in my speech. (Duncan, 1949, p. 258)

The conflict in the first involves the boy's approach-avoidance urges to say "dirty" words and not to say them; that in the second and third involves a disturbance in the mother-child relationship; and that in the fourth involves a desire to speak before having adequate breath support to do so fluently.

According to Van Riper (1992), emotional conflicts that have been reported to precipitate stuttering occur on three levels: word, situation, and relationship. Those on the *word level* to which the onset of the disorder has been attributed include conflicting urges to say something and not to say it, trying to say unfamiliar words, and trying to think of and say the "right" word without being sure that it is the right (appropriate) one.

Events resulting in emotional conflicts on the *situation level* that have been reported to precipitate stuttering initially cause the disorder to manifest itself in (be confined to) only one situation. In one case, for example, the situation was talking on the telephone and in another it was talking to a puppy (Van Riper, 1982, p. 77).

Conflicts on the *relationship level* that have been reported to precipitate stuttering involve a disturbance in the relationship between the child and someone else. Most often the "someone else" is reported to be the child's mother. The excerpts in this section from the case studies by Harle and Wyatt illustrate such conflicts.

Emotional conflicts on word, situation, or relationship levels that have been reported to precipitate stuttering may not have actually done so. The fact they occurred at the time the disorder was thought to have begun may have been a coincidence. Also, children who stutter do not appear to differ from their normal-speaking peers with regard to the number of emotional conflicts that they have (Andrews & Harris, 1964; Johnson & Associates, 1959). Finally, many children experience emotional conflicts similar to those reported to precipitate stuttering without developing the disorder.

While emotional conflicts, by themselves, may not precipitate many cases of stuttering, they may contribute to doing so by making a child more disfluent. As Van Riper (1982, p. 79) has stated, "It is at least tenable that the motor sequencing of speech breaks down when communication is overloaded by stress of any kind. . . ." Certainly, conflicts on word, situation, and relationship levels can produce a great deal of stress. Hence, while experiencing such conflicts some children may tend to be more disfluent than they were previously. This would increase the probability that someone would become concerned about their speech fluency and communicate this concern to them. According to the diagnosogenic theory, such an expression of concern can contribute to precipitating stuttering. This same scenario could result in communicative stress contributing to precipitating the disorder.

Demand for fluency exceeding capacity

This hypothesis has been referred to as the "demands and capacities" model. According to Starkweather (1987):

> In this model, the capacities for fluent speech—the motoric, cognitive, and linguistic skills that make easy speech possible for most chil-

dren—interact with demands for fluency placed on the child by the
external communicative environment and by the child himself. As the
capacity for fluency grows, the expectations of parents and of the
child will also increase. Very young children are expected to be hesi-
tant and stumbling in speech. Older children are expected to produce
more words more quickly and more easily. In this way, capacities and
demands for fluency are simultaneously increasing. If the environment demands more fluency than the child can produce, stuttering
will begin. Whether the stuttering will continue or remediate
depends on whether a growing capacity to produce fluent speech can
catch up with the world's accelerating demands. (p. 144)

Some implications of this model are explored in a special section of the
2000 Volume of the *Journal of Fluency Disorders* (pp. 317–383), and in
Starkweather (2002).

Reduced ability to generate temporal patterns

Kent (1983) has posited that stuttering results (at least in part) from a
central nervous-system disturbance, the nature of which "is a reduced
ability to generate temporal patterns, whether for sensory or motor
purposes, but especially the latter" (p. 252). Stutterers, according to
this hypothesis, do not have as much ability as their nonstuttering
peers to "smoothly" sequence the movements (gestures) of which spoken words consist. While the reason for their deficit is physiological
(possibly genetic), the degree to which their capacity for temporal reg-
ulation is reduced at a particular moment while speaking is likely to
be a function of social and psychological variables. This hypothesis,
like the preceding one, being of relatively recent origin, has not been
evaluated sufficiently on an empirical level to judge its cogency.

Linguistic and paralinguistic components being dyssynchronous when the speaker is under time pressure

Perkins, Kent, and Curlee (1991) have proposed a theory of neuropsycholinguistic function to explain the production of fluent speech, normal disfluency, and moments of stuttering. They have summarized
their theory as follows:

> Speech involves linguistic and paralinguistic components, each of
> which is processed by different neural systems that converge on a
> common output system. Fluent speech requires that these compo-
> nents be integrated in synchrony. When they are dyssynchronous,
> the result can be either nonstuttered disfluency or stuttering,
> depending on time pressure. Time pressure is defined as the
> speaker's need to begin, continue, or accelerate an utterance. Non-
> stuttered disfluency results when the linguistic and paralinguistic
> components are dyssynchronous and the speaker is not under time
> pressure. Stuttering results when the speaker is under time pressure
> and is relatively unaware of the cause of dyssynchrony. Both of these

factors are necessary for the identification of the phenomenon of stuttering. Stuttering is defined as a disruption of speech that is experienced by the speaker as a loss of control. (p. 734)

There is considerable evidence that stuttering severity tends to increase when a stutterer speaks while experiencing time pressure (see chapter 2). While this hypothesis appears to explain the moment of stuttering, at least in part, it is of relatively recent origin and has not been tested sufficiently to judge its overall cogency and heuristic value.

WHY DO PEOPLE CONTINUE TO STUTTER?

Thus far in this chapter, two of the three levels at which attempts have been made to explain the etiology of stuttering have been explored: those dealing with the predisposing cause and with the precipitating cause. In this section the third of these levels is explored: that dealing with the *maintaining* cause of stuttering. Specifically, we will consider "answers" that have been given to the following questions:

- Why do moments of stuttering occur when they do, and what is their nature?
- Why do people continue to stutter after they have begun doing so?

Hypotheses are categorized as done previously, on the basis of whether they indicate some type of *breakdown, repressed-need,* or learned *anticipatory-struggle* response. For further information about these and other hypothesis about maintaining causes of stuttering see Bloodstein (1987), Freund (1966), and Van Riper (1982).

Breakdown Hypotheses

While these hypotheses are concerned primarily with predisposing and precipitating causes of stuttering, some do offer answers to the questions posed in this section. Some of those who attribute the moment of stuttering at onset to some type of physiological breakdown probably would assume that people continue to stutter because the physiological anomaly in speech motor-control processes is still present. Further, they probably would regard moments of stuttering as being a symptom of this physiological anomaly, the occurrence of which may be influenced by stress and variables that are not physiological, such as sociocultural and behavioral ones (Smith, 1990b).

Repressed-Need Hypotheses

These hypotheses view the moment of stuttering as a *symbolic* expression (symptom) of a repressed emotional need. It is symbolic in the sense that movements that occur during moments of stuttering communicate the nature of this need. For example, those who believe that the repressed need involves fixation at the oral stage of infantile sexual development as a consequence of inadequate mothering interpret movements that occur during moments of stuttering as symbolizing infantile sucking behavior (Glauber, 1982). According to these hypotheses, people continue to stutter after they have begun doing so (at least in part) because the repressed need that precipitated the disorder has not been adequately met.

Anticipatory-Struggle Hypotheses

These hypotheses view the moment of stuttering as learned behavior that is somehow precipitated by it being anticipated and feared. They indicate that what maintains the disorder is *anticipating* stuttering and *struggling* to avoid it. Some of those who advocate such hypotheses (such as Bloodstein, 1987) refer to the moment of stuttering as "struggle behavior." Theoretically, if a person who had the disorder stopped fearing and desiring to avoid stuttering (could develop a "don't care" attitude about it), he or she would become more fluent, perhaps even normally fluent. Better yet, if such a person could be made to *want* to stutter (somehow to be made to view it as advantageous to do so), he or she would be even more likely to experience increased fluency.

While many persons knowledgeable about stuttering agree that anticipation of stuttering contributes to both precipitating moments of stuttering and maintaining the disorder, there is no general agreement on the nature of the mechanism by which this occurs. Specifically, there is no agreement on the answer to the following question: How do events associated with the anticipation and occurrence of moments of stuttering serve to reinforce (maintain) the behavior? Among the answers that have been suggested are the following:

- The "unpleasantness" of stuttering reinforces the desire to avoid it and, thereby, reinforces the behavior (Van Riper, 1982).

- Because the presence of a stimulus (words or situations) that tends to give rise to anticipation of stuttering is not always followed by stuttering, the behavior is reinforced on a *partial reinforcement schedule* (Brutten & Shoemaker, 1967). As a consequence, the experience of being fluent a number of times in the presence of such a stimulus (words or situation) does not extinguish the fear of stuttering when encountering it. This may partially explain why some persons who have recovered from the disorder relapse after months, or even years, of being normally fluent. That is, relatively long periods of being normally fluent may not extinguish the fear of stuttering, nor do they necessarily result in an unshakable anticipation of fluency. The occurrence of only a few instances of disfluency that the person judges to be abnormal may be sufficient to cause him or her to again anticipate stuttering and precipitate a relapse.

- The success that most persons who stutter experience when communicating reinforces the struggle behavior (Silverman, 1976a). Even while stuttering severely, they usually are able to make themselves understood.

TO WHAT EXTENT IS STUTTERING LEARNED BEHAVIOR?

Many types of behaviors can occur during, or accompany, moments of stuttering (see chapter 2). Which of these are learned, and how are they learned? Is there more than one type of learning involved? These questions are addressed here.

Perhaps the first question we should ask here is: How well do authorities agree that at least some behaviors associated with moments of stuttering are learned? They appear to agree fairly well. In a review of factors in the etiology of stuttering, Smith (1990a) stated:

> For many years the debate raged whether stuttering was a "learned" or "organic" disorder. Happily this debate has passed, and at present I do not think anyone would argue with the statement that learning plays a role in the development of stuttering. (p. 43)

In the previous section we discussed hypotheses that regard stuttering as anticipatory-struggle behavior. Those who accept these hypotheses view the moment of stuttering—at least in part—as learned behavior. However, these hypotheses are not accepted by everyone who believes aspects of stuttering are learned.

There are behaviors associated with moments of stuttering that almost everyone agrees are learned. These are the so-called secondary behaviors, or secondary symptoms (see chapter 2). They include facial grimaces, "starters," and lack of eye contact (Van Riper, 1982). Facial grimaces consist of gestures that the person uses to avoid or reduce the severity of moments of stuttering. These become habitual by the time they cease being effective.

"Starters" are gestures and/or words that are used before moments of stuttering to either avoid them or reduce their severity. They are thought to have been learned initially because at the times when they occurred before words on which stuttering was anticipated, the stuttering either did not occur or its severity was judged by the person to have been considerably less than expected. The outcome, of course, could have been the same if the "starter" had not been used. Nevertheless, the person's belief in at least the occasional efficacy of the starter may cause him or her to continue using it, even when he or she regards it as not having been effective for a while. This is particularly likely to happen if there were periods in the past during which it did not seem to "work" followed by ones during which it did.

A third type of behavior associated with moments of stuttering that most persons knowledgeable about the disorder agree is learned is poor eye contact. Embarrassment and shame are signaled in our culture by looking away (Atkins, 1988). The person has *learned* to be embarrassed or ashamed about stuttering.

While there appears to be fairly good agreement among persons knowledgeable about stuttering that secondary symptoms are learned, this is not the case for the disfluency behaviors themselves (the primary symptoms). Some believe that these behaviors are learned either because they can be *manipulated* in the same manner as behaviors that are known to be learned, or because they are *distributed in a nonrandom manner* that can be explained by learning theory. For example, some believe they are learned because their frequency of occurrence can be manipulated by response-contingent reinforcement in a manner that would be expected if they were learned. That is, they would be expected to be reduced by response-contingent punishment. Some persons do not accept this as proof that stuttering is learned, either because they feel that the available data are not sufficiently compelling to support this conclusion or that there are other possible explanations for the variations in stuttering severity that occur after response-contingent reinforcement.

A second reason why people may believe that disfluencies occurring during moments of stuttering are learned is because they are distributed in the speech sequence in a manner that can be explained by learning theory (Starkweather, 1987). They are, for example, more likely to occur on words on which moments of stuttering have occurred previously than would be expected by chance (see the discussion of the consistency effect in chapter 2). A plausible explanation for this phenomenon is that they have learned to stutter on these words.

Thus far, we have addressed the question of which behaviors associated with moments of stuttering are learned. Assuming that some are learned, how are they learned? Is there more than one type of learning involved, or are they all learned in the same way? Persons knowledgeable about the disorder who believe that some behaviors are learned do not agree very well on how they are learned. This is unfortunate, because the strategy a clinician would use to modify a behavior (response) would be based, at least in part, on his or her assumption about how it was learned (Williams, 1968).

One particularly influential answer to the questions raised in the preceding paragraph utilizes a two-process theory to explain how behaviors associated with moments of stuttering are learned (Brutten & Shoemaker, 1967). It stipulates that some are *classically conditioned* responses and others are *instrumental*. According to this theory, the disfluencies (repetitions, disrhythmic phonations, and tense pauses) that occur during moments of stuttering are probably classically conditioned responses and most of the other behaviors that do so (e.g., poor eye contact) are likely to be instrumental. The stronger a person's desire to avoid a classically conditioned response, the *more* likely it is to occur. On the other hand, the stronger his or her desire to avoid an instrumental response, the *less* likely it is to occur. If, for example, a person is told before performing a speaking task that he or she will be administered an electric shock after completing the task for each time he or she evinces a particular behavior during the task (e.g., syllable repetitions), the effect of this information on the frequency of occurrence of the behavior will be determined by whether it is a classically conditioned response or an instrumental one. The behavior would tend to occur *more frequently* if it was a classically conditioned response, and it would tend to occur *less frequently* if it was instrumental.

For a lively discussion of the implications of learning theory for explaining and modifying stuttering, see the papers in the March 1993 issue of the *Journal of Fluency Disorders.*

IS STUTTERING TRULY A DISORDER OF SPEECH?

Stuttering traditionally has been viewed as a disorder of speech. It is not particularly surprising, therefore, that most of the theorizing about its etiology has focused on the speech mechanism. People have attempted to explain why the speech mechanism malfunctions to give rise to moments of stuttering. Proponents of breakdown hypotheses have theorized about physiological anomalies that either alone or in combination with stress could disrupt the functioning of the speech mechanism. Proponents of repressed-need hypotheses have theorized about how certain psychological anomalies can disrupt its functioning, and proponents of anticipatory-struggle hypotheses have theorized about how anticipating stuttering and desiring to avoid it can do so.

In this section stuttering is considered from a somewhat different perspective. Rather than viewing it as a disorder of speech per se, we are going to view it as *one member of a class of disorders* that are characterized by the anticipation of "difficulty" increasing the likelihood of occurrence. This perspective, therefore, is a generalization of the anticipatory-struggle hypotheses.

The notion that stuttering is a member of a class of disorders characterized by fearful expectancy of "difficulty" causing its occurrence is not a new one. Approximately one hundred years ago the kinship of stuttering with a great many similar disturbances in other areas was detected (Denhardt, 1890) and later, as a consequence, stuttering was classified by some psychiatrists as an *expectancy neurosis* (Freund, 1966). According to Freund, expectancy neuroses are:

. . . disturbances of learned and automatized skills, of simple motor and vegetative functions, and even of elementary perceptual acts, manifesting themselves as "stuttering," e.g., in the playing of any musical instrument, as stutter-like disturbances in artistic singing, . . . writer's cramp, erythrophobia, stage fright, . . . some forms of sexual impotence, etc. . . . All these forms of expectancy neurotic disturbances have as a common characteristic that they are based upon actual "primary" traumatic experiences of failure in the performance of a learned skill or a simple motor or sensory act, often though not necessarily, in socially embarrassing situations. The anticipation of their dreaded recurrence leads then . . . to the establishment of a *vicious spiral* [italics mine]. . . . A further common feature is that dread, anticipation and the whole hypercompensatory mechanism are in the beginning on a completely unconscious level, and that awareness and conscious anticipation are usually later developments. (pp. 37–38)

The vicious spiral (or vicious circle) referred to in the preceding paragraph is displayed graphically in figure 5-2. The experience of "failure" leads to anticipating the recurrence of "failure," which leads to the recurrence of "failure," which leads to again anticipating its recurrence, et cetera. As long as the person continues to anticipate, with dread, the recurrence of failure in the performance of the skill or act, the vicious circle/spiral will not be broken. A similar expectancy/anticipation phenomenon has been reported by psychologists (see Miller & Turnbill, 1986, for a review of the psychological literature on this phenomenon).

Is the expectancy neurosis viewed by psychiatrists as being learned behavior? The answer to this question appears to be "yes." According to Freund (1966), the terms *neurosis* and *learned maladjustive behavior* define the same set of phenomena.

Are some persons more likely than others to develop the type of "learned maladjustive behavior" disorder referred to as an expectancy neurosis? Some authorities believe that there are genetic-constitutional, psychodynamic, psychosocial, and/or psychophysiological factors that make some persons more likely than others to develop such a disorder (Freund, 1966). These, then, would function as predisposing causes for them.

Is stuttering a member of the class of learned maladjustive behavior disorders that can be referred to as expectancy neuroses? This question probably would not be answered in the same way by all persons who are knowledgeable about stuttering. The answer would be determined, at least partially, by their belief regarding the precipitating and maintaining causes of the disorder. A person who accepted an anticipatory-struggle explanation probably would be more willing to classify stuttering as this type of disorder than one who accepted a breakdown or repressed-need explanation. The answer to this question also would be influenced by their belief regarding the degree of similarity between the symptomatology and phenomenology of stuttering and that of other disorders looked upon as being precipitated and maintained by the type of vicious spiral depicted in figure 5-2. These *may* include the following:

- *Stutter-like disruptions in the playing of a musical instrument.* Several investigators (Freund, 1966; Meltzer, 1992; Nadoleczny, 1926; Packman & Onslow, 1999; Silverman & Bohlman, 1988) have reported disruptions in "fluency" during the playing of such musical instruments as the flute, French horn, piano, violin, and trumpet that there is reason to believe were precipitated and maintained by such a vicious spiral.

- *Stutter-like disruptions in manual communication.* Silverman and Silverman (1971) surveyed teachers at residential schools for the deaf in the United States to determine whether they had ever observed "disruptions" during manual communication that appeared to be similar to stuttering during speech. Several responded that they had seen such cases and from their descriptions of them there is reason to believe that they could have been precipitated and maintained by such a vicious spiral. Montgomery and Fitch (1988), in a survey of schools for the hearing impaired, also received reports of stutter-like disruptions in manual communication.

Figure 5-2 Vicious spiral (circle) associated with the type of "learned maladjustive behavior" disorder that has been referred to as an expectancy neurosis.

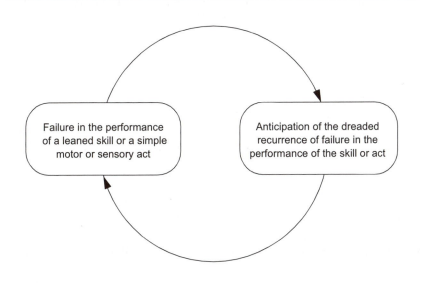

- *Agoraphobia.* Most persons with this disorder have "anxiety attacks" if they stray too far from their home, and these attacks are thought to be precipitated (at least in part) by their recurrence being anticipated with dread.

- *Diarrhea.* Some persons precipitate episodes of diarrhea by anticipating their recurrence with dread.

- *Headaches.* Some persons develop severe headaches by anticipating their recurrence with dread.

- *Impotence.* Some men frequently are unable to achieve or maintain erection because they anticipate, with dread, being unable to do so.

- *Insomnia.* Some persons, at times, are unable to sleep because they anticipate, with dread, being unable to do so.

These are only a few of the disorders that are thought to be precipitated by anticipating and dreading their recurrence. Since almost any aspect of functioning can be disrupted in this manner, the list probably is quite long.

What would be the implications—both theoretical and clinical—of viewing stuttering as a member of this class of disorders rather than as a disorder of speech per se? Theoretically, it would present a challenge to those who attribute stuttering to a physiological anomaly specific to the functioning of parts of the speech mechanism (such as the larynx), because comparable breakdowns in performance can occur that do not involve these structures. It also could add to our understanding of the symptomatology, phenomenology, and etiology of stuttering because information about other disorders in this class may provide some valuable insights into them.

Viewing stuttering in this way may also have clinical implications. For example, it could enable our clients to benefit from the clinical research and experience on other disorders in this class. That is, intervention strategies that have been helpful to persons who have one of these disorders also may be helpful to persons who stutter.

IS THE MYSTERY OF STUTTERING SOLVABLE?

After hundreds—perhaps thousands—of years of attempts to determine the cause of stuttering, there is still no general agreement. The prevailing view has cycled periodically between constitutional and environmental explanations (see Perkins, 1994). For at least two reasons it is particularly surprising that there is still no consensus about its etiology. A huge amount of information about the symptomatology and phenomenology of the disorder and about persons who have it has been gathered and published during the past 70 years. And fantastic advances have been made in establishing the etiologies of many other disorders during this period.

While the reason for our lack of success in determining the etiology of stuttering is uncertain, it may be—at least in part—a consequence of the approach that has been used to test theories about it. There are two basic strategies that can be used for this purpose. The first is to gather evidence to prove a theory "true," and the second is to do so to prove a theory "false." Almost all investigators who have attempted to test theories of stuttering have used the first strategy, and almost all of those who have been successful in explaining other phenomena—including other disorders—have used the second.

While it is possible to prove that a theory is false, it is impossible to prove that it is true (Perkins, Kent, & Curlee, 1991). Even if a theory can explain everything that is known about a phenomenon, it is possible that something will be learned about it in the future that the theory cannot explain. On the other hand, one fact about a phenomenon that a theory cannot explain proves it to be false.

Almost all attempts that have been made to prove a theory about the etiology of stuttering true consist of reports of data that are consistent with it. These data may have been generated by the person testing the theory, taken from the literature, or both. Data that were not consistent with the theory were either ignored; declared to be uncertain with regard to validity, reliability, and/or generality; or interpreted as indicating that stuttering does not have a single cause and, consequently, there are one or more subgroups of stutterers to which the theory does not apply. In most scientific fields such data would cause a theory to be rejected. If it becomes fashionable to be more exacting when evaluating theories about the etiology of stuttering—that is, to do it like it's done in other scientific fields—perhaps the mystery of stuttering will be solved! For other discussions of this issue, see Perkins (1994) and Perkins, Kent, and Curlee (1991).

ETIOLOGY OF CLUTTERING

There appears to be a high level of agreement among those who have written about cluttering that its etiology is usually a genetic/organic condition. According to Myers and St. Louis (1992),

> All of the well-known reviews of the literature on cluttering conclude from the available anecdotal and experimental evidence that cluttering is frequently associated with physiological, perhaps inherited, conditions. (p. 16)

The physiological condition to which its etiology has been attributed most often is heredity because of the strong tendency for it to occur repeatedly in certain families.

ETIOLOGY OF NEUROGENIC ACQUIRED STUTTERING

Neurogenic acquired stuttering can result from damage to either the right or left hemisphere of the brain. According to Lebrun (1997),

> The causal lesion may be cortical, subcortical or both. It is sometimes focal and sometimes diffuse. It may be vascular, traumatic, neoplastic, toxic or degenerative. Stuttering may also occur after brain concussion. Focal lesions are not invariably confined to a particular cerebral area, but may be found in various parts of the encephalon. Thus, the nature and the localization of the cerebral injury that causes acquired stuttering lack specificity. (p. 121)

Conditions with which the types of brain damage that can precipitate neurogenic stuttering are associated include stroke, head trauma, Parkinson's syndrome, tumors, dementia, and drug usage. Neurogenic stuttering, incidentally, can be a side effect of a prescription drug (Brady, 1998).

ETIOLOGY OF PSYCHOGENIC ACQUIRED STUTTERING

The cause of psychogenic acquired stuttering is psychopathology. That said, it would not be unreasonable to ask what is meant by the term *psychopathology* in this context. Unfortunately, there doesn't appear to be a consensus about this. Baumgartner (1999) has suggested that perhaps the best way to answer this question at present is by means of the explanation suggested by Dr. Arnold Aronson of the Mayo Clinic for the etiology of psychogenic (hysterical) voice disorders—i.e., psychological distress or disequilibrium.

ASSIGNMENTS

Cause Survey

Survey at least five young adults who have not had any training in speech-language pathology about what they believe to be the cause of stuttering. Did they tend to view the disorder as primarily a physiological or a psychological one? Did any of them mention causes that are no longer widely accepted, such as imitation? If they were the parents of children who stutter, would any of their beliefs be likely to impede therapy? Why?

Relaxation

Several times when you are feeling tense or anxious, tell yourself to relax within the next 10 seconds. What effect did doing this have on your tension or anxiety level? If it did not reduce, what do you think was the reason?

6

Evaluation
Principles and Methods

INSTRUCTIONAL OBJECTIVES

By the end of this chapter, you should be able to:

▸ Specify five reasons why a speech-language pathologist may be asked to evaluate a child's or adult's speech fluency.

▸ Specify an answerable question.

▸ Describe three strategies that, singly or in combination, can be utilized during an evaluation to answer answerable questions.

▸ Describe seven cultural considerations that could affect the conducting of evaluations for fluency disorders.

▸ Describe some strategies for determining whether a preschool-age child is beginning to stutter.

▸ Describe some strategies for determining whether a school-age child or adult has a fluency disorder when his or her fluency during the evaluation seems normal.

▸ Describe some strategies for determining whether a child is at risk for stuttering or for developing a stuttering overlay on another fluency disorder.

▸ Describe some strategies for determining which of the four types of fluency disorders a client evinces.

> ‣ Specify some answerable questions for identifying a client's impairments, disabilities, and/or handicaps.
>
> ‣ Specify some strategies for answering answerable questions that pertain to a client's impairments, disabilities, and/or handicaps.
>
> ‣ Describe several strategies for assessing a client's motivation for therapy.
>
> ‣ Specify seven factors to consider when making a prognosis for whether a client who has a fluency disorder is likely to benefit from therapy.
>
> ‣ Specify five reasons for not scheduling a client who has a fluency disorder for therapy.
>
> ‣ Describe using a computer to make communicating ques-

In this chapter, I provide a methodology for determining whether a client has a fluency disorder and, if he or she does, whether it is stuttering, cluttering, neurogenic acquired stuttering, psychogenic acquired stuttering, or some combination of these. I also provide a methodology for identifying the set of behaviors that define a particular client's fluency disorder(s). This methodology consists of asking questions that are both relevant and answerable and then making the observations needed to answer them. While you can use this methodology with both children and adults who have any of these disorders, the specific questions you would ask and the tasks you would use to make the observations needed to answer them would, of course, be at least partially determined by the disorder(s) you suspect a client of having as well as by his or her age and cultural background. Other clinically relevant topics that are discussed in this chapter include determining whether a client is at risk for stuttering, assessing a client's motivation for therapy, making a prognosis, and drafting an evaluation report.

REASONS FOR EVALUATING SPEECH FLUENCY

There are a number of reasons why a speech-language pathologist may be asked to evaluate a child's or adult's speech fluency. The most common ones are discussed in this section.

To Determine Whether the Client Has a Fluency Disorder or Is at Risk for Developing One

One reason for undertaking such an evaluation is to determine whether the amount of repeating (or being disfluent in other ways) that a client is doing is abnormal. A clinician is more likely to be asked to evaluate a preschool-age or elementary-school-age child than he or she would an older child or adult. One reason is that such children often must be evaluated to assess the need for developing an Individualized Training Program (IEP) (Cooper, 1978). This determination is often difficult to make for preschool-age children because many of them who are normally fluent do a lot of repeating (see chapter 4). Guidelines have been developed to assist clinicians in making such assessments. Riley and Riley (1989), for example, have devised a data-based screening protocol—*Physician's Screening Procedure for Children Who May Stutter*—that can be used by physicians and others (including speech-language pathologists) for assessing the degree of abnormality of a child's disfluency and reactions to it (see Appendix C).

If a child is currently stuttering, the clinician must decide if the child is likely to recover without therapy. Many children have been reported to do so (see chapter 4). One device that is helpful when making this decision is the *Stuttering Prediction Instrument for Young Children* (Riley, 1984). It yields a score that is based on both parental responses to a questionnaire and clinician observations of selected aspects of the child's disfluent speech. If a child's score is 9 or lower, he or she would be judged likely to stop stuttering without intervention. For further information about this device and other measures that have been proposed for making this determination, see Yaruss and Conture (1993).

If a person's speech fluency appears to be within normal limits, the clinician should then attempt to determine if the person is at risk for developing a fluency disorder. That is, the clinician will attempt to determine whether there are any existing conditions that could directly or indirectly precipitate such a disorder. If, for example, a clinician believed that stuttering could be precipitated in the manner posited by the diagnosogenic theory (see chapter 5), he or she probably would regard persons at risk if they were reacting negatively to their hesitations and attempting to avoid them. Persons who do not have a fluency disorder but are at risk for developing one may be in need of intervention (see chapter 7).

A discussion of considerations and procedures for determining whether a preschool-age child is beginning to stutter appears later in the chapter.

To Determine the Type of Fluency Disorder

After a clinician has determined that a client has a fluency disorder, he or she usually will attempt to identify its type. This is important, in part because intervention programs for the various types are not the same (see chapter 7).

To Identify the Set of Behaviors
that Define the Client's Fluency Disorder

A client's fluency disorder is defined by a set of behaviors. (The term *behavior*, as used here, includes what traditionally have been referred to as attitudes and feelings because both have behavioral components.) The set for a particular client is likely to include some that are not components of his or her abnormal disfluency behavior, including behaviors associated with (motivated by) attitudes and feelings toward speaking abnormally.

Information about this set of behaviors can be used clinically in several ways. First, it can be used to judge the severity of both a client's *abnormal disfluency behavior* and his or her *fluency problem*. For example, scales for rating stuttering severity in specific situations—such as the *Iowa Scale of Severity of Stuttering* (see Appendix C)—use information about behaviors that occur during moments of stuttering that are a part of this set.

A second way this information can be used clinically is to establish a prognosis for achieving specific goals. The presence and/or absence of certain behaviors can influence how likely goals are to be achieved. For example, the absence of a strong desire to conceal stuttering from a client's set should result in the client being more willing than otherwise to "work on" his or her speech outside of the clinic environment, which should increase the likelihood of achieving goals that necessitate him or her doing so (Van Riper, 1973).

A third way such information can be used clinically is to establish goals for therapy. To reduce the severity of a client's fluency problem it is necessary to eliminate or modify behaviors in the set that defines the problem. Since the goals for a particular client are determined by the behaviors in this set, it is essential that they be identified.

To Assess Progress

Clients are reevaluated periodically to determine whether there is any change in the set of behaviors that define their problem. They are judged to have improved if there are fewer behaviors in this set or if some of them in it have been modified in desirable ways. If there has been little or no change, the clinician is likely to do further evaluation to determine the reason. Among the possibilities that he or she is likely to consider are:

- The assumption being made about why the client is exhibiting the behavior(s) is *wrong* and, hence, the intervention (which is based on it) is *inappropriate*.
- The assumption being made about why the client is exhibiting the behavior(s) is *correct*, but the intervention is *inappropriate*.

- The assumption is *correct* and the intervention is *appropriate*, but the client is not sufficiently motivated to do what is necessary to improve.

To Assess the Severity of the Problem for Funding Eligibility, Litigation, and Other Purposes

Speech-language pathologists occasionally are asked to evaluate speech fluency for a reason other than rehabilitation. They may be asked to testify as an expert witness about the severity of a person's disorder and/or the extent to which he or she is handicapped by it (Silverman, 1999a). Such an expert opinion may be requested by an attorney, an insurance company, or an organization to which the person has applied for funding. For example, persons who stutter have applied to and received funding from state vocational rehabilitation agencies for educational purposes. Expert opinion also may be requested by a court in a criminal case (see Shirkey, 1987; Bloodstein, 1988).

AN OVERVIEW OF THE EVALUATION PROCESS

The evaluation process for persons who have a fluency disorder consists mainly of *asking and answering questions*. The clinician formulates "answerable" questions and then makes the observations (gathers the data) needed for answering them. Answerable questions are those that can be answered by making observations and that indicate the observations needed to answer them (Johnson, 1946). These questions differ in the extent to which they are answerable. Consider the following questions:

1. Has the client improved during the past six months?

2. Have any of the behaviors in the set that define the client's stuttering problem been eliminated or changed "for the better" during the past six months?

The second is more answerable than the first because it indicates the observations needed to answer it less ambiguously.

While the specific questions asked during an evaluation are determined by the reason it is being conducted, there are several that are likely to be asked regardless of the reason:

1. Does the client have a fluency disorder?

2. If the client has a fluency disorder, what type is it?

3. How severe is the disorder? (The answer to this question would be based on answers to more specific ones, such as these two:)

   - To what extent does the client's fluency disorder interfere with communication (i.e., cause him or her to be disabled)?

• How much impact does the disorder have on the client's life (i.e., to what extent is he or she handicapped because of it)?

4. What is the prognosis for a meaningful reduction in the severity of the disorder?

These questions probably should be answered whenever a client is being seen for the first time, even if he or she has recently been evaluated by another clinician and a report is available. There are at least two reasons for doing so. First, all clinicians do not use the same data to answer these questions and, hence, they could arrive at different answers (Van Riper, 1982). Second, some answers could have changed since the last time the client was evaluated. Behaviors could have been eliminated from or added to the set that defines the client's fluency problem, or behaviors still included in it could have changed in some way. Some of the questions clinicians attempt to answer during an evaluation are formulated before it is begun. Others are formulated during the evaluation from information they obtain.

Thus far, we have addressed the "question-asking" part of the evaluation process. We will now discuss the "question-answering" part.

There are three approaches used for gathering data to answer questions. The first is observing the client's behavior under conditions that were purposefully created, or structured, by the clinician. The clinician asks the client to do a task and observes certain aspects of his or her behavior while it is being done. The behaviors that are observed, or attended to, may be related to the client's speech, body language, physiological functioning, something he or she has written, or some combination of these. An example of a task in which the behavior attended to is likely to be an attribute of speech is reading in chorus: The clinician would observe the effect of this condition on the client's speech fluency.

An example of a task in which a behavior attended to is likely to be an attribute of body language is asking the client questions: the clinician could observe whether the client maintained normal eye contact while answering them. An example of a task in which the behavior attended to could be an aspect of physiological functioning is having the client say syllables on command and observing through the use of instrumentation whether his or her phonatory initiation and termination times are abnormally long (see chapter 3). An example of a task in which the behavior attended to would be an attribute of what a client has written is having him or her complete a questionnaire: certain of the responses would be analyzed.

The second of these data-gathering approaches is observing aspects of a client's behavior under conditions that were *not* created (structured) by the clinician. In this situation, he or she does not attempt to manipulate the behavior. With the first, the clinician does attempt to do so by having the client perform a task. For example, if a clinician wanted to use the first method to observe behaviors that occur during moments of stuttering, he or she could ask the client to do the "job task" (Johnson, 1961)—have the client talk for a few minutes about his or her present job or one for which he or she is being trained. On the other hand, if the clinician wanted to use the second method for this purpose, he or she could observe the client while the client is conversing with someone.

The third of these approaches is interviewing an informant— either the client or someone (such as a parent, spouse, or teacher) who has information about particular aspects of the client's behavior. The interview could be conducted face to face, on the telephone, or in response to written questions (such as a case-history questionnaire). This is the most frequently used approach for obtaining information about the symptomatology and phenomenology of the disorder outside of the therapy room. Since the abnormal disfluency exhibited by a client during an evaluation may not be typical of that in most other situations (Silverman, 1975), it is necessary to establish whether it was by asking the client and/or another informant who was present.

After the necessary data have been gathered, the questions are answered, the answers are interpreted, and recommendations are made. This information is usually communicated in a written report that may consist of a paragraph or two in a client's chart, or it may be a formal, multipage document. It usually includes information about the reason for the evaluation, the questions asked, how they were answered, the answers obtained and interpretations made of them, and recommendations for future action ("Where do we go from here?"). Its purpose is communication—both to other professionals and to the person who wrote it. Without a written report to jog your memory, you are unlikely to remember very much about an evaluation you did even a month or two earlier.

CULTURAL CONSIDERATIONS

There are a number of ways that the successful completion of an evaluation for a fluency disorder can be jeopardized by a clinician's failure to recognize differences between what is acceptable/unacceptable and believed/not believed in both the clinician's culture and that of the client and/or the client's family, including:

- Beginning the evaluation (e.g., history taking) before taking time for social amenities (i.e., establishing rapport). This is considered impolite in many cultures and can alienate a client and/ or his or her family to the point where completing the evaluation becomes difficult, if not impossible.
- Addressing case history questions to a child's mother when both parents are present and the cultural expectation is that the

husband will be the spokesperson for the family. The best way to cope with this expectation is to address the questions to both parents and let them decide who will respond. Addressing both parents is, in fact, worth doing routinely. Husbands may be better able to answer some questions than their wives.

- A female clinician assuming an authority role when interviewing either a male client or a client's father from a culture in which the female is subservient to the male. Her doing so is likely to be deemed both insulting and threatening.

- The clinician doing the evaluation being of a different sex than the client, particularly if the client is an adult. This is particularly likely to impede communication between client and examiner if the client is from a Middle-Eastern Moslem culture.

- Insisting on answers to questions about family matters (e.g., to complete a case history form) when the family is from a culture in which family matters are considered private and not to be shared with strangers.

- Ridiculing clients or family members about their beliefs concerning the cause of the client's fluency disorder when their beliefs are not consistent with those in your culture. Such beliefs can range from God's will and possession to imitation. They tend to be strongly held and you're most likely to cope with them successfully by working around them rather than challenging them.

- If you are a male, insisting that a female client be alone with you during the evaluation. This could be a taboo in a Moslem culture.

- Touching the client (e.g., patting him or her gently on the head or shoulder). In some cultures, touching of someone (even a child) by a person who is not related by blood is taboo.

Cultural considerations are discussed further in chapter 7 in the context of treatment, and in chapter 8 in the context of prevention.

DETERMINING WHETHER A CLIENT HAS A FLUENCY DISORDER

It isn't safe to assume that someone who is scheduled for an evaluation for a fluency disorder does, in fact, have one. Consequently, one of the first questions (perhaps *the* first question) that you must answer during any such evaluation is: "Is the client's speech fluency within normal limits?" In some instances, particularly with adults whose disorder is stuttering or neurogenic acquired stuttering, this question can be answered affirmatively by merely having a few minutes of informal conversation with the client and observing his or her speech fluency. In other instances, however, answering it is more time consuming because the client either doesn't exhibit any abnormal hesitation phenomena during the evaluation session or exhibits hesitation phenomena that could be either normal or abnormal. The latter is often the case for preschool children who are referred for a fluency evaluation because of someone's concern that they may be beginning to stutter. Some strategies are presented here for coping with this situation and others in which the presence or absence of a fluency disorder isn't obvious.

Determining Whether a Preschool Child Is Beginning to Stutter

Determining whether a young child—particularly one of preschool age—is beginning to stutter may be very difficult. This is because the part-word and single-syllable word repetitions of children who are beginning to stutter (see the description of Bloodstein's Phase I stuttering in chapter 4) are often quite similar to those of children who are not developing the disorder—particularly those who are at the *upper end of normal limits* with regard to the amount of these disfluencies they produce.

When deciding whether a child is beginning to stutter you can make two kinds of errors: You can conclude that a child who is beginning to stutter is being normally disfluent, and you can conclude that a child who is being normally disfluent (perhaps at the upper end of normal limits) is beginning to stutter. While both kinds of errors are undesirable, one can have more serious consequences than the other. If you accept the diagnosogenic theory for the onset of stuttering (see chapter 5), the second kind of error—diagnosing normal disfluency as being abnormal—would be more likely to have undesirable consequences than would the first.

I use the following approach: Because I accept the diagnosogenic theory as being the most likely explanation for most cases of stuttering, I try hard not to make the second kind of error. Consequently, I will only label a child's repetitions "abnormal" if there is considerable evidence to support such a diagnosis. I would not, however, label a child's repetitions as "normal" if he or she had the characteristics of Bloodstein's Phase II, III, or IV stuttering (see chapter 4). Incidentally, labeling a child's repetitions as "normal" when they are really "beginning stuttering" could be therapeutic if it caused persons (especially the child's parents) to stop reacting to them in undesirable ways.

My decision about whether a child's disfluencies are abnormal is based both on information about them from informants (usually parents) and on my observations of the child's speech. If the child has moments of stuttering while in the therapy room, it is likely that he or she will have them elsewhere also. However, if he or she does not have them while in the therapy room, it is still possible that he or she will in other environments. At the end of the diagnostic session, I ask the parents whether the child produced the disfluency behavior that concerned them during the session. If they indicate that they didn't hear any instances of the behavior, I ask them to tape-record the child's speech in situations in which he or she had exhibited it in the past and to make an appointment to see me when they have some instances of it on tape. During the session, we listen to the tape and I let them know whether the disfluencies they recorded suggest that their child has a disorder.

One factor that I consider when deciding whether a child's fluency level requires intervention is the child's awareness of and concern about his or her disfluencies. If a child is concerned about them, some intervention is likely to be needed regardless of whether they are normal or abnormal. Based on the diagnosogenic theory, such concern could precipitate stuttering if the disfluencies were normal or could make the disorder more severe if they were abnormal (see chapter 5).

One way to determine whether a child is concerned about being disfluent is to ask the parents whether he or she has ever said anything to them that would suggest such concern. Another way to determine it is to have the child do the three-wishes task (described later in the chapter).

Determining Whether a Client Has a Fluency Disorder When His or Her Fluency during the Evaluation Seems Normal

It isn't safe to assume that a client who is normally fluent during an evaluation session doesn't have a fluency disorder. Persons who stutter can be quite fluent during such a session, particularly if they are relaxed, aren't motivated to avoid stuttering, or are doing things to conceal their stuttering. Persons who clutter may be monitoring their speech more carefully than usual and, consequently, are speaking more slowly and being more fluent than usual.

If an older child or adult seems to be normally fluent during an evaluation that he or she sought, at the end of the session I ask the person whether he or she exhibited in my presence any of the behavior that caused him or her to seek the evaluation. If the client answers affirmatively, I ask him or her to imitate it. If it's unclear whether the behavior is abnormal after the person imitates it, or if the client indicates that he or she didn't exhibit any of the behavior during the session, I tell the client to make tape recordings at times when he or she is likely to exhibit the behavior, and when there are samples of it on tape, to make an appointment to see me and bring the recording.

If a client isn't self-referred, I try to arrange to have the person making the referral present at the evaluation session (either in the same room or behind a one-way mirror). If I don't hear any abnormal disfluency during the session, I ask the person if he or she heard any and if they did, to imitate it. If it's unclear whether what the person was reacting to is abnormal or if the person indicates that he or she didn't hear any of the abnormal behavior during the session, I have the person do the tape recording task described in the previous paragraph.

DETERMINING WHETHER THE CLIENT IS AT RISK FOR STUTTERING OR DEVELOPING A STUTTERING OVERLAY ON ANOTHER FLUENCY DISORDER

If a client doesn't appear to be stuttering at present or a client has another fluency disorder, the next question to answer would be: "Does the client appear to be at greater than normal risk for beginning to stutter or for developing a stuttering overlay on his or her existing fluency disorder?" If parents or others are pressuring the client to avoid being disfluent and/or the client is pressuring himself or herself to do so, the client is probably at greater than normal risk for either beginning to stutter or for developing such an overlay. Some strategies for reducing this risk are outlined in chapter 8.

DETERMINING THE TYPE OF FLUENCY DISORDER

Once it's established that a client has a fluency disorder, the next step is answering the following question: "Is the client's disorder stuttering, cluttering, neurogenic acquired stuttering, psychogenic acquired stuttering, or some combination of these?" Information is presented here that often can facilitate making this determination.

Distinguishing Stuttering from Cluttering

In older children and adults, a disorder is more likely to be *cluttering* than stuttering if:

1. The client's speaking rate is quite rapid.
2. Because the client is unaware that his or her speaking rate is excessive and that he or she is being abnormally disfluent, he or she is not concerned about it. Consequently, the client neither avoids talking nor does "things" to avoid being disfluent—there are no secondary behaviors.
3. The client does not become more disfluent when he or she feels it is important to speak well. In fact, the opposite may be true. The client may be *more fluent* at these times than he or she is at other times because the act of carefully formulating speech results in a slower speaking rate.

Distinguishing between stuttering and cluttering in young children can be quite difficult because the second and third conditions listed above are also true for children who are beginning to stutter. Furthermore, determining whether a young child's speaking rate is excessive may be difficult.

Daly (1993a) has developed a 33-item checklist "which presents features that numerous clinical researchers believe are indicative of cluttering" (see Appendix C). Each item is rated 0 to 3—the total number of points possible being 99. Daly suggests that a score of 60 or above is usually sufficient to support a diagnosis of cluttering and one between 30 and 60 a diagnosis of cluttering-stuttering. The checklist items that Daly indicates are the most indicative of cluttering are 2, 3, 7, 9, 10, 12, 14, 20, 25, and 33.

Distinguishing Stuttering from Neurogenic Acquired Stuttering

In older children and adults, a disorder is more likely to be neurogenic acquired stuttering than stuttering if:

1. The onset was after the age of 10.
2. An event occurred immediately before the onset of the disorder that resulted in damage to the central nervous system.
3. The amount of abnormal disfluency *does not vary* from day to day and from situation to situation in the same manner as it does in stuttering. There probably is no situation in which the client is completely fluent.
4. Abnormal disfluency is not reduced significantly or eliminated by reading in chorus. Consequently, if a client exhibits little or no abnormal disfluency while reading in chorus, the disorder is more likely to be stuttering than neurogenic acquired stuttering.

Distinguishing between stuttering and neurogenic acquired stuttering in children younger than ten is likely to be quite difficult unless it can be established that there is damage to the central nervous system that could result in excessive disfluency and that this damage occurred before the onset of the fluency disorder.

Evaluations of older children and adults for stuttering should routinely include a short choral reading task (Silverman, 2000). Parts of the passages in Appendix C can be used for this purpose. If the disorder is stuttering, moments of abnormal disfluency will be almost or completely eliminated. On the other hand, if the disorder is neurogenic acquired stuttering, reading in chorus will have little or no effect on the abnormal disfluency.

I treated a woman in her 40s a number of years ago whose moderately severe fluency disorder had been labeled stuttering, and had been treated as such, since childhood. She did not become more fluent on the choral reading task, and her "stuttering" didn't appear to vary much in severity from day to day and from situation to situation. Both aspects of the phenomenology of her disorder suggested that it was neurogenic acquired stuttering rather than stuttering. Since previous therapists had told her that her lack of improvement was due to not trying hard enough, this misdiagnosis caused her to have a poorer self-concept than she probably would have had otherwise. Even if routinely doing a short choral reading task during evaluations for stuttering results in preventing only one such misdiagnosis during your professional career, in my opinion it will have been time well invested!

Distinguishing Psychogenic Acquired Stuttering from Neurogenic Acquired Stuttering

In older children and adults, the disorder is more likely to be psychogenic acquired stuttering than neurogenic acquired stuttering if:

1. The onset was after the age of 10.

2. No event occurred immediately prior to the onset of the disorder that could have resulted in damage to the central nervous system.

3. An event occurred immediately prior to the onset of the disorder that could have resulted in severe psychological trauma.

4. The amount of abnormal disfluency *does not vary* from day to day and from situation to situation in the same manner as it does if the disorder is stuttering. There may be no situation in which the client is completely fluent. Abnormal disfluency is not reduced significantly or eliminated by reading in chorus. Consequently, if a client exhibits little or no abnormal disfluency while reading in chorus, the disorder is more likely to be stuttering than psychogenic acquired stuttering.

5. The client is aware of but *not particularly concerned about* his or her abnormal disfluency. A person who has neurogenic acquired stuttering is likely to be both aware of and concerned about it.

Distinguishing between neurogenic acquired stuttering and psychogenic acquired stuttering in children younger than ten is likely to be quite difficult unless the child has been diagnosed as having a psychiatric disorder that could produce abnormal disfluency. Such cases probably are extremely rare, judging by the lack of reports of them in the literature.

IDENTIFYING THE BEHAVIORS IN THE SET THAT DEFINES A CLIENT'S FLUENCY DISORDER

The set of behaviors that defines a client's fluency disorder can include impairments, disabilities, and handicaps. These are entities that if eliminated, modified, or compensated for would tend to reduce, at least a little, the negative impact that the disorder is having on the client's life. The overall goal of therapy for a particular client, therefore, would be to eliminate, modify, or compensate for as many of the behaviors in the set that defines his or her fluency disorder as possible (see chapter 7 for strategies for doing so).

To identify the behaviors in the set that defines a particular client's fluency disorder, you would ask a series of questions and then make the observations needed to answer them. Following are some of the questions that you might want to ask.

- *Amount of disfluency.* Is the client ever normally fluent? How frequently does the client usually exhibit abnormal disfluency behavior? To what extent does the amount of disfluency exhibited by the client vary on a *situational* basis—that is, are there some situations in which the client almost always is more fluent than in others? To what extent does the amount of disfluency exhibited by the client vary on the basis of *content* (e.g., is the likelihood of the client being disfluent greater during oral reading than during spontaneous speech)? To what extent does the amount vary on the basis of the client's *emotional state* (for example, whether the client tends to hesitate less frequently than usual when angry)?

  To what extent does the amount vary on the basis of *how important it is for the client to be fluent*—that is, does the client tend to be most disfluent when he or she wants to be most fluent? Does the client become more fluent when he or she speaks in a *nonhabitual manner* (for example, at a slower than usual rate)? Is the client normally fluent while reading in chorus? Does the client tend to be less fluent while talking to someone on the telephone than while conversing face-to-face? Does the client tend to be more fluent while talking to some persons than while talking to others? If the answer to the preceding question is "yes," who are the persons with whom the client tends to be most and least fluent?

  Has the level of the client's fluency in most situations changed since the onset of the disorder? If the answer to the preceding question is "yes," has it decreased or increased? Does the client do things to avoid being disfluent? If the answer to the preceding question is "yes," what does the client do? How much confidence does the client appear to have in his or her fluency-enhancing capability? Has a speech-language pathologist or other clinician ever suggested to the client specific techniques or strategies for becoming more fluent? If the answer to the preceding question is "yes," what techniques or strategies were suggested and how well does the client feel that they have worked? How important does it appear to be to the client to become more fluent? How confident does the client appear to be in his or her ability to achieve this goal?

• *Behaviors that occur during moments of abnormal disfluency.* Does the client tend to repeat sounds, syllables, and/or single-syllable words more often than his or her peers? If the answer to the preceding question is "yes," approximately how much more often? What is the average and maximum number of units of repetition (the number of times a particular sound, syllable, or word is repeated)? Are there instances in which the phonemes (particularly vowels) repeated during syllable repetitions are not appropriate for the word that follows? How often are the repetitions accompanied by tension? How aware does the client appear to be of his or her repetitions?

Does the client ever exhibit blocks (prolonged sounds, "broken" words, tense pauses, and/or abnormally long silent pauses)? If the answer to the preceding question is "yes," how often do they occur? What are the average and longest times that blocks tend to last? Do the majority of the client's blocks tend to be audible or silent? Do the behaviors that occur when the client "blocks" almost always tend to be the same? If the answer to the preceding question is "yes," in what sequence do they tend to occur? Do both repetitions and blocks ever occur on the same word? How aware does the client appear to be of his or her blocks?

Do extraneous movements and vocalizations (secondary symptoms) ever occur while the client is being disfluent? If the answer to the preceding question is "yes," describe them and indicate approximately how often each occurs. Why does the client appear to be making them? How aware does the client appear to be of them?

Does the speed of the client's speech appear to be excessive? If the answer to the preceding question is "yes," does the client appear to be aware that it is? Does the amount of disfluency tend to decrease when the client speaks at a rate that is slower than his or her habitual one?

Is there any evidence of word-finding difficulty, dysarthria, or apraxia while the client is being disfluent? If the answer to the preceding question is "yes," does a slower-than-habitual speaking rate affect his or her disfluency behavior, and if it does, how?

Does the client exhibit the "consistency" effect (see chapter 2)? If the answer to the preceding question is "yes," what words or sounds (if any) does the client report being particularly difficult for him or her to say?

Does the client usually maintain normal eye contact while being disfluent? If the answer to the preceding question is "no," can the client do so for at least a few minutes if requested? To what extent does this lack of normal eye contact appear to result from feelings of shame and/or embarrassment about being disfluent?

- *Avoidance of disfluency.* Does the client ever reduce verbal output (not talk) to avoid being disfluent? If the answer to this question is "yes," in what situations and with what persons is he or she most likely to do it? Does the client appear to avoid using the telephone for this reason? Are there persons from whom the client has been able to conceal his or her disorder by doing so? If there are, what does the client believe would happen if they learned "the truth?" Does the client appear to have considered the possibility that his or her interpersonal relationships are hurt more than they are helped by avoiding talking?

Can the client predict with better-than-chance accuracy some of the words on which he or she is going to be disfluent? If the answer to the preceding question is "yes," what strategies, if any, does the client use to avoid being disfluent? Does the client ever substitute words for ones on which disfluency is anticipated? If the client does this, are the words substituted ever inappropriate? Does the client ever answer questions incorrectly or incompletely to avoid being disfluent? Does the client ever choose not to revise errors (mispronunciations and "wrong" words) because of fear of being disfluent while doing so? Does the client ever use circumlocution as a device to avoid being disfluent? If the client does so, are the phrases (utterances) substituted ever inappropriate?

Does the client ever use devices (e.g., syllables, words, and/or gestures) that function as "starters?" If the answer to the preceding question is "yes," which ones does the client use? What devices does the client report having used in the past for this purpose? Are any behaviors observable while the client is being disfluent that in the past could have been "starters?"

- *Client's attitude toward his or her disfluency.* To what extent does the client react negatively to his or her disfluency? Does the client react more negatively to it than most listeners are likely to?

Does the client appear to feel ashamed or embarrassed about speaking disfluently? Does the client behave in a manner that is likely to signal listeners that he or she is ashamed or embarrassed about doing so (such as having poor eye contact)? To what extent does the client judge his or her performance in speaking situations on the basis of how fluently he or she spoke rather than on how well he or she communicated? Has anyone previously attempted to encourage the client to base such decisions more on the latter?

How strong is the client's desire to conceal his or her fluency disorder? If it is relatively strong, how does the client believe people would react differently if they were aware of it? Does the client ever purposely bring his or her fluency disorder "out into the open"? If the answer to the preceding question is "yes," how does the client do it? In what ways does the client appear to be handicapped by the fluency disorder? How frequently does it keep the client from being understood?

If the fluency disorder were to disappear tomorrow, how much impact does the client appear to believe it probably would have on his or her life? What things would the client begin doing that he or she does not do now? Does the client appear to believe that he or she would have more friends? That dating would be more enjoyable? That his or her marriage probably would be better? That he or she probably would be happier? Respected more by people? Better off financially? More outgoing and/or have a better self-concept? More effective as a communicator? Would the client be likely to change jobs? If the answer to this last question is "yes," what field(s) might the client enter (or go to school to get the training to enter)? Does the client appear to believe that his or her speech at present is not good enough for entering these fields? Is the client's present job one that does not require him or her to talk much? Does the client appear to believe that becoming more fluent might, in some way, be disadvantageous?

- *Impact of the disorder on the client's self-concept.* In what ways (if any) has the disorder adversely affected the client's self-concept? Is the client a "people pleaser"? Is the client chronically depressed? Is the client suicidal? Does the client often appear to be a "wimp"? Do the client's body language, grooming, and/or clothing frequently suggest that he or she has a poor self-concept? Does the client tend to be more fluent when he is feeling good about himself? Does the client openly express anger when she feels it, or is the client usually passive aggressive? How assertive is the client? Does the client's orientation toward life tend to be optimistic or pessimistic? Does the client tend to be a risk taker? What are some things that make the client feel good about himself or herself? Achieving what goals, other than fluency, does the client believe would improve his or her self-concept?

Does the client appear to overvalue fluency? Does the client's orientation toward it tend to be two-valued ("success" is perfect fluency and "failure" is anything else)? Do the client's disfluencies tend to call less adverse attention to him or her than he or she seems to believe?

After the clinician has identified at least some of the behaviors in the set that defines the client's fluency disorder, the next task is to formulate a tentative hypothesis (explanation) for each. Such hypotheses are likely to influence both the goals for therapy and the intervention strategies (therapies) selected for accomplishing them (Williams, 1968).

Clinicians are unlikely to have the same degree of confidence in the accuracy of all their hypotheses about why clients are behaving in particular ways. In some cases, they are likely to regard them as being no more than "hunches." Such hunches are more likely to be based on observations than the persons making them may assume. This phenomenon has been referred to as *tacit knowing* (Polanyi, 1967). According to Polanyi:

> *We know more than we can tell.* This fact seems obvious enough; but it is not easy to say exactly what it means. Take an example. We know a person's face, and can recognize it among a thousand, indeed among a million. Yet we usually cannot tell how we recognize a face we know. (p.4)

ANSWERING QUESTIONS

We have focused thus far in this chapter primarily on the first part of the evaluation process—asking answerable questions. We'll now focus on the second part of this process—making the observations needed to answer such questions.

There are three general approaches that can be used, alone or in combination, for making the observations (collecting the data) needed for answering the questions asked during an evaluation. These approaches (described earlier in the chapter) are informal observation, questioning an informant, and having a client perform a task. The approach or combination that is most likely to yield the information needed at low cost with adequate levels of validity, reliability, and generality is used.

What is meant here by yielding data that have adequate levels of validity, reliability, and generality? An approach (or combination of approaches) would yield data that possessed an adequate level of validity if it allowed you to observe *what* you needed to observe to answer a question.

An approach (or combination) would yield data that possessed an adequate level of reliability if it allowed you to observe what you needed to observe to answer a question in a way that is *repeatable*. Repeatable here could have two meanings. First, it could mean that two or more persons viewing an event (for example, a behavior) would describe it similarly enough that they would answer a question about it the same way. If, for example, a group of clinicians rated the severity of the stuttering in a videotaped sample of a client's speech, their ratings probably would be adequately reliable if the majority indicated that the severity was "mild" and none indicated that it was "severe."

A second meaning of repetition with an adequate level of reliability in this context is that the client behaves in the same way during repeated observations that occur too close together in time for it to be likely that he or she has changed. If, for example, a client read in chorus with a clinician a number of times and during none of them did he or she stutter, the conclusion that the client does not do so under this condition would appear to be reliable.

An approach (or combination) would yield data that possessed an adequate level of generality if it allowed you to observe what you needed to observe in order to *infer* how the client would be likely to behave under a particular set of circumstances outside of the clinic environment. A client's behavior in the therapy room is not necessarily representative of that in other situations. This is particularly likely to be true for stuttering severity. Many clients, particularly children, tend to be more fluent in the therapy room than they are in most other situations (Silverman, 1975). For this reason, it usually is necessary to determine how representative the sample of a client's fluency observed during an evaluation is of fluency in other situations. This can be done by questioning the client and/or another informant (e.g., a parent) or by obtaining samples of his or her speech in other situations.

Now that we have considered the concepts of validity, reliability, and generality in this context, we will consider that of *cost*. Cost here refers to both the amount of time it takes to gather the data needed for answering a question and the expense involved in doing so. If two approaches are likely to yield data that possess adequate levels of validity, reliability, and generality and one takes less time and/or involves less expense than the other, that one usually would be selected.

What Types of Information Can Be Obtained by Informal Observation?

The data needed for answering some questions can be obtained through informal observation. Aspects (attributes) of speaking behavior about which information can be acquired in this manner include:

- speaking rate
- verbal output (including avoidance of talking)
- amount of disfluency
- types of disfluency behaviors
- sequence of behaviors that tend to occur during moments of abnormal disfluency, particularly stuttering
- duration of moments of disfluency
- amount of tension accompanying disfluency

- extraneous movements (gestures) accompanying disfluency
- use of devices (such as starters, word substitution, and circumlocution) for avoiding disfluency
- eye contact while being disfluent
- level of awareness of disfluency

Information also can be acquired by informal observation about aspects (attributes) of a client's functioning other than speech, including:

- physical health
- mental retardation or other types of cognitive deficits
- the presence of depression
- self-concept
- attitudes toward the fluency disorder (such as feelings of shame or embarrassment)
- willingness to acknowledge the disorder openly ("bring it out into the open")
- willingness to be assertive
- tendency to be a "people pleaser"
- relationships with one or more significant others (such as parents)

Information acquired in this manner can be written down immediately after it is obtained or at some future time from tape recordings of the evaluation session. Some clinicians routinely tape-record their initial evaluation sessions with clients who have fluency disorders. While audiotapes can be used for this purpose, videotapes may be better, particularly if it is desirable to describe visual behaviors (such as eye contact while being disfluent) as well as auditory ones.

Abstracting information from a recording rather than writing it down immediately after it occurs can have several advantages. First, it makes it unnecessary to interrupt the flow of the evaluation repeatedly while you record information on a pad or form. As a consequence, you can pay more attention to (be in better rapport with) the client. Second, it may allow you to record information more reliably. You can listen to and/or watch segments of the evaluation as many times as required to describe behaviors accurately. Third, it may allow you to record information more completely. At certain times during an evaluation session, a number of relevant events may be occurring almost simultaneously. In addition, certain events that did not appear to be significant when they occurred may take on significance later in the session. If the session was recorded, the clinician could evaluate the segments containing this information.

The main disadvantage associated with abstracting information from a recording rather than writing it down immediately is that doing so is more time consuming. The amount of time that a clinician can devote to an evaluation may not be sufficient to do this routinely. One compromise would be to tape-record the evaluation session, but to use the recording only when it is absolutely necessary.

What Types of Information Can Be Obtained from an Informant?

Information needed for answering some questions can be obtained most efficiently from an informant. This is particularly likely to be the case for questions concerning behaviors that cannot be observed in the clinic and for questions concerning the representativeness of behaviors that can be observed there. Information needed for answering questions about events that occurred in the past (such as those related to the development of the disorder), of course, can only be obtained in this way. The informant would either be the client or someone who has observed him or her (such as a parent or a teacher).

This approach differs from the other two in that it uses the observations of someone other than a clinician, usually someone who has had no training in speech-language pathology. A person who has not had such training is apt to perceive events differently than one who has. He or she, for example, may not abstract some attributes of the client's speaking behavior that a clinician would be likely to, and vice versa. While this does not invalidate the use of information about speaking behavior from informants, it does suggest that it is not safe to assume that an informant's description of such behavior would be the same as yours.

Types of information that can be obtained from an informant include:

- the reason(s) why an evaluation is being sought at this time
- the circumstances under which the fluency disorder began
- how the disorder has developed since onset
- previous attempts to ameliorate the disorder
- the extent to which the client tends to be disfluent in specific situations
- the types of disfluency behaviors about which the client and/or others are concerned
- the client's level of awareness of the disfluency
- the client's attitude toward the disfluency
- how those with whom the client interacts react while he or she is being disfluent
- the amount of talking the client does
- the client's use of word substitution and other devices to avoid stuttering

- the extent to which the client's disfluency usually interferes with communication
- the extent to which the client avoids using the telephone
- the client's willingness to bring the disorder "out into the open"
- the client's physical and emotional health (For example, does he or she tend to be chronically depressed?)
- the client's self-concept and personality attributes
- ways in which the client is handicapped by the disorder
- the client's level of motivation to invest in therapy
- the client's educational history
- the client's motor, cognitive, and social development
- the client's receptive and expressive speech/language development
- the family history of fluency and other communicative disorders

What Types of Information Can Be Acquired by Having the Client Do a Task?

The data needed for answering some questions can be acquired by having the client perform a task and analyzing aspects of his or her behavior. The types of tasks that a client who has or is suspected of having a fluency disorder may be asked to do include:

- talking about a specified topic or reading a particular passage
- speaking under a particular condition (such as reading in chorus with the clinician)
- responding to the items on a questionnaire
- taking a test

Representative tasks of each type are described in this section.

Talking about a specified topic or reading a particular passage
While you can generate a spontaneous speech sample of adequate length (at least one hundred words) by having a client talk about any number of topics, certain topics have been used frequently. There are several reasons why a clinician may want to adopt these topics for his or her purposes: They are likely to generate a sample of adequate length; "normative" data are available for various disfluency behaviors; and it is unnecessary in reports to describe them in detail because one can refer to a book or journal article in which this is done.

One task that has been used with adults for generating spontaneous speech samples is known as the *job task* (Johnson, 1961). The client is asked to talk for approximately three minutes about his or her present or future vocation. Specifically, the client is told to describe the vocation and indicate why he or she chose it. If the client has not decided on a vocation, he or she is asked to talk about previous jobs. The client is allowed a minute or so to think about what to say. If the client stops speaking before the end of two minutes, the clinician can encourage him or her to continue by asking further questions. An effort should be made, however, to avoid formal structuring of the speaking performance. Data on the frequency of occurrence of various types of disfluency behaviors on this task, for male and female adults who stutter as well as for normal speakers of both sexes, are presented in table 4 of Johnson's (1961) paper.

Another type of task that has been used for generating spontaneous speech samples with adults who have fluency disorders is telling a story about the events depicted in a drawing. The *TAT task* (Johnson, 1961) is representative of this type. The client is shown Thematic Apperception Test (Bellak, 1954) card number 10 (see figure 6.1) and told to develop a dramatic story based on the picture. The client is told to speak for about five minutes about what is happening at the moment in the pictured situation, what events preceded those shown in the picture, and what the outcome is likely to be. The client is allowed up to a minute to prepare the story. If the client stops talking before the end of three minutes, he or she can be encouraged to continue by asking leading questions. Data concerning the frequency with which various types of disfluency behaviors occur during this task, for both adults who stutter and normal-speaking peers, are presented in table 5 of Johnson's (1961) paper.

The *CAT task* provides another way to elicit a spontaneous speech sample by having the client talk about the action depicted in drawings (Silverman, 1974). It differs from the preceding method in that it can be used with both children and adults and more than one drawing usually is used. The client is presented with the ten Children's Apperception Test (CAT) cards (Bellak, 1954), one after the other, and asked to make up a "once-upon-a-time" story about each. The specific instructions are as follows (Silverman, 1974):

> I want you to imagine that you are helping to take care of a very young child. One way to keep a small child sitting still is to tell him or her a story. I am going to show you some cards with pictures on them. I would like you to make up a story, a once-upon-a-time kind of story, about each one that you could tell to a young child. Here is the first card. Let me know as soon as you think of a story and I'll turn on the recorder. (p. 33)

After the client finishes telling a story about the first card, he or she is handed the second. If the first few stories are relatively short (consist of only a few sentences), the client is encouraged to make subsequent ones longer. On the other hand, if the first few stories are relatively long (yield at least a three-minute speech sample), it

Figure 6-1   Drawing used for the TAT (Thematic Apperception Test) task.

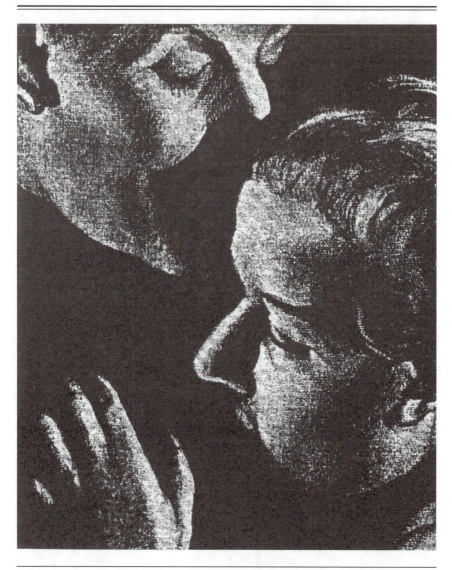

may not be necessary to use the other cards. Data on how frequently various types of disfluency occur during the performance of this task for male elementary-school-age children who stutter and their normal-speaking peers are presented in table 2 of Silverman's (1974) paper. Somewhat comparable data for male and female preschool-age children who stutter and their normal speaking peers are presented on pages 206 and 207 in *The Onset of Stuttering* (Johnson & Associates, 1959).

A third type of task that has been used for eliciting spontaneous speech samples is answering a series of questions. An example that is intended to be used with young children is the *Stocker Probe Technique*. According to Stocker (1980):

> A probe consists of a series of ten questions or requests about two different common objects presented to the child. The questions are presented in random order and represent five graduated *levels of demand* on the speaker. The first five questions relate to the first object presented and the second five questions to the second object. . . .
>
> The different *levels of demand* involve different degrees of creativity on the part of the child, and the *level of demand* associated with each question/request is reflected in the type of response the child ordinarily gives.
>
> A *Level I* question elicits a short repetition response of a few words to the examiner's question. For example, if you hand the child a ball and ask, "Is it hard or soft?" the answer is implicit in the question and is a low-level verbal task.
>
> A *Level II* question also elicits a short response requiring the name of a common object that is present in the examining situation but the name of the object is *not* given in the question, e.g., "What is it?"
>
> A *Level III* question elicits a response usually consisting of a propositional phrase, where the referents are *not* present in the examining situation and are not named in the question, e.g., "Where would you keep one?"
>
> A *Level IV* request elicits a series of attributes *not* named in the request. In this task, the child typically responds as follows: "The ball is red, round, bouncy." Furthermore, unlike *Levels II* and *III*, the syntactic form of the response is *not* constrained by the nature of the question, e.g., "Tell me everything you know about it."
>
> At *Level V*, the highest *level* of the *probe*, the child is asked to "Make up a story about the object." (p. 11)

The type of speech sample generated by this task at *Level V* is likely to be similar to that generated by the CAT and TAT tasks.

We have considered thus far in this section tasks for eliciting spontaneous speech samples. A speech sample generated by reading a passage may also be secured.

Why might a clinician want an oral reading speech sample in addition to a spontaneous speech sample? One reason is that some persons who have fluency disorders, particularly those who stutter, use word substitution and circumlocution to avoid doing so (see chapter 2). Hence, an estimate of the amount of disfluency based solely on a spontaneous speech sample could be too low. Since clients cannot substitute words or use circumlocution while reading a passage, they may be more disfluent while doing so than while speaking spontaneously.

Almost any passage that contains at least 150 words with which the client is likely to be familiar can be used for this purpose. The client should be told to read the passage aloud as he or she ordinarily would do. Do not give any more detailed instructions than this. If the client asks specific questions about how it should be read, simply repeat the instruction to read it as he or she ordinarily would.

Two passages have been used clinically for a number of years with clients who have fluency disorders. Both are loaded with the types of words on which stuttering tends to occur. The first, the 330-word "Rainbow Passage" (see Appendix C), is intended for adults. The second, the 180-word "Arthur the Young Rat" passage (also in Appendix C), can be used with most adults and children above the sixth-grade level.

If a client cannot read, you can elicit a speech sample free from word substitution and/or circumlocution by having him or her repeat a series of fairly short sentences that contain many of the types of words on which moments of stuttering tend to occur (see chapter 2). A set of such sentences, which total 100 words, is reproduced in Appendix C.

After a speech sample has been elicited, the abnormal disfluency behavior in it is analyzed both quantitatively and qualitatively. Based on the amount (both frequency and duration) and the degree of tension and extraneous behavior accompanying it (see chapter 2), a judgment is made on its severity. A number of rating (scaling) methods have been used for this purpose. Two that have been used a great deal clinically are the Iowa Scale of Severity of Stuttering (Darley & Spriestersbach, 1978) and the Stuttering Severity Instrument (Riley, 1972). Both are reproduced in Appendix C.

The Iowa Scale of Severity of Stuttering has a range from zero to seven, with zero indicating "no stuttering" and seven indicating "very severe" stuttering. Each point on the scale is a composite of several variables, including stuttering frequency and duration, amount of muscle tensing, and conspicuousness of facial grimaces and other extraneous body movements. This scale can be used fairly easily for rating the severity of some persons' stuttering. However, it is difficult to use for rating that of others because each of the behavioral variables used for defining specific points on the scale may not be the same in degree for all stutterers (Van Riper, 1982). For example, a person who stuttered on only one percent of words, but whose blocks usually lasted for more than four seconds and were accompanied by very conspicuous facial grimaces, could be rated either a two or a seven on this scale.

One approach used for accommodating behavioral variables that do not all increase in the same amount for all stutterers is to rate the variables individually. With the Stuttering Severity Instrument, for example, frequency of stuttering, duration of moments of stuttering, and physical concomitants (including distracting sounds, facial grimaces, and extraneous movements of the head and extremities) are rated separately. Ratings for frequency can range from zero to eighteen, those for duration from zero to seven, and those for physical concomitants from zero to twenty. Also, the individual scores can be totaled and an overall severity rating assigned. A total of zero to five would be labeled "very mild," six to fifteen "mild," sixteen to twenty-three "moderate," twenty-four to thirty "severe," and thirty-one to forty-five "very severe" (Riley, 1972, table 1).

Another instrument used for individually rating behavioral variables is the Profile of Stuttering Severity (Van Riper, 1972, chapter 9). It is a revision of the Iowa Scale of Severity of Stuttering, in which ratings for individual variables—including frequency of stuttering, duration of moments of stuttering, and degree of tension—are plotted on a chart (see figure 6-2). Such charts can be quite useful for measuring change during therapy.

The devices described thus far for analyzing the abnormal disfluency in speech samples yield quantitative data. They indicate how often in a speech sample abnormal disfluency occurs, how long individual instances tend to last, and the degree to which they are accompanied by tension and extraneous movements. Devices also are available for cataloging the behaviors that occur in a speech sample during moments of abnormal disfluency. One such device, the Checklist of Stuttering Behavior (Darley & Spriestersbach, 1978), allows you to describe the presence or absence of twenty-six behaviors during six such moments (see Appendix C). While it may be possible to make such judgments reliably while the client is speaking "live," it probably would be easier to do so from a videotape.

Speaking under a particular condition

These tasks allow you to observe how the frequency of disfluency varies under certain conditions. The information yielded by them can be used in several ways. One is to differentiate stuttering from other types of abnormal disfluency. Persons who stutter tend to behave differently on several of these tasks than do those with other fluency disorders. Another is to assess the ability of certain intervention strategies to reduce a client's disfluency.

Tasks are described in this section that allow you to observe how the amount of abnormal disfluency varies under certain conditions. While these are not the only tasks that can be used for this purpose, they include those that have been used most often.

- *Reading in chorus.* The clinician hands the client a reading passage and reads it in chorus (unison) with him or her. This appears to be one of the best ways to differentiate "ordinary" stuttering from neurogenic acquired stuttering. While persons who stutter usually become normally fluent under this condition, those who have neurogenic acquired stuttering do not.

Figure 6-2   Profile of Stuttering Severity showing changes as a result of therapy.

Profile of Stuttering Severity

Scale	Frequency	Tension-Struggle	Duration	Postponement-Avoidance
1.	Under 1%	None	Under 1/2 sec.	None
2.	1 - 2%	Rare but present	Average 1/2 sec.	Less then 5%
3.	3 - 5%	Usual but mild	Average 1 sec.	5 - 10%
4.	6 - 8%	Severe	Average 2 sec.	11 - 20%
5.	9 - 12%	Very severe	Average 3 sec.	21 - 31%
6.	13 - 25%	Overflow to eyes and limbs	Average 4 sec.	31 - 70%
7.	More than 25%	Overflow to trunk	Longer than 5 sec.	More than 70%

Name: _Joe P._   **Date:** _____   **Speaking Situation:** _TAT Pictures_

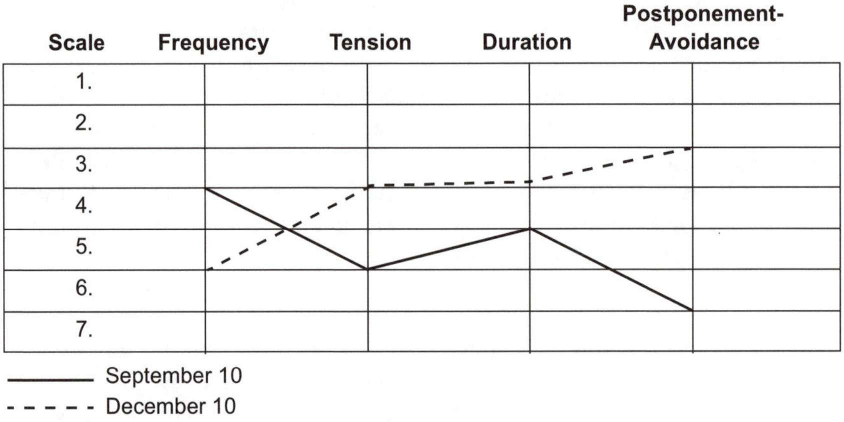

Scale	Frequency	Tension	Duration	Postponement-Avoidance
1.				
2.				
3.				
4.				
5.				
6.				
7.				

————— September 10
- - - - - December 10

Reproduced with permission from Van Riper, 1982, p. 201.

- *Singing.* The client is told to sing a song, such as our national anthem or a hymn. Almost all persons who stutter become normally fluent while doing so (regardless of how well they sing). If a client does not become normally fluent while singing, he or she probably has some other fluency disorder.
- *Speaking at a slower than usual rate.* The client is told to speak or read aloud at a rate that is slower than usual. Some persons who have a fluency disorder become significantly more fluent while doing so. They may be helped by intervention strategies that result in a reduction in speaking rate (see chapter 7).
- *Speaking while listening to masking noise.* Masking ("white") noise is presented to the client binaurally through headphones

at a level of approximately 90 dB above threshold, and he or she is told either to read aloud or to do a spontaneous speech task. The masking-noise generator on many audiometers can be used for this purpose. Some persons who stutter are more fluent than usual while speaking under this condition (see chapter 2). They may benefit from using a miniature, voice-activated masking-noise generator, such as the Edinburgh masker (Ingham, Southwood, & Horsburgh, 1981).

- *Speaking under delayed auditory feedback.* The client is inter-faced with a delayed auditory feedback device and told either to read aloud or to do a spontaneous speech task. Some persons who stutter become more fluent under this condition (see chapter 2). They may benefit from the use of intervention strategies for reducing stuttering severity that utilize these devices to teach a slow rate of speech through prolongation of syllables (Craven & Ryan, 1984; Kalinowski, 2003; Muellerleile, 1981).

- *Pacing speech with a metronome.* The client is told to pace his or her speech while reading aloud or doing a spontaneous speech task with the beats of a metronome—usually one word per beat. Some persons who stutter become more fluent while speaking in this manner (see chapter 2). There have been attempts to treat such persons by fitting them with miniature electronic metronomes (Silverman & Trotter, 1973a, 1973b, 1974, 1975).

- *Talking on the telephone.* The client is told to make a telephone call—to a store, for example, to find out if they have particular items in stock. Since many persons who stutter do so more severely than usual while talking on the telephone (see chapter 2), this task is likely to elicit a sample of the client's stuttering that is at the *upper end* of his or her severity range. It is partic-ularly likely to yield useful information if the client does not stutter or does so very little while talking face-to-face during the evaluation session.

- *Attempting to modify behaviors that occur while being disfluent.* The client is told to read aloud or to do a spontaneous speech task and while doing so to try to change a specific behavior that tends to occur while he or she is being disfluent. For example, a client who has poor eye contact while being disfluent might be asked to modify this behavior. This task provides information about the client's ability to modify certain behaviors. It also pro-vides information about whether these behaviors (assuming they are learned) are instrumental or classically conditioned (Brutten & Shoemaker, 1967).

- *Predicting moments of stuttering.* The client is told to predict whether he or she is going to stutter on certain words before saying them. A person who is able to predict a high percentage of his or her moments of stuttering probably would benefit more from an intervention program that stressed modification of moments of stuttering while they occur than would a person who is not able to do so (Van Riper, 1973).

Several tasks have been used for this purpose. In one, the client is handed a copy of a reading passage and asked to underline the words on which he or she expects to stutter. The client then reads the passage and the clinician determines the accuracy of his or her predictions. In another, the client is shown a series of words one at a time and asked to signal before saying each whether he or she expects to stutter while doing so. After making each prediction, the client says the word, and the clinician judges whether it was stuttered. A set of fifty words (nouns, verbs, adverbs, or adjectives) that begin with consonants, are five letters or more in length, and are in the client's reading vocabulary) that have been typed on cards can be used here (Silverman & Williams, 1972a). This task may provide more useful information than the first about the feasibility of teaching the client to modify moments of stuttering while they occur because it assesses the ability to predict them a few seconds (rather than a few minutes) before they occur.

- *Trying to stutter.* The client is told to stutter "for real" as severely as possible while reading aloud or doing a spontaneous speech task. If the client becomes considerably more fluent, he or she may be a good candidate for a fluency-enhancing strategy known as *paradoxical intention* (Frankl, 1985, pp. 145–152), described in chapter 7.

Responding to items on a questionnaire

Questionnaires are useful for gathering information. They can reduce the amount of time it is necessary to spend during an evaluation session asking questions and writing down answers.

It may be desirable for some questionnaires to be completed and returned before the evaluation session because doing so could help the clinician identify questions that need to be answered during the session. These questions could either be answered incompletely or unclearly, or could be suggested by answers to original questions on the questionnaire.

There are several types of information that usually can be obtained through the use of questionnaires. One is information about the client and the history of his or her disorder. Included here would be information about the client's birth and development during childhood, family, medical history, educational history, and social history, as well as a description of the onset and development of the disorder.

Another type of information that can usually be gathered in this manner is relevant to the client's abnormal speaking behavior, such as his or her attitudes toward it, and the manner in which he or she attempts to cope with it. A number of questionnaires intended for gathering such information have been published. Those described below are representative.

- *The Stuttering Problem Profile.* This task (see Appendix C) can be used both for identifying the set of behaviors that define a client's stuttering problem and establishing goals for therapy (Silverman, 1980b). Clients are presented with 86 first-person statements that reflect behaviors that could be in the set defining their stuttering problem. They are told to circle the numbers of those statements that they would like to be able to make at the termination of therapy but that they do not think they could make now. The following are typical of the types of statements included in the profile:

  1. I am usually willing to stutter openly.

  6. I am usually willing to use the telephone.

  17. I have learned to live with my problem.

  38. I have expanded my activities, both business and social.

  86. I recite in the classroom as much as most students.

The statements in the Stuttering Problem Profile were abstracted from the responses of 108 adults who stutter, from 17 speech clinics representing various theoretical orientations, to the following: "Would you describe the ways in which you feel your stuttering problem has improved during the past five years?" (Silverman, 1980a). While these persons may not have changed in the ways they indicated, it is reasonable to assume that they considered the behaviors mentioned to be components of their stuttering problem.

The statements a client selects refer to behaviors in the set that defines his or her stuttering problem. If the behavior referred to by a statement is not obvious, the clinician questions the client about what he or she had in mind when selecting it. A set that is defined solely in this manner is likely to be incomplete. Some of the behaviors in it may not be mentioned in any of the statements, and some of the statements that do refer to them may not have been selected.

The statements a client selects also suggest goals for therapy that he or she is interested in achieving. This Profile application is discussed in chapter 7.

- *The S-Scale.* This questionnaire provides information about the attitudes of persons who have fluency disorders toward interpersonal communication (Erickson, 1969, pp. 717–718). It consists of 39 statements (see Appendix C) that the client rates as either true or false. A client's score on the S-Scale is the number of the 39 statements to which he or she responded in the manner indicated by the bracketed responses. Hence, S-Scale scores can range 0 to 39; and the higher the score, the poorer the attitude toward interpersonal communication. Based on Erickson's (1969) data, a score of more than 25 suggests that the client's interpersonal relationships are being affected adversely by his or her attitudes. An item-by-item analysis of a client's responses may also provide useful information.

• *Stutterer's Self-Ratings of Reactions to Speech Situations.* This questionnaire (see Appendix C) can be used for gathering information about a client's avoidance of speaking situations, particularly from young adults (Shumak, 1955; Darley & Spriestersbach, 1978). The client is asked to give four ratings (between 1 and 5) to each of 40 speaking situations. These ratings relate to the amount he or she *avoids* speaking in the situation, *enjoys* speaking in the situation, *stutters* (or is otherwise abnormally disfluent) while speaking in the situation, and *encounters* the situation. The numbers of 1s, 2s, 3s, 4s, and 5s on each of the four scales can be totaled and the mean on each can be compared to that in the normative data reported by Shumak (1955)—which are reproduced in Appendix C.

• *Inventory of Communication Attitudes.* This questionnaire (see Appendix C), which examines affective, cognitive, and behavioral components of attitudes, consists of 13 subscales representing a variety of types of speaking situations. For each of these subscales, there are three representative examples—a total of 39. Each of these is rated on five scales. These are judgments concerning (1) the client's enjoyment of speaking in the situation, (2) the client's speech skills in the situation, (3) other persons' enjoyment of speaking in the situation, (4) other persons' speech skills in the situation, and (5) the frequency at which the client encounters the situation (Watson, Gregory, & Kistler, 1987). While this questionnaire appears to have been developed primarily for research purposes, responses to it could be used clinically for such purposes as assessing the extent to which a client's enjoyment of speaking in a particular situation is related to his or her fluency level while doing so.

• *Problem Profile for Elementary-School-Age Children Who Stutter about Talking.* This questionnaire (see Appendix C) consists of a series of questions about seven aspects of "talking" intended to provide information about the child's awareness of stuttering, people's reactions to the child's speech, and his or her feelings about them (Williams, 1978, pp. 68–70). The questions are asked by the clinician and the child's responses are either written down immediately or recorded.

Williams (1978) also suggests the following questions that can be asked of the parents and teachers of elementary-school-age clients to obtain information about their attitudes toward and reactions to the child's stuttering problem and the effect they perceive it has had on the child:

> Why do you believe that he continues to stutter? How serious a problem is it to you or to him? How do you handle it and how do you think it should be handled by other people? In what ways do you feel it has affected your child? What kind of child is he now? In what ways do you think he would be different if he had not stuttered? How does he get along with boys and girls his own age while at school or playing? To what degree has stuttering influenced his relationships with children or with adults (teacher, grandmother, others)? How has it limited what he has achieved socially or educationally? How much help does he need in meeting new situations or new problems? What special allowances do you think he should receive because of his stuttering? How independent is he in comparison with other children? How has he reacted to his stuttering? How has he reacted to your help and concern about it? (p. 68)

· *"Three Wishes" Task.* This task (Silverman, 1970b) can be used to determine whether young children are aware of and concerned about their speech disfluency without inadvertently suggesting to them that they should be concerned about it. Clients are asked to imagine that they have a fairy godmother who tells them that she will grant any three wishes. They are asked to tell what their wishes would be. If the client does not make a wish for speech fluency, this general three-wishes task is followed by a second (more structured) one. The client is told to imagine that his or her wishes were granted and that the fairy godmother returned and said the client could wish to *change any three things* about himself or herself. The client is then asked to tell what his or her wishes would be.

If a client makes a speech-improvement wish on either of these tasks, this would suggest that he or she is both aware of and concerned about being abnormally disfluent and would, incidentally, provide an opportunity to explore his or her feelings about it more directly. On the other hand, if a child does not make such a wish, his or her level of concern is less certain. While the absence of such a wish would suggest that he or she is not highly concerned about the disorder, it would not by itself establish this.

- *Speech Locus of Control Scale.* This task (McDonough & Quesal, 1988) is intended to determine whether a client tends to believe in an internal or external locus of control for speech. According to McDonough and Quesal (1988):

  An individual with an internal locus of control believes that his/her own behaviors, abilities, and attributes determine "reinforcements." Those individuals with an external locus of control believe that reinforcements are under the control of "luck," "chance," "good days," "bad days," "powerful others," etc., rather than under their personal control. (p. 98)

  The task consists of eight questions or statements that are either answered "yes" or "no" or to which degree of agreement is expressed. McDonough and Quesal have speculated that clients who score at the "internal" end of the locus-of-control continuum may be able to maintain therapy gains better than those who score at the "external" end: Kroll and De Nil (1994) provide some support for this speculation.

- *Perceptions of Self Semantic Differential Task.* This task (see Appendix C) can be used to assess clients' self-perceptions (Kalinowski, Lerman, & Watt, 1987). It is based on a semantic differential that was devised by Woods and Williams (1976). Clients' ratings of themselves on each of the 25 nine-point, bipolar, adjectival scales can provide information about their self-concepts.

- *Southern Illinois University Speech Situation Checklist.* This questionnaire (see Appendix C) is intended to identify speech-related anxiety (Brutten & Shoemaker, 1974). It consists of 51 situations that the client rates on a five-point scale with regard to the amount of negative emotion he or she currently experiences. The higher the total for the ratings, the higher the degree of speech-related anxiety.

- *Disfluency Descriptor Digest.* The goal of this task (see Appendix C) is to determine which of six fluency-initiating gestures might be used most advantageously with a particular stutterer (Cooper, 1982). These gestures are:

  (1) *Slow Speech,* characterized by a reduction in the rate of speech involving the equalized prolongation of syllables; (2) *Easy Onset,* characterized by the initiation of phonation with as little laryngeal area tension as possible; (3) *Deep Breath,* characterized by a consciously controlled inhalation prior to the initiation of phonation; (4) *Loudness Control,* characterized by a conscious and sustained increase or decrease in the volume of the client's speech; (5) *Smooth Speech,* characterized by a reduction in phonatory adjustments and by light articulatory contacts with plosive and affricate sounds being modified to resemble fricative sounds; and (6) *Syllable Stress,* characterized by conscious loudness and pitch variations. (Cooper, 1982, pp. 355–356)

The digest consists of 20 statements describing behaviors that occur frequently during moments of disfluency. A checkmark is placed in the box preceding each behavior observed in the client's speech. Following the 20 of the statements that appear predictive of the successful utilization of each. By transferring the checkmarks from the statements at the top of the form to the table at the bottom, a clinician can identify gestures that may be helpful for reducing the client's stuttering severity.

- *Communication Attitude Test.* This is a 35-item questionnaire (see Appendix C) designed to assess the speech-associated beliefs of children (Vanryckeghem & Brutten, 1992). Children respond to the items by circling either the word True or False next to each item. About half the items are indicative of a negative attitude toward speech if the respondent circles the word "true" for them. The score is the total number of statements marked in a way that suggests negativity. This questionnaire has been administered to children as young as six. An attitude modification program—Think-Wise!—that is based partially on this test was developed at the University Hospital Dijkzigt Rotterdam in the Netherlands (Nagel & van Eupen, 1994).

- *The Cooper Chronicity Prediction Checklist.* This checklist (see Appendix C) was designed to assist clinicians in differentiating between those children who are likely to recover without intervention and those who are not (Gordon & Luper, 1992). It consists of 27 questions that can be answered "yes" or "no." The probability of recovery without intervention is estimated from the number of "yes" responses—the higher the number, the lower the probability of recovery. The authors caution users not to make chronicity judgments solely on the basis of the checklist (Cooper & Cooper, 1985b).

Taking a test

Tests have been used to acquire information about a client's *overall functioning* and the possible impacts of the disorder on it. They have been utilized with clients who have fluency disorders to acquire information about their personality, intelligence, educational achievement, speech/language functioning aside from fluency, and hearing. Many clinicians routinely screen children that they are evaluating for fluency disorders for other speech, language, and hearing disorders.

ASSESSING MOTIVATION

To be successful, rehabilitation almost always requires the active participation of the client and/or his or her family. They must be willing to *invest* whatever is necessary to maximize the likelihood that the client will be helped. For any rehabilitation process to have a reasonable chance of being successful, they must to be willing to make investments of money and time, and they must be willing to be uncomfortable. A necessary condition for them to make such investments is having a high level of motivation to accomplish rehabilitation goals.

Encouraging a client who lacks adequate motivation to achieve at least one rehabilitation goal to begin therapy can be harmful in several ways. It obviously does a little harm by wasting both the client's and clinician's time and someone's money. Such harm, though regrettable, usually isn't serious enough to warrant discouraging a client from beginning therapy. There is, however, a kind of harm that can result from unsuccessful therapy that is serious enough to warrant doing so—reinforcing the client's certainty that he or she can't change.

It is rarely justifiable to consider therapy successful unless the client changes in some way, at least a little. With a client who is an older child or adult, change is unlikely unless the client believes strongly that change is possible. If a client doesn't believe this or, worse yet, believes the opposite, a type of self-fulfilling prophesy is likely to be triggered that some psychologists refer to as a negative placebo effect.

Therapy that a client regards as having been unsuccessful can cause him or her to expect future therapy to be unsuccessful, thereby reducing the likelihood that future therapy will succeed. The more therapy experiences a client has had that he or she deems unsuccessful, the stronger the client's expectation of failure is likely to be.

The mechanism responsible for such harm is one that you may have experienced. Suppose that you felt you needed to lose some weight and decided to lose it by dieting. If this was your first diet and it was recommended by somebody whom you regarded as an authority on dieting (e.g., your doctor), you would probably expect the diet to be successful. However, if you either didn't lose a significant amount of weight while on the diet or you lost it but almost immediately put it all back on, what would your expectation be the second time you tried to lose weight by dieting? Would you be as certain of success as you were the first time? Now, let's suppose that your current diet is your 25th, and the previous 24 yielded either no significant weight loss or only a temporary weight loss. What would your expectation be for diet number 25? Most likely, you would hope for a different outcome but wouldn't really expect one. Moreover, because you would be anticipating failure, you would probably go off of the diet at the first indication it wasn't working, thereby contributing to produce a self-fulfilling prophesy.

For clients and their families to be likely to be willing to make the investments of time, money, and comfort needed to benefit from rehabilitation, they must believe strongly that the potential changes it can produce will significantly improve their lives. Few clients will be willing to make such an investment if they don't anticipate (realistically or unrealistically) a substantial payoff from making it. That is, their motivation will be determined, at least in part, by the size of the benefit they anticipate. Clients who don't expect to benefit substantially from rehabilitation are unlikely to invest much in it and, consequently, are unlikely to improve. All they are likely to take away from therapy is a strengthening of their certainty that they can't change.

Older children and adults should not be encouraged to begin therapy if they appear to lack sufficient motivation to make the necessary investments. Encouraging them to do so will reduce the likelihood that they'll benefit from therapy if at some future time they do have adequate motivation, because they'll probably be entering therapy with a weaker expectation of success than they would otherwise. Consequently, they will have been harmed by the therapy experience.

Three tasks are described in this section for assessing motivation for stuttering therapy. Of course, they are not the only ways possible to determine a child's or adult's level of motivation for rehabilitation. The first of these—which can be used with even very young children—is the *three-wishes task* (see Silverman, 1970b, 2000). Its use is discussed for a different purpose (i.e., assessing awareness of being abnormally disfluent) earlier in the chapter. The task involves two steps, the first being traditional. The child is told to imagine that his or her fairy godmother came and said she would grant three wishes. The child is asked what his or her wishes would be. If the child gives an impairment-related wish, this could indicate concern and in all likelihood a willingness to invest in rehabilitation.

If a child doesn't give an impairment-related wish, he or she is told to imagine that the fairy godmother had granted the three wishes and offered to grant three more wishes to the child, this time to change any three things about himself or herself. The child is given an example of such a wish that is unlikely to be one of his or hers. If the child isn't overweight, the example given could be to become thinner. The child is then asked in what three ways he or she would wish to change. An impairment-related wish could indicate concern and in all likelihood a willingness to invest in rehabilitation. Unfortunately, the failure to give such a wish wouldn't necessarily indicate a lack of concern. Consequently, this task is only interpretable if a child responds in a particular way.

The second of these tasks—which would be used with older children and adults—requires the client and/or members of the client's family to answer one or more *hypothetical questions* (see Silverman, 2000). You'd begin by asking the following hypothetical question: "If you [or the client] woke up tomorrow and were no longer as disabled or handicapped by the impairment, what effect would it have on your [or the client's] life?" If the answer didn't indicate that there would be a significant impact, you would follow up with specific questions such as:

- What would you [or the client] begin doing that you don't [or the client doesn't] do now?
- What would you [or the client] cease doing that you do [or the client does] now?
- Would you [or the client] be able to get a better job?
- How would it affect your [or the client's] relationships with others?
- Would you [or the client] pursue hobbies or other interests that you [or the client] avoid now because of your [or the client's] impairment?

A judgment would be made from a client's [or a family member's] responses to these questions about the amount of benefit that would be anticipated from such an outcome. A client or family member who doesn't believe that reducing the disability or handicap resulting from the client's impairment would change his or her life substantially would be unlikely to invest very much in rehabilitation and, consequently, the client would be unlikely to benefit very much from rehabilitation. Such a belief could be realistic, particularly if the client had reached the acceptance stage in the grieving process and had gotten on with his or her life. Such a person may not be severely disabled or handicapped by his or her impairment.

The third of these tasks is the *Problem Profile*. It can enable older children and adults to have input into goal selection and to alert their clinician to goals they are genuinely interested in achieving. It consists of a set of first-person statements that describe ways in which the disability and handicap resulting from an impairment can improve through rehabilitation. Clients are told that to assist themselves and their clinicians in defining therapy goals, they are to circle the numbers of those statements *they would like to be able to make at the termination of therapy that they don't think they could make now.* They are also told to write on the last page of the profile booklet any statements not included in the list that they would like to be able to make. Circled statements indicate changes that clients would like to be able to make and, consequently, aspects of their disability and handicap they are likely to be motivated to modify. A copy of the Problem Profile for stuttering can be found in Appendix C.

MAKING A PROGNOSIS

After it has been established that a client has a fluency disorder, the type has been determined, the set of behaviors that defines it has been identified, and tentative hypotheses have been formulated concerning the etiology of the behaviors, the next step is to decide whether the client is likely to be helped by therapy and if so, to what extent. There are at least two reasons for this. First, it is a violation of the Code of Ethics of the American Speech-Language-Hearing Association to accept a client for therapy who is highly unlikely to benefit from it.

Second, the client needs this information in order for his or her *consent* to participate in therapy to be an *informed* one (Silverman, 1999a). It is important that it be "informed" both for the legal protection of the clinician (Silverman, 1999a) and to maximize the probability that the client's expectations when entering therapy will be realistic.

A number of factors can influence the likelihood that a client will benefit from therapy. Some are mentioned in this section. The order in which they are discussed is not intended to indicate their importance for establishing a prognosis.

The Length of Time the Client Has Had the Disorder

The longer the client has had the disorder, the poorer the prognosis tends to be. For example, the prognosis for significantly reducing stuttering severity in young children tends to be better than that for adults (Cooper, 1987). According to Freund (1966):

> Age seems to limit the chances for a complete cure. We have as yet not seen an adult who, after successful self-treatment or treatment by a therapist, has lost every trace of stuttering or who has never experienced any relapse, even if brief or minute, or any anticipatory dread of impending stuttering (internal stuttering), though this is not necessarily noticeable to others. (p. 183)

This does not mean that adults who stutter are unlikely to benefit from therapy. However, they appear less likely to be "cured" than young children.

Level of Motivation

The more a client "invests" in therapy, the more likely he or she is to improve (Van Riper, 1973). Consequently, the prognosis for significant improvement tends to be better for highly motivated clients than for less motivated ones.

Previous Therapy Experiences

The more the client regards previous therapy for the disorder as having been successful, the better the prognosis. As Sheehan (1970; quoted in Barbara, 1982) has indicated:

> Being enrolled in therapy raises hopes and when nothing results, hopes are dashed, and future motivation is diminished. . . . Moreover, many stutterers acquire an attitude of hopelessness, give up the search, and deny themselves the possibility of future therapy that might really help them. (p. 74)

If the client does not believe that it was helpful, he or she is likely to enter therapy hoping it will work but not really expecting it to. Such an "expectation" can reduce the effectiveness of almost any intervention program.

Intervention Goals

The prognosis for modifying behaviors in the set that defines a client's fluency disorder is likely to be better for some behaviors than for others. Hence, the prognosis for a particular client is a function, in part, of what the clinician hopes to accomplish.

therapy to fit their attitude

Personality Attributes and Emotional Status

Aspects of a client's personality and emotional state can influence the likelihood that he or she will benefit from therapy (Van Riper, 1979). For example, a client who is an extreme perfectionist or chronically depressed probably is less likely to benefit than one who is not.

Attitudes of Family Members and Significant Others

The attitudes of family members and friends toward both the fluency disorder and the client can influence the prognosis. If their attitudes are such that they do not cause the disorder to become worse, and they are supportive of the client's desire to seek therapy for it, the prognosis is likely to be better than if the opposite were true.

Presence of the Chronic Perseverative Stuttering (CPS) Syndrome

Cooper (1993) has suggested that for approximately one of every five individuals who stutter, "maintaining an acceptable level of fluency may require a *lifetime* [italics mine] of coping." He uses the label *chronic perseverative stuttering (CPS) syndrome* for their disorder. According to Cooper (1993):

> Because the CPS syndrome consists of multiple coexisting and interacting affective, behavioral, and cognitive components coalescing over a period of years, the hope for a complete cure or a total remission of symptoms appears remote. However, the outlook for these individuals is not bleak. With assistance, these individuals typically are able to develop and maintain a feeling of fluency control that enables them to communicate successfully in even the most challenging speech situations. The abundant number of professionally and personally successful individuals who are chronically disfluent testifies most tellingly to an optimistic outlook for those experiencing the CPS syndrome. (p. 13)

As a person who has had this syndrome for more than 60 years and has treated persons who had it for more than 40 years, I can testify both to the reality of the syndrome and to an optimistic outlook for those who have it.

What information is needed to determine if a person has the CPS syndrome? This information can be gleaned from the items in the *CPS*

Syndrome Checklist that Cooper developed as an aid for making this determination. The checklist is reproduced below (Cooper, 1993):

- The individual's fluency disorder developed concomitantly with the development of language and speech.
- The individual's fluency disorder has persisted for 10 or more years.
- The individual's disfluencies are, or have been, accompanied by a fleeting but generalized feeling of loss of control.
- The individual has experienced periods of normal fluency accompanied by the feeling of control.
- The individual experiences a persistent fear of a catastrophic loss of fluency although, in fact, such occurrences are extremely rare.
- The individual has identified one or more adjustments in speech production that generally, but not always, enhance fluency.
- Although capable of predicting the level of fluency to be experienced in most situations, the individual continues to experience unpredictable fluency failures.
- The individual has experienced fluent periods after a heightened or sustained period of psychic and physical concentration on attaining fluency but has been unable to maintain that level of concentration or fluency.
- The individual's predominant self-perception is that of being a stutterer.
- The individual experiences periods of obsessive absorption in striving for normal fluency. (p. 13)

Not every stutterer who has the CPS syndrome will evince every characteristic in the checklist. However, the more of them a stutterer does evince, the more confident one can be that the diagnosis is correct.

A diagnosis of CPS syndrome does not necessarily mean that a speech-language pathologist can be of little help to the person. To the contrary, many can be helped by them to reduce both the severity of their stuttering and the extent to which it interferes with their lives. In some cases, the diagnosis itself can be therapeutic. It can enable a stutterer to stop being obsessively absorbed with striving for normal fluency and to get on with his or her life.

REASONS FOR NOT SCHEDULING THERAPY FOR A CLIENT WHO HAS A DISORDER

Once it has been established that the client has a fluency disorder, some type of intervention *usually* is recommended. There are several reasons, however, why it may not be advisable to do so. These include the following: the client is coping successfully with the disorder; the client lacks adequate motivation; the client is unable to make the necessary investments; the client's intervention needs can be better met by somebody else; or the clinician does not believe that the client's goals are achievable.

If the client appears to be coping successfully with the disorder, therapy may not be recommended because he or she has been functioning and seems capable of continuing to function as his or her own therapist. A second reason why it may not be advisable to recommend therapy is insufficient motivation. A client is unlikely to make the investments necessary to achieve therapy goals unless he or she is highly motivated to do so. Clients who do not invest sufficiently to benefit from therapy waste their time and possibly their financial resources. In addition, as a result *they may develop (or reinforce) a certainty that they cannot be helped by therapy.* Consequently, when they enter therapy in the future, they may have less confidence in it than they had previously. This can reduce the probability of it being effective.

Why might past unsuccessful therapy experiences make future successes less likely? According to an old saying, "Nothing succeeds like success or fails like failure." Your previous experiences of success or failure when trying to make a particular type of change influences your *expectation* of success or failure when trying again. This expectation can become a self-fulfilling prophesy. Let's return to the example of weight. If this was the first time you attempted to do so and the weight-loss program was recommended by your physician, you probably would begin expecting the program to be successful. On the other hand, if this was your tenth such program and you believed that the previous ones had not been successful, you probably would begin it being less certain of success than you were the first time. While you would hope the result this time would be different, on a gut level you probably would expect it to be the same. As a consequence, after the first few times you stepped on a scale and concluded that you had not lost enough weight, you would be likely to assume the program was not working and go off of it. Perhaps it would have been successful if you had stayed with it longer! Regardless of what the outcome would have been, this additional "failure" experience probably would reinforce your certainty that you cannot lose weight, which would make success at doing so even less likely in the future.

A third reason why it may not be advisable to schedule a client for therapy is that he or she is unable at present to make the necessary investments. The client may, for example, be a full-time student who has a part-time job and must spend a great deal of time studying in order to survive academically. Such a person, even if highly motivated, probably would be unable to make therapy a priority.

A fourth reason is that a client's intervention needs can be better met by someone else, most likely another speech-language pathologist or a psychotherapist. There are several reasons why a client who has a fluency disorder may be referred to another speech-language pathologist: first, because this clinician has had more experience with the particular type of fluency disorder the client has; second, because it would be more convenient and/or affordable for the client to receive therapy from someone else (a speech-language pathologist at a university clinic, for example, may refer a child to one at his or her school); and third, because he or she feels that the clinician to whom the referral is being made is likely to be more effective. (A male clinician, for example, may feel that a client is more likely to establish a productive therapeutic relationship with a woman.)

If a speech-language pathologist refers a client who has a fluency disorder to a psychotherapist (a psychiatrist, psychologist, or psychiatric social worker), the reason may or may not be directly related to the fluency disorder. Some clients have emotional problems that do not appear to be directly related to their disorders (Van Riper, 1979). They may, for example, be chronically depressed—perhaps suicidal. Also, there are persons whose abnormal disfluency behavior is thought to be a symptom of psychopathology (see chapter 5).

Finally, it may not be advisable to schedule a client who has a fluency disorder for therapy if the clinician does not believe that his or her goal or goals are attainable. The client, for example, may be seeking a complete "cure," and the clinician may not believe that this would be a likely therapy outcome.

COMMUNICATING QUESTIONS, ANSWERS, AND RECOMMENDATIONS

The final step in the evaluation process is communicating what was learned and what was decided (see, e.g., Ingham & Riley, 1998). The persons to whom this may be communicated are the client, members of the client's family (such as his or her parents or spouse), and other professionals (including other speech-language pathologists). The clinician who did the evaluation may also be included because few clinicians can remember for more than a few weeks all that they learned during an evaluation.

Questions, answers, and recommendations usually are communicated both orally and in written form. They are likely to be communicated in an oral summary at the end of the evaluation. They also may be communicated face to face or over the telephone at some later time. In addition, they are likely to be communicated in a written report.

Most, if not all, clinicians currently write evaluation reports using a personal computer with word-processing software. Preparing reports in this manner has many advantages. Changes can be easily made, the software identifies spelling errors and "typos," and sections can be written in the most convenient sequence and later rearranged (e.g., the "Recommendations" section can be written first and later inserted at the end of the report without having to retype it).

Another way that a computer with word-processing software can facilitate report writing is to make it possible to use standard (boiler-plate) sentences and paragraphs (see Appendix A). These may or may not require "blanks" to be filled in. Their use can facilitate the report-writing process by making it unnecessary for clinicians to re-create and retype some sentences and paragraphs each time they write a new report.

ASSIGNMENTS

The three assignments at the end of chapter 2 may be more relevant here than they are for the earlier chapter. They were presented in chapter 2 so that you would have more time during the course to become proficient in doing disfluency identifications, descriptions of moments of stuttering, and stuttering severity ratings.

7

Intervention
Principles, Goals, and Strategies

INSTRUCTIONAL OBJECTIVES

By the end of this chapter, you should be able to:

▶ Describe 14 ways that a clinician can inadvertently harm a client who stutters or has another fluency disorder.

▶ Describe nine attributes of an appropriate therapeutic relationship.

▶ Specify several cultural factors that can affect therapy outcome.

▶ Describe four factors that it's important to consider when selecting goals for therapy.

▶ Describe five generic (general) intervention goals that could be helpful to a client, regardless of the specific nature of his or her fluency disorder.

▶ Provide several illustrations for formulating the wordings of specific intervention goals appropriately.

▶ Provide guidelines for devising strategies to achieve specific goals for coping with fluency-related impairments, disabilities, and handicaps.

▶ Describe using the interaction-frame model to reduce stuttering severity.

▶ Describe 15 strategies that are reportedly successful in directly modifying moments of stuttering.

> ▸ Describe at least three strategies for modifying negative reactions to a client's abnormal speech disfluency.

> ▸ Describe seven strategies for modifying clients' reactions to their stuttering and the reactions of others.

> ▸ Describe a strategy for reducing stuttering relapse following termination of therapy.

> ▸ Describe a strategy for reducing the degree to which clients are disabled and/or handicapped by stuttering or another fluency disorder.

> ▸ Clarify, at least a little, what constitutes recovery from stuttering.

> ▸ Describe selecting and implementing intervention for cluttering, neurogenic acquired stuttering, and psychogenic acquired stuttering.

> ▸ Describe benefits that persons who stutter (or have another fluency disorder) often derive from participating in a self-help group.

After it has been established that a client has a fluency disorder and some of the behaviors in the set that defines it have been identified, intervention usually begins. This almost always includes an attempt *to assist the client and/or his or her parents and teachers* in either eliminating, modifying, or compensating for certain behaviors in this set. The italicized words appear in the preceding sentence because, regardless of the strategy used, the primary responsibility for implementing intervention is usually with the client, or in the case of a young child, with his or her parents and teachers. The role of the clinician is to be *helpful*—that is, to provide the client and/or his or her parents and teachers with at least some of the information and support needed for making the desired changes. This role could involve providing information about the disorder as well as techniques for modifying certain behaviors associated with it. It also could involve providing counseling for better coping with the disorder and offering the client support for attempting to change or for "accepting oneself and getting on with one's life." The clinical relationship can serve as a *catalyst* for change, but the client or parent (or possibly the classroom teacher) has to assume the primary responsibility for change outside of the therapy room.

Older children or adult clients should be informed at the beginning of the intervention process that they will have to function as their own therapist and that the clinician will do whatever possible to facilitate their doing so. They should also be told that the roles the clinician will assume in this process are those of consultant, teacher, and coach. Clients will be unlikely to improve if they do not assume this responsibility and will be unlikely to maintain any gains if they do not continue doing so. This appears to be the reason why some persons who have fluency disorders—particularly those who stutter—relapse after therapy is terminated (Perkins, 1983b).

While clients have the primary responsibility for changing their behavior, it is not necessarily their fault if they are unsuccessful in doing so. They may have failed because the behavior they tried to eliminate could not, at that time, be eliminated or the intervention that was used was inappropriate (Perkins, 1983b). According to Cooper (1986):

> My research as well as my thirty years of experience with hundreds of stutterers of all ages convinces me that a significant number of disfluent stutterers will remain disfluent despite anything they might do or have done to them. Certainly, we all hope that the day will arrive when we have the ability to cure stuttering in everyone. Realistically, however, we know that such a time may never come. Until it does, I trust that our practitioners will communicate to those for whom normal fluency is an unrealistic goal the real sense of success that comes from being able to modify fluency. I have never known disfluent individuals unable to alter their fluency. (pp. 324–325)

Cooper's final statement about "never having known disfluent individuals unable to alter their fluency" refers to stuttering.

Our focus, thus far, has been on being helpful to persons who have a fluency disorder. We may also have to be helpful to their significant others—e.g., their spouses or parents. The following comment by a STUTT-L participant illustrates rather dramatically why doing so may be necessary:

> As the parent, I have experienced a rollercoaster of emotions. I have felt failure when I wasn't able to "fix" the problem. I have felt lonely when I wasn't able to have a decent conversation with my son because he stuttered so badly that he only ever answered in one-word sentences. I have felt desperation about his future and how he will manage. And I have also felt great love for my son, but somehow the stuttering seemed to get in the way.

The better you are able to understand the problems your clients will encounter as they try to change, the more able you will be to help them do so. One way to gain such understanding is to try to change an aspect of your own behavior (e.g., to exercise on a more regular basis, procrastinate less on keeping up with assignments, or reduce your intake of junk food). For a number of years I have required this assignment for students in my fluency disorders course. Judging from their comments, most have found the assignment to be a valuable—though not necessarily enjoyable—experience. If you decide to do it, you may find Lay's (1982b) suggestions helpful.

"Do No Harm"

The Code of Ethics of the American Speech-Language-Hearing Association requires us as clinicians "to hold paramount the welfare of persons served professionally." One of the ways that we fulfill this obligation is by doing them no harm. This injunction appears in the ethical codes of all healthcare professions and is even present in the *Oath of Hippocrates* (paraphrased here):

> I will carry out regimen for the benefit of the impaired according to my ability and judgment; *I will keep them from harm* [italics mine] and injustice.

It isn't customary in fluency disorder textbooks to begin the chapter on therapy by discussing this injunction. Consequently, you may wonder why I chose to do so. The reason, quite frankly, is that speech-language pathologists and other healthcare professionals have harmed as well as helped persons who stutter or have another fluency disorder. The ways in which harm is most frequently caused (judging by comments from clients) are discussed here. Fortunately, most (if not all) such harm can be easily prevented by using common sense.

Giving Stutterers the Message (Directly or Indirectly) That They Could Stop Stuttering If They Really Desire It

While clinicians have conveyed this message to children and adults who stutter directly (including me), they've usually done it indirectly. There are two basic themes. One is that the person chooses to stutter, in at least some situations, to satisfy some psychological need—for example, as a passive-aggressive way to make listeners uncomfortable or as an attention-getting device. The second theme is that the person chooses not to do what is necessary to improve his or her speech because of a psychological deficit—a character weakness. If a stutterer believed this message, his or her self-concept would most likely be affected adversely. The available research, incidentally, provides practically no support for such a "repressed need" explanation for the maintenance of stuttering (see chapter 5).

Those of you who doubt that a speech-language pathologist would give a stutterer such a message directly may find this comment by a STUTT-L participant illuminating:

> Teach your young clients that just because they stutter does not make them bad people, and it doesn't reflect on their families. My first speech therapist spent my elementary school years (3rd through 6th grades) telling me that I was bad for stuttering and it made my family look bad also.

I suspect that one reason for a clinician having such a belief is that he or she does not really understand how stuttering differs from almost all of the other disorders that a clinician may treat. Suppose that a clinician observed a client speaking without stuttering at least half the time. The clinician may assume what it would be reasonable for him or her to assume—for example, if a client who had a w/r sound substitution produced /r/ correctly half the time, it would seem reasonable to assume that if the client tried harder, he or she could learn to produce /r/ correctly almost all the time. Unfortunately, as we've discussed, stutterers tend to stutter most when they want to stutter least (see chapter 2). Consequently, a stutterer who is trying harder to stutter less will probably end up stuttering more.

Diagnosing Secondary Stuttering in Preschoolers as Normal Disfluency

While deciding whether a young child has begun to stutter can be difficult (see chapter 8), there are times when it's obvious that a child's disfluency isn't normal. Such a child may be evincing an awareness and fear of being disfluent, avoidance of talking, and/or secondary behaviors. None of these are attributes of normal disfluency behavior, and consequently their presence necessitates some form of intervention. Clinicians have used Wendell Johnson's diagnosogenic theory (see chapter 5) as justification for diagnosing stuttering in preschoolers as normal disfluency behavior. This is *not* an appropriate application of Johnson's theory. If a child is exhibiting secondary stuttering, ignoring it is highly unlikely to make it go away!

Failing to Consult Clients When Setting Therapy Goals

Clients can be harmed in at least two ways if their goals for therapy and those of their clinician are not the same. First, they'd be less likely to achieve their goals than they would otherwise; and second, they'd be unlikely to achieve their clinicians' goals because of a lack of motivation to achieve them. In either case, they'd be likely to terminate therapy believing that it hadn't been particularly helpful, thereby reducing the likelihood (at least a little) that they'll expect to benefit from therapy in the future. This could, of course, become a self-fulfilling prophesy and an additional source of harm. It's crucial, therefore, that you negotiate therapy goals with clients. The Stuttering Problem Profile (see Appendix C) can provide a structure for doing so with clients whose disorder is stuttering, cluttering, neurogenic acquired stuttering, and possibly even psychogenic acquired stuttering.

Making Clients Feel Bad about Themselves because They Aren't Highly Motivated to Learn to Control Their Speech

While a fluency disorder is an impairment, it doesn't necessarily disable or handicap a person sufficiently to make controlling it a priority for him or her. Consequently, if a client isn't highly motivated to learn to control his or her speech for this reason, the client's decision not to invest in doing so should be validated by the clinician. The most likely outcome from failing to validate it is a poorer self-concept for the client. Such validation is particularly likely to be necessary when a client is not self-referred.

The following comment by a STUTT-L participant communicates quite eloquently why such motivation can be low:

> Stuttering is acceptable to me. It's a quirk that I've grown to like about myself. I've put so much energy in trying to become fluent throughout my life that I've missed out on many other things that needed my energy. I can be a happy person and still stutter.

Encouraging Children or Adults Who Stutter to Try to Avoid Stuttering

This practice can be harmful in at least two ways. First, it can result in an increase rather than a decrease in stuttering severity. (Remember that stutterers tend to stutter most when they want to stutter least!) Second, it can reinforce feelings of guilt, shame, and embarrassment about stuttering.

Encouraging Stutterers to Speak in Ways that Call More Adverse Attention to Them than Does Their Stuttering

Clinicians have encouraged stutterers to modify their stuttering in ways that call more adverse attention to them than does their stuttering. For example, this can result from the use of such techniques as light articulatory contact, an abnormally slow speaking rate, the "bounce," pacing speech with the beats of a miniature metronome, and using pull-outs (e.g., Manning, Burlison, & Thaxton, 1999), described later in this chapter. Encouraging the use of such techniques is more likely to be harmful to clients whose stuttering tends to be at the lower half of the severity continuum than to those whose stuttering tends to be relatively severe.

Giving Clients Unrealistic Assignments

Giving clients assignments that they aren't adequately motivated to complete can be harmful to them in at least two ways. First, it can make them feel guilty; and second, it can discourage them, thereby reducing their motivation to invest in trying to change.

Placing Stutterers and Others
on Unrealistic Maintenance Programs

A long-term maintenance program is a component of many of the approaches that focus on training clients to control their stuttering (e.g., fluency-shaping approaches). Clients are likely to be expected to spend some time each day (e.g., 30 minutes) working on their speech. For many (perhaps most) stutterers such an expectation is probably unrealistic. The following comments on STUTT-L by two moderately severe stutterers provide some support for this assertion:

> The amazing thing to me never ceases to be how difficult it is for me to have the discipline to do the work. Here's this condition— stuttering—that I dislike so much. Yet in my entire adult life I doubt I have ever been able to do speech practice for even half an hour, religiously, every day, for even six months.

> I know what you mean about not being able to do the "fluency enhancing" exercises everyday. I talk about it a lot, but I often stop doing them after a while. It's very difficult for me to make it a priority on a daily basis. And I like doing the exercises, too!

A client who fails to follow through on a maintenance program is likely to feel guilty. Worse yet, if the client relapses, the clinician is more likely to blame it on the client's failure to follow through than on the unrealistic expectations engendered by the maintenance program. Consequently, the client is likely to end up being no more fluent and having a poorer self-concept than at the beginning of therapy.

Blaming Stutterers and Others for Failing to
Utilize Techniques Outside the Therapy Room

Techniques that yield fluency in the therapy room will not necessarily do so in a client's environment. There can be at least three reasons. First, the therapy room environment is probably more likely to facilitate a client remembering the use of a technique than is his or her home and work environment. Second, in the therapy room, practicing a technique can be given a higher priority than communicating, which is not usually the case in a client's environment. Third, if the client is a stutterer, he or she is likely to be less highly motivated to avoid stuttering in the therapy room than in at least some situations in his or her environment. This would tend to translate into less severe stuttering in the therapy room, which would tend to make it easier for the client to use a technique there than in some other environments. A clinician's failure to recognize these and possibly other significant differences between using a technique in and out of the therapy room can cause a client to feel guilty and/or embarrassed.

The following comment from a STUTT-L participant underlines the significant difference between utilizing a technique within and

outside of the therapy room and the harm a clinician can do by failing
to recognize this difference:

> It seems to me that a lot of SLPs really don't understand stutter-
> ing. When they see greater fluency in the clinic room where there
> is less communicative stress, they immediately think quickie fix—
> that all that's involved is generalizing that happy state of affairs
> using some "technique." When that doesn't work, they blame the
> client for not working hard enough with the "technique."

Using Techniques with Stutterers that Yield Temporary Fluency by Having Them Speak in a Nonhabitual Manner

Clinicians who don't stutter, particularly those with less experience,
are likely to be impressed by the instantaneous, dramatic increase in
fluency that usually results from using any of the techniques
(described later in the chapter) that cause a stutterer to speak in a
nonhabitual manner. The improvement can be so dramatic that it
almost seems like a miracle. And it can even last for a while. However,
as soon as the nonhabitual way of speaking becomes habitual and the
client loses confidence in its ability to facilitate fluency, he or she will
probably relapse. Perhaps the greatest harm likely to result from the
use of such techniques is that when relapse occurs, the client will again
have to go through the grieving process for his or her disorder and consequently will again experience depression because of having it.

Focusing Insufficiently on the Disabilities and Handicaps Yielded by Clients' Fluency Disorders

Based on 60+ years of personal experience and 40+ years of clinical
experience, I can attest to the fact that the disabilities and handicaps
yielded by a fluency disorder can adversely affect a person's life as much
or more than the disfluency per se. Consequently, having disfluency
reduction as the primary goal for therapy is likely to be inappropriate,
particularly for clients for whom the prognosis for achieving long-term
normal fluency is poor. Even if it were possible to reduce abnormal disfluency almost completely, the residual disfluency could still yield disabilities and handicaps that needed to be addressed. The following
comment by a STUTT-L participant is enlightening in this regard:

> With lots of practice I could reduce the tension of my voice and the
> number of disfluencies, but never to the point where I could say I
> am no longer a stutterer or even feel that when I spoke I likely
> would not stutter. So with all the practice, I'd still be a stutterer
> and, consequently, perceived as that by the world (with all the
> results, "the look," etc.) and thus perceived as that in myself.

Ignoring the disabilities and handicaps yielded by a client's fluency
disorder would be failing to abide by the requirement of the American

Speech-Language-Hearing Association (ASHA) Ethical Code "to hold paramount the welfare of persons served professionally" and would, therefore, be doing harm to him or her.

It can be uncomfortable for a clinician, at first, to focus on disabilities and handicaps rather than on fluency. As one STUTT-L participant commented:

> As a speech-language pathologist trained to teach fluency, it has been a long hard road to understanding that speech therapy is not only about fluency. It is about life. Still, as I work to change my approach during a session, a little devil is sitting on one of my shoulders saying, "But what are you DOING?" Then, the angel on my other shoulder is saying, "You are BEING, you are LIVING, you are showing someone how to LIVE and BE."

Failing to Make Appropriate Referrals, Particularly to Self-Help/Support Groups

To satisfy the ASHA ethical requirement "to hold paramount the welfare of persons served professionally," speech-language pathologists do not have to meet all of their clients' disorder-related needs themselves. However, they do have a responsibility to do what they can to facilitate their clients' disorder-related needs being met. This may entail making referrals to nonprofessional entities—for example, self-help/support groups and Toastmasters International. Some clinicians resist making such referrals, even when they would be likely to benefit their clients significantly. By not doing so, they are harming their clients by limiting their potential for improvement.

Some clients, incidentally, will resist participating in such a group because being with other persons who have a fluency disorder makes them feel uncomfortable. As one STUTT-L participant commented:

> My relationship to stuttering has changed a lot in recent years, but up until maybe four years ago, for my whole life, I HATED talking to other people who stuttered. I'm sure it had a lot to do with having my self-delusion shattered, being confronted with the fact that this was how I looked and sounded to other people, and being so uncomfortable with that.

Using Intervention Strategies That Are Counterintuitive

If you're unable to rationalize intuitively that an intervention strategy is appropriate for achieving a goal, it is unlikely to facilitate achieving that goal for at least two reasons. First, it may be inappropriate, even though it may have been recommended by an authority for achieving that goal. The authority's conceptualization of the cause of the impairment, disability, or handicap that you are seeking to modify may differ from yours. Second, you'd be likely to communicate your lack of enthusiasm for the strategy to the client, which would tend to reduce the likelihood of it being effective.

Wasting Clients' Time

A clinician can waste a client's time in a number of ways, including:

- unnecessarily prolonging the session. If you can accomplish the goal of a session in 10 minutes, it makes little sense to prolong the session for 45 minutes.
- Scheduling unnecessary sessions. Scheduling a fixed number of sessions every week for a semester is likely, for example, to be more appropriate for a client who has a language disorder than for one who has a fluency disorder.
- working toward goals that a client isn't highly motivated to achieve.
- failing to prepare adequately for sessions.

Failing to Encourage Clients to Assume the Primary Responsibility for Managing Their Disorder

Clients are likely to have to cope with stuttering and most other fluency disorders for many years, perhaps for as long as they live. There are likely to be a number of persons and resources from which they can derive some benefit, including individual or group therapy from speech-language pathologists and/or psychologists, self-help groups, books, audiotapes, videotapes, workshops, and the Internet. Thus, it makes most sense for the primary responsibility for managing a client's fluency disorder to be assumed by the client (unless, of course, the client is a young child or an older child or adult who is cognitively impaired). Consequently, the client should be encouraged to function as the leader of his or her rehabilitation team. Membership on the team would, of course, change from time to time depending on the client's needs.

THE THERAPEUTIC RELATIONSHIP

The first step in the intervention process is to establish a good therapeutic relationship with the client and, possibly, some of his or her significant others, including parents, teachers, or spouse (Gootwald & Hall, 2003). The nature of this relationship can profoundly influence the effectiveness of any intervention strategy. A good relationship can enhance it, and a poor one can practically guarantee its being ineffective.

What are the characteristics of a good therapeutic relationship? Some of those that are particularly important to consider when working with clients who have fluency disorders are listed below. For further information about these and others, see chapter 11 in Silverman (1995), Van Riper (1979), and Lay (1982a).

The characteristics of a productive clinical relationship include:

- *Mutual respect.* The client respects the clinician for his or her training, experience, and expertise. The clinician respects the client and manifests this respect by treating him or her as a person of worth, whom he or she wants to help.

- *Trust.* The client trusts the clinician to treat whatever he or she is told as confidential. Also, the client trusts the clinician not to recommend goals that are unattainable or intervention strategies that could be harmful or useless.

- *Honesty.* Both the client and clinician are honest with each other. They tell each other the truth, which may not be what one or the other wants to hear. For example, in a good relationship clients will not tell clinicians that they are improving or that they have done what was recommended when they have not; and clinicians will not tell clients that it's O.K. to avoid doing what they dislike doing if they know this to be untrue. Some of the assignments that clinicians give to clients who have fluency disorders (such as bringing their disorder out into the open) tend to make clients feel uncomfortable; hence, they are likely to dislike doing them.

- *Empathy.* To be helpful to clients who have fluency disorders, clinicians need to have some insight into what they experience, both while they are being abnormally disfluent and while they are trying to change. One strategy clinicians can use for developing such empathy is to perform the simulation assignment described in chapter 1 and the behavior modification assignment at the end of this chapter.

- *Communication.* The client and clinician communicate reasonably well with each other in spite of the client's fluency disorder. Communication is the medium through which the clinician attempts to influence the client and the client attempts to make the clinician aware of his or her needs.

- *Hope.* While the clinician cannot guarantee that the client will improve, he or she can continually offer hope to the client (and his or her significant others) that this is possible. The client's beliefs concerning his or her ability to change can significantly affect the outcome of therapy.

- *Success.* The clinician gives the client the opportunity to experience success whenever possible. "Nothing succeeds like success or fails like failure." You will recall that some clients who have fluency disorders enter therapy with the belief that they cannot be helped because of previous therapy experiences they regard as not having been successful. One way to help them cope with this belief is to give them the opportunity to experience success.

- *A contract.* The contract (which may be either written or oral) specifies what each promises to contribute to the relationship. The clinician usually promises to contribute his or her time and expertise, and the client usually promises to follow through on the clinician's recommendations. A client who enters therapy without understanding the terms of the contract (what will be expected from him or her) will be less likely to meet the clinician's expectations than one who does. Also, such a client will be less likely to conclude, after a period of therapy, that he or she has benefited from it.

- A *"positive" placebo effect.* What clients believe about the efficacy of their treatment can influence the impact it is likely to have on them (Shapiro, 1964). If they do not expect it to be effective, it probably will be less likely to succeed than otherwise ("negative" placebo effect). On the other hand, if they do expect it to be effective, it probably will be more likely to be so than otherwise ("positive" placebo effect).

  How might clinicians behave in order to bring about a "negative" placebo effect? One way is to signal clients verbally or nonverbally that they do not have a high degree of confidence in the therapy they are using—for example, continually changing intervention strategies without giving the client a reasonable explanation for doing so. Such behavior is particularly likely to result in a negative placebo effect if intervention strategies tend to be changed whenever clients express concern about their progress.

  Another behavior that could result in a negative placebo effect is to give clients a choice of intervention strategies—in particular, suggesting that if they have not tried a particular one yet, they may want to. This is unlikely to create a high degree of confidence in their clinicians' ability to help them. From the client's perspective, why would he or she be given a choice if the clinician knew which strategy is most likely to be effective?

CULTURAL CONSIDERATIONS

Cultural factors can affect the outcome of therapy as well as the outcome of an evaluation. Some of the same factors can, in fact, affect both, including the gender of the clinician, a male clinician being alone with a female client, and touching a client (see chapter 6).

One cultural factor that can significantly impact therapy is clients' and their families' beliefs about the cause of fluency disorders. If, for example, they believe strongly that their cause is punishment from God for something they've done, they are also likely to believe just as strongly that a fluency disorder can only be alleviated by atoning for their sins. Such an attitude would have to be addressed (possibly by a clergy member) before a client or client's family would be likely to follow through on therapy recommendations.

Another cultural factor that can impact therapy for stuttering and possibly other fluency disorders is the acceptability of maintaining eye contact. In some cultures, maintaining eye contact is considered an aggressive or even hostile behavior (Leith, 1986). A client from such a culture is likely to resist his or her clinician's attempts to encourage maintaining good eye contact while stuttering.

For further information about the types of cultural values, practices, and beliefs that can affect the clinical relationship, see Bebout and Arthur (1992), Cooper and Rustin (1985), Hammer (1994), Leith (1986), Maestas and Erickson (1992), Matsuda (1989), and Shames (1989).

ESTABLISHING GOALS

One of the first tasks a clinician must accomplish when trying to be helpful to a client who has a fluency disorder is to establish goals and to communicate them *unambiguously* to him or her. If clients do not understand what their clinician wants them to accomplish, they obviously will be less likely than otherwise to succeed in doing so.

Therapy goals are derived from behaviors in the set that was identified during the evaluation as defining the client's fluency disorder. Achieving these goals eliminates or modifies these behaviors, thereby reducing—at least a little—the severity of the disorder.

Since there usually will be more than one possible goal, the clinician will have to decide which to work toward first. There are a number of factors that he or she should consider when doing so, including:

- the ease with which each goal can be achieved. It usually is desirable to select those goals at the beginning of therapy that the client is likely to be able to achieve fairly quickly, particularly if he or she believes that previous therapy experiences were not successful. Having a client succeed in attaining a goal is probably the best way to convince him or her that change is possible.

- how interested the client is in achieving each goal. The client is likely to be more highly motivated to achieve some goals than to achieve others. If a client were highly motivated to achieve a particular goal, he or she probably would invest more to do so than otherwise. If there are several goals toward which a client could work, the amount of interest he or she would have in achieving each of them should be considered when deciding.

- the impact that achieving each goal would have on the severity of the client's disorder. Everything else being equal, the goals selected should be those that, if accomplished, would significantly reduce its severity.

- the number of behaviors that are likely to be affected by achieving each goal. Accomplishing a goal may affect more than one behavior. If, for example, the disorder is stuttering, "bringing it out into the open" can both make a client feel more comfortable (less anxious or embarrassed) and cause him or her to stutter less frequently (Van Riper, 1973).

The following comment by a STUTT-L participant highlights the value of bringing stuttering out into the open:

> When I give formal talks, I usually speak briefly about my stuttering before I begin. This has been an ENORMOUS help to me and to my audience. The ability to talk about my stuttering was a long time in coming, and I still find it difficult to do it at times in spite of the fact that it has always been well-received.

Since in most cases it is desirable for a client to participate in the goal-setting process, how can this be accomplished? One way is to have him or her complete the *Stuttering Problem Profile* (Silverman, 1980b). This task (described in chapter 6 and reproduced in Appendix C) enables clinicians to identify goals that clients are interested in achieving.

Some General Intervention Goals

What can a clinician attempt to accomplish that is likely to be helpful to a client with a fluency disorder? Several general goals are discussed in this section that may or may not be appropriate for and achievable with a particular client.

To "cure" the client's fluency disorder

While this is the goal that both clinicians and clients regard as being the most desirable, it appears more likely to be attainable for young children than for adolescents and adults (Cooper, 1987; Freund, 1966; Wingate, 1976). For a client's fluency disorder to be regarded as "cured," it seems reasonable to require that the following conditions be satisfied:

- The amount of disfluency in the client's speech is within normal limits.
- The client's fluency level has been within normal limits for at least five years.
- The client no longer believes that he or she has a fluency disorder or will again develop one.

The first of these conditions does not require the client to be almost completely fluent—it only requires that his or her disfluency level be somewhere in the normal range. The second is important because research indicates that a high percentage of those who are normally fluent at the termination of therapy relapse within five years (Boberg, 1981; Boberg et al., 1979; Craig, 1998; Conture & Guitar, 1993; Craig

& Calver, 1991; Freund, 1966; Perkins, 1983b; Silverman, 1981). The third condition is important if the disorder is stuttering because of evidence suggesting that fear of relapse can precipitate it (Bloodstein, 1987; Freund, 1966; Prins, 1993; Silverman, 1981; Van Riper, 1973).

Which clients who have fluency disorders will be most likely to attain this goal? Perhaps preschool-age children who are beginning to stutter. There are reports (such as Starkweather, Gottwald, & Halfond, 1990) that suggest that many such children recover completely. While there are reports in the literature of persons of all ages being cured of stuttering, the probability of this occurring appears to be negatively related to the length of time the person has had the disorder (Bloodstein, 1987; Cooper, 1987, 1993; Freund, 1966). In other words, the longer a client has had a disorder, the poorer the prognosis is for that client being cured.

To reduce the severity of the client's fluency disorder
This goal should be attainable by almost any client who has a fluency disorder if:

- the client believes his or her severity can be reduced or, at least, has a "wait and see" attitude
- the client is sufficiently motivated to make the changes needed
- the behaviors the clinician is encouraging the client to change are modifiable
- the intervention strategies used by the clinician are appropriate
- the client receives positive reinforcement from his or her significant others

The first of these factors requires the client not to believe that therapy will fail. Unfortunately, as you will recall, clients who had therapy experiences they regarded as unsuccessful may have developed a "certainty" that they cannot be helped. This attitude, which has been referred to in the psychological literature as *learned helplessness* (see Maier & Seligman, 1976), needs to be changed—at least to one of "wait and see"—before such clients are likely to benefit from any attempt at intervention. The second factor requires the client to assign a high priority to reducing the severity of the disorder. If the client does this, he or she should be more willing than otherwise to make the investments required to attain this goal.

The third factor requires that the client be capable of doing what he or she is being asked to do. Not all behaviors may be modifiable (Cooper, 1987) and not all clients may be capable of modifying those that are (Van Riper, 1979). The fourth factor requires that the intervention strategies used be appropriate for the particular client being treated. Using strategies that are appropriate for most clients but not for yours is one of the main reasons for intervention being unsuccessful.

The fifth factor requires most persons with whom the client interacts (particularly those whose opinions he or she values) to respond positively to his or her attempts to change. If they do not—or worse yet, respond negatively to these attempts—the client will be more than likely to stop trying to modify his or her behaviors (Boberg & Boberg, 1990).

Why might such persons respond negatively to a client's attempts to change? They may feel that the client's "new" way of talking calls more adverse attention to him or her than the "old" way. They could be right! For example, after stutterers were encouraged to pace their speech with a miniature metronome (Brady, 1971), it was discovered that doing this tended to make the speech of persons with relatively mild stuttering less acceptable to listeners than their "old" way of talking, even though they stuttered less frequently while doing so (Silverman & Trotter, 1973c).

A second reason why such persons may react negatively is that they have adapted to the clients' "old" way of talking but not yet to their "new" way. If persons who have fluency disorders are not constantly signaling listeners that they are embarrassed about it, listeners are likely to attend to, or abstract, their abnormal disfluency behavior less frequently than they did initially (Trotter & Kools, 1955). However, if clients change how they speak, listeners are again likely to attend to their disfluency and, as a consequence, may conclude that it has gotten worse. It is important that clients be made aware of this phenomenon at the beginning of therapy so that if it occurs they will be less likely to become discouraged and stop trying to change.

A third reason for negative reactions is that a client's attempt to change is adversely affecting relationships with significant others because the client is no longer willing to play his or her "old" role. The client may, for example, develop a better self-concept and, as a consequence, become less dependent and more assertive. While such changes are almost always desirable, they may be regarded as "threatening" by one or more of the client's significant others. For example, in his or her marriage the client may have played the submissive role and the spouse the dominant one. If the client becomes less willing to be dominated, the spouse may try to discourage him or her from changing further. If the clinician suspects that such a scenario is being acted out, both the client and those who are being threatened should be referred for counseling.

To reduce the extent to which the client is disabled and/or handicapped by his or her fluency disorder

The amount of abnormal disfluency in a client's speech does not necessarily determine how much he or she will be disabled or handicapped because of it. Some who have relatively little disfluency are more disabled and/or handicapped than some who have a great deal. The amount clients are disabled and handicapped is a function of how much the disfluency keeps them from doing what they want to do—

how much it adversely affects their lives. One determinant of this is client attitude toward the disfluency. Consequently, for some clients with fluency disorders an appropriate goal is developing a less negative (or more objective) attitude toward the disorder, thereby reducing the amount it disables and handicaps them. The goal is not to get clients to the point at which they do not care that they have a fluency disorder. No sane person would want to have one, particularly considering the negative personality traits that tend to be "projected" on those who do. Rather, the goal should be to persuade clients to accept the fact that they have the disorder and get on with their lives!

To determine whether it is possible to reduce the severity of the client's fluency disorder

A clinician may not know at the beginning of therapy whether he or she can be helpful to a particular client. There can be a number of reasons—including uncertainty about the client's level of motivation to invest in therapy. An initial goal in such a case would be to assess his or her potential for improvement.

To get the client to accept a referral

Some clients with fluency disorders need to be evaluated and possibly treated by professionals other than speech-language pathologists. The reason may or may not be directly related to their fluency disorder. The most common type of referral that speech-language pathologists are likely to make for these clients is for psychotherapy. The practitioner to whom a client would be referred could be a psychiatrist, a clinical psychologist, or a psychiatric social worker. Among the reasons for making such a referral are chronic depression and poor social adjustment.

Clients and/or members of their families may regard a referral as threatening—particularly if it is to a psychotherapist—and, as a consequence, they may not accept it. If you feel it is necessary or desirable for a client to be seen by another professional and the client (or a member of his or her family) refuses to accept the referral, one of your goals probably would be to persuade him or her to do so (Van Riper, 1979).

To increase the client's motivation

Clients are unlikely to benefit from therapy if they are not sufficiently motivated to make the investments required. It is sometimes possible to increase their motivation. If, for example, the reason for the lack of motivation was that the client did not expect therapy to be effective because of previous unsuccessful therapy experiences, proving that change is possible could result in an increase in the client's motivational level. An initial intervention goal for such clients could be to prove to them that they can change, by engineering it so that they *do* change some aspect(s) of their behavior.

Some Specific Intervention Goals

In the preceding section we considered some general intervention goals for clients who have a fluency disorder. We will consider some specific goals here.

What specific intervention goals might be established for a client who has a fluency disorder? This would be determined by the behaviors in the set that defines his or her problem. This section illustrates the types of goals one might have as well as how they are worded. The wording of a goal can influence how likely a client is to regard therapy as having been successful. Consider the following two versions of a specific goal:

1. The client will no longer avoid contributing to class discussions.

2. The client will not avoid contributing to class discussions *as often as he or she did previously.*

A client would more likely feel that he or she had achieved the goal if it was worded like the second version. If the first wording were used, avoiding speaking in class only once could cause a client to believe that he or she had "failed."

A clinician may find it advantageous to specify a specific minimum amount that a client should seek to change. The goal in the preceding paragraph, for example, could be rewritten as follows: "The client will reduce the amount he or she avoids contributing to class discussions *by about 10 percent.*" This would permit the client to do a lot of avoiding yet still experience "success"!

One problem that a clinician may encounter when setting specific goals is that the client may have a *two-valued orientation* (Johnson, 1946). Such persons judge their performances as being either good or bad; successful or unsuccessful. For a performance to be regarded as a success, they must judge it to be almost perfect—any significant deviation from perfection is likely to cause them to regard it as a failure.

How might having a two-valued orientation interfere with therapy? It could cause a client to fail more often than succeed. A client with such an orientation is likely to evaluate his or her performance in this manner regardless of how goals are worded. It is desirable, therefore, that the orientation be changed from two-valued to *multivalued.* With the latter there can be degrees of success and failure. While some clients will require psychotherapy to change their orientation, others will be able to do so by studying an appropriate self-help book, such as Wendell Johnson's *People in Quandaries.*

Following are *examples* of specific goals that might be established for a client who has a fluency disorder.

- The client will not avoid talking in specific situations as often as he or she did previously.

- The client will reduce the frequency of a specific behavior that occurs during moments of abnormal disfluency in a particular situation by 10 percent.

- The client will bring his or her fluency disorder "out into the open" (acknowledge it to listeners) more often than previously.

- The client will reduce his or her feelings of shame and embarrassment because of having the disorder.

- The client will judge his or her speech less often based on how fluent he or she was and more often based on how successfully he or she communicated.

- When angry, the client will communicate more often how he or she really feels (the client will reduce his or her tendency to be a "people pleaser").

- The client will develop a better self-concept.

- The client's knowledge about (understanding of) the disorder will increase.

- The client will become more confident that he or she can do something about the disorder and the impact that it is having on his or her life (that is, the client will not as frequently view himself or herself as "a giant in chains").

For further information about establishing goals for therapy, see Starkweather (1993).

SELECTING AND IMPLEMENTING INTERVENTION STRATEGIES

Factors Affecting the Choice of Strategy

After one or more goals have been formulated, the next step is selecting strategies for achieving them. A number of factors should be considered when doing so, including:

- the specific behaviors (including attitudes) that have to be modified

- the clinician's beliefs (hypotheses) about the causes of the behaviors

- the clinician's beliefs about how to modify behaviors having the hypothesized causes

- economic and time constraints

- the client's therapy history

- the client's age and level of motivation to invest in therapy
- the clinician's faith in and competency with alternative strategies
- the attitudes of the client's significant others toward alternative strategies

Some possible impacts that each factor could have on the selection process are described in this section.

The intervention strategies a clinician selects obviously will be influenced both by what he or she is trying to accomplish and the specific behaviors that have to be modified. A single strategy may be appropriate for accomplishing more than one thing. For example, encouraging a client to bring his or her stuttering problem out into the open could accomplish several goals, including:

- putting the client more at ease in speaking situations
- putting those with whom the client communicates more at ease
- reducing the severity of the client's stuttering
- reducing the extent to which the client signals listeners that he or she is ashamed or embarrassed about stuttering
- reducing the extent to which the client avoids speaking because of his or her stuttering

Another factor that is likely to influence the choice of intervention strategy is the clinician's beliefs (or hypotheses) about the cause(s) of the behaviors he or she seeks to modify. The program you develop for modifying a behavior should be based on your "best guess" as to why the client is exhibiting it. If your hypothesis is correct, you are more likely to be successful than otherwise (Williams, 1968).

A clinician's beliefs about the best way to modify behaviors having a particular cause is also likely to influence his or her choice of intervention strategy. Authorities do not agree about what strategies are most likely to be successful for modifying some of the behaviors exhibited by persons who have fluency disorders, particularly the abnormal disfluency exhibited by stutterers. As a result, a relatively large number of strategies for reducing stuttering severity have been advocated and used by at least a few clinicians.

Two other factors that can influence the choice of intervention strategy are economic and time constraints. A clinician may reject a strategy that is otherwise likely to be effective because it is not practical for one or both of these reasons. It may require the client to invest more time in therapy sessions and/or daily practice than he or she is willing or able to. Or it may require the client to make a financial investment that he or she cannot afford.

A client's therapy history also can influence the choice of intervention strategy. If a client has tried a particular approach and has concluded rightly or wrongly that it was not effective, it *may* not be advisable to try that approach again, particularly if there is a viable alternative. The reason is that if you do so, the client is likely to expect it not to "work," which could reduce the likelihood of it being effective.

In addition, a client's age and level of motivation to invest in therapy can influence the choice of intervention strategy. Some strategies that are appropriate for use with adults may not be appropriate for use with young children. Also, some strategies appropriate for clients who are highly motivated would not be so with others. Voluntary stuttering is an example of such a strategy.

Thus far in this discussion of factors that influence the choice of intervention strategy the focus has been primarily on the client. A clinician's awareness of, confidence in, and competence to use alternative strategies can also influence this choice. Obviously, if a clinician is not aware of a particular strategy, it will not be considered. Also, the more confidence a clinician has in a particular strategy, the greater the likelihood that he or she will select it. Finally, a clinician is unlikely to select strategies that he or she does not feel reasonably competent to use, particularly if there are alternatives.

The choice of an intervention strategy may be influenced not only by factors pertaining to the client and clinician, but also by those pertaining to persons with whom the client frequently interacts. The attitudes of a client's family, friends, teachers, employer, and others toward a strategy and the impacts that it has on him or her can influence the choice, particularly if the client is a child. If a client does not receive positive reinforcement from these persons for trying to change in a particular way, he or she is less likely to succeed.

Strategies for Reducing Stuttering Severity

Most persons who stutter consult a speech-language pathologist because they either want to reduce the severity of their stuttering or want to "cure" it. Many strategies have been recommended for curing stuttering during the past 2,000 years, and there is anecdotal evidence suggesting that most of them enabled at least one person to succeed (Van Riper, 1973).

All of these strategies are not mentioned in this section. Rather, a scheme is presented here for conceptualizing their impacts on stuttering severity, and brief descriptions are included of most of those currently advocated and/or used in the context of this scheme. My intent is to provide you with the information needed to *select* a strategy—not the information needed to *use* it. Providing such information in depth would considerably increase the length (and cost) of this book. Furthermore, it is unnecessary to provide in-depth information about each of these strategies because it is available from other sources. Several sources for information about a strategy should be consulted before attempting to use it. A single source is apt to be incomplete and/or reflect its author's biases.

The interaction-frame model

This scheme (see figure 7-1) was adapted from one proposed by Wendell Johnson (1946). Although it originally was promulgated in the context of a specific theory about the etiology of stuttering (in this case, the anticipatory-struggle hypothesis; see chapter 5), it appears to be usable regardless of whether you believe the cause of this disorder is physiological, psychological, or some combination of the two. This is because it has been established unequivocally that the severity of a client's stuttering is likely to be influenced by the reactions of persons in his or her environment as well as his or her own reaction to it (see chapter 2). There is no agreement, however, on the amount of influence that these are likely to exert on stuttering severity. Those who view stuttering, at least in part, as anticipatory-struggle behavior probably would ascribe a greater influence to the reactions than those who view its etiology as physiological.

According to the interaction-frame model, it is possible to reduce stuttering severity by targeting the behavior itself, the reactions of others to the behavior, and/or the client's own reactions to it. By modifying one of these, the other two are likely to be modified (which is the "interaction" aspect of the scheme). For example, by helping a client eliminate behaviors that occur during his or her moments of stuttering, you are likely to reduce negative reactions from listeners to the stuttering and, thereby, reduce the client's desire to avoid or conceal it. This, in turn, should result in a further reduction in stuttering

Figure 7-1   The interaction-frame model.

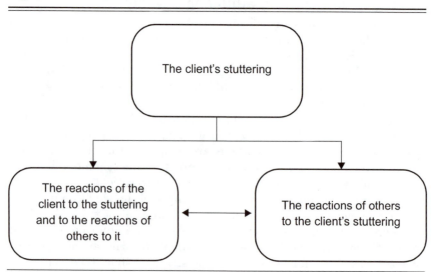

severity (assuming that the desire to conceal stuttering tends to increase its severity) and a further reduction in negative reactions from listeners, and so forth. Consequently, this scheme indicates that we can reduce (not necessarily eliminate) undesirable reactions from listeners to a client's stuttering and undesirable reactions of a client to his or her own stuttering by focusing on modifying it—that is, by reducing its severity.

One important implication of the interaction-frame model is that it is possible to reduce a client's stuttering severity by modifying his or her attitude toward stuttering. Such modification may not only improve his or her self-concept and enable him or her to lead a more rewarding and productive life, but may also reduce the amount that he or she stutters! Following are examples of attitudinal changes that, based on the model, would be likely to result in a reduction in stuttering severity:

- having less desire to avoid stuttering.
- being more willing to bring the stuttering problem out into the open—that is, to acknowledge it openly.
- judging performance in a speaking situation *less* on the basis of fluency level and *more* on that of success level in communicating.
- developing a better self-concept through recognition. Such recognition may be directly related to speaking—for example, a high school or college student may be regarded as a good debater in spite of the fact that he or she stutters (Silverman, 1960).
- developing a stronger belief that he or she can cope with stuttering if it occurs and possibly desiring to have it occur in order to be able to practice "controlling" it.
- anticipating fluency more frequently than previously. Just as anticipation of stuttering is likely to lead to increased stuttering, anticipation of fluency is likely to lead to increased fluency (Van Riper, 1982).
- becoming less embarrassed or ashamed about stuttering. This should result in a reduction in the desire to avoid it and, as a consequence, a reduction in its severity.
- becoming less two-valued or less of a perfectionist when evaluating one's performance and, as a consequence, experiencing "success" more often in speaking situations.
- feeling less of a need to overcome stuttering before going on with one's life. Gaining a greater realization that a person can succeed in life in spite of the fact that he or she stutters (Carlisle, 1985; Tillis & Wager, 1984), no longer feeling as much like "a giant in chains" (the "chains" being stuttering).

- having more of a "what you see is what you get" attitude toward self and, hence, feeling less of a need to impress people by being relatively fluent.

- having more of a sense of humor about stuttering—perhaps even being able to laugh at "Porky Pig" cartoons.

- being less likely to assume that people will think less of you if they know you stutter.

Obviously, some overlap occurs between these changes in attitude, and all are likely to lead to the same outcome: less desire to avoid stuttering. Such a reduction would be expected to result in increased fluency, at least temporarily (see chapter 2).

One STUTT-L participant, incidentally, made the following comment that provides a little anecdotal support for the ability of an attitude change called for by the interaction frame model to reduce stuttering severity:

> Really, what helped me the most was changing my attitude towards my stuttering. The more comfortable I became with my stuttering, the less I stuttered.

Another made a comment that reinforces the need for stutterers to develop a sense of humor about their stuttering:

> Once in high school Spanish class the teacher called on me to do a question-response and my one-sentence response took a full 20 minutes. My friends in the class were cracking up laughing when I finished—not so much at me as at the absurdity of the whole situation.

Strategies for modifying moments of stuttering directly

Many strategies have been advocated and used for *directly* modifying behavior that occurs during moments of stuttering. Judging by reports in the literature, most appear to have helped at least one stutterer, at least temporarily. One problem frequently encountered with all these strategies is clients being reluctant to practice and use them outside of the clinical environment. This may be partially due to the fact that they and their listeners tend not to regard the resultant "stutter-free" speech as sounding completely normal (Franken, Boves, Peters, & Webster, 1992).

Following are some intervention strategies that have been used alone or in combination during the past 50 years for reducing the frequency of moments of stuttering and/or for making them appear less abnormal. The order in which they are described is not intended to indicate their effectiveness, nor are the books and articles cited necessarily the best or only ones for learning about them. They are, however, a good starting point.

Voluntary stuttering. Clients are told to speak disfluently. Specifically, they are told to do one of the following: imitate their own stuttering behavior, produce a relatively effortless repetition of the initial sounds of words (this has been referred to as the "bounce," described in detail later in this section), or simulate stuttering that is more severe than usual for them (Van Riper, 1973). Which approach to take would be determined by what the clinician hoped to accomplish. If, for example, the goal was to increase client awareness of behaviors that occur during moments of stuttering, they probably would be told to imitate their own stuttering behavior. On the other hand, if the goal was to desensitize them to their stuttering or to encourage them to bring their stuttering out into the open, any of the three could be used, though for desensitization the third might be most effective (Freund, 1966).

Clients usually are encouraged to try voluntary stuttering first in the clinic environment on a relatively small number of words. If this strategy were being used solely for increasing their awareness of what they do during moments of stuttering, they probably would not be encouraged to do it outside of the clinic environment. However, if it were being used (at least in part) for desensitizing them to their stuttering and/or for bringing their stuttering problem out into the open, they probably would be encouraged to do it on at least a few words outside of the clinic environment.

Most clients will find it difficult to do voluntary stuttering (particularly outside of the clinic environment), at least initially. For years their goal has been to stutter as little as possible. Now they are being told to do something that is likely to make their stuttering appear to be more severe than it would otherwise. In fact, if their stuttering is extremely mild, they probably are being asked to reveal their stuttering to at least a few persons who were not previously aware of it. They may benefit from doing so, both because it could help to convince them that they can be accepted in spite of the fact that people are aware they stutter, and because it could allow them to make use of at least some of the energy they usually devote to concealing their stuttering for more life-enhancing proposes. Clients who understand and accept their clinician's rationale for recommending voluntary stuttering probably will be more likely to try it than those who do not. There is a need, therefore, to make clients aware of this before encouraging them to try it.

One variation of voluntary stuttering, the *bounce*, has been used as a technique for reducing stuttering severity. Clients are trained to repeat in a relatively effortless manner the initial syllables of words on which they do and do not expect to stutter. On those on which they expect to stutter, they are told to continue repeating the initial syllable until they either can say the word without stuttering or with only minimal stuttering. While this technique has been reported to be effective in reducing stuttering severity (Bryngelson, 1952), there is a potential "danger" associated with its use. Some who use it will develop the habit of repeating the initial syllables of words and will continue doing so even if the strategy is no longer effective for reducing the severity of their stuttering. This would tend to cause listeners to perceive their speech as being more abnormal than otherwise (Berlin & Berlin, 1964).

"Light" consonant contact. This strategy—also referred to as ventriloquism speech (Froeschels, 1950)—differs from the previous one in that the goal is to *reduce stuttering severity voluntarily* rather than increase it. It is intended to provide clients with a tool for "breaking" (or reducing the tension in) blocks in which there are hard contacts involving one or more articulators (Ham, 1990b). During such a block, for example, there could be a hard, prolonged contact between the upper teeth and lower lip (if, for example, the word contained an /f/ phoneme). Clients are taught both to produce consonant sounds on which they *anticipate having* a hard block with an extremely light contact and to try to change the strength of the contact between articulators to a light one while they *are having* such a block. While consonants produced in this manner may be perceived by listeners as distorted or even absent, such distortions and omissions are unlikely to impede communication seriously because of the redundancy present in language. Though it has been used mainly with older children and adults (Ham, 1990b), a few attempts to use it with young children have been made (Ramig & Wallace, 1987). This strategy's ability to reduce stuttering severity may not be permanent (Ham, 1990b; Perkins, 1983b).

Another problem frequently encountered when using approaches such as this one in which clients are instructed to modify moments of stuttering while they occur is that the moments are of such short duration that modification is extremely difficult, if not impossible. Zebrowski (1994), for example, found that for the stuttering children in her sample the duration of sound prolongations and sound/syllable repetitions was typically 750 milliseconds or less.

Cancellations, pull-outs, and preparatory sets. This set of techniques, developed by the late Dr. Charles Van Riper of Western Michigan University, enables clients to reduce the severity of their moments of stuttering—allowing them to stutter more fluently (Van Riper, 1973). While they can be used for the same purpose as the light-consonant-contact technique, they differ from it in several ways, including that the theoretical foundation on which they are based is stronger and a systematic program has been developed for teaching their use (see Van Riper, 1973).

The *cancellation technique* usually is taught first. After clients block on a word, they are supposed to (at least some of the time) pause briefly and think about what occurred during the block and then try to say the word again. The goal is not to say the word without stuttering, but to reduce, at least a little, the amount of abnormality that previously occurred while blocking on it.

There are several reasons why it seems reasonable to believe that the cancellation technique could contribute to reducing stuttering severity. First, it could help to convince clients that they can learn to reduce the severity of their moments of stuttering. Second, it can reduce their desire to avoid stuttering, which is likely to result in reduced stuttering. To practice this technique it is *necessary* to stutter. Third, this technique can enable them to bring their stuttering problem out into the open. Listeners' curiosity about the cancellation technique would give stutterers an opportunity to talk about or acknowledge their stuttering. Doing so should reduce its severity, at least a little (see chapter 2).

The *pull-out technique* usually is taught after the client has made some progress mastering cancellation (Van Riper, 1973). It differs from cancellation in that it is used during a block rather than after one has occurred. It is referred to in this way because it is a technique for "pulling out" of blocks. Clients are taught to finish a word after they have begun blocking it—to terminate the block—with a relatively smooth, controlled prolongation of sounds. This aspect of the Van Riper approach is the most similar to the light-consonant-contact strategy (Ham, 1990b). Since much of the abnormality that occurs during moments of stuttering results from a frantic struggle to terminate blocks, terminating them in this manner would be expected to produce less abnormality and, hence, the blocks should be perceived as being less severe than they would have been otherwise.

The *preparatory-set technique* usually is taught after the client has made some progress in mastering the other two. It is intended to be used immediately *before* moments of stuttering. Van Riper (1973) based this technique on his observation that persons who stutter frequently exhibit certain abnormal behaviors—assume a particular kind of tense *preparatory set*—as they prepare themselves to begin saying words on which moments of stuttering occur. These abnormal behaviors include: tensing the musculature of the speech mechanism; saying the first sound of the word with a fixed position of the articulators rather than with a normal (coarticulatory) movement leading into the next sound; and initiating phonation before beginning to say the first sound of the word. He felt that this preparatory set was responsible for much of the abnormality that occurs during moments of stuttering (Van Riper, 1973). He recommended, therefore, that clients be taught to assume different—more relaxed—preparatory sets before beginning to say words on which they expect to stutter. Specifically, he recommended beginning with the articulators in a state of rest, saying the first sound as a movement leading into the next sound, and initiating air flow and phonation when beginning to say the first sound of the word (not before it).

After clients are proficient in all three techniques, they are told to use them in the reverse order in which they were learned (assuming that the order in which they were learned was the usual one). Before saying a word on which they expect to stutter, they should attempt to assume the "new" *preparatory set.* If they are not successful and begin to block with a great deal of abnormality, they should attempt to *pull out* of the block. If they are not successful in pulling out of the block, they should use *cancellation* immediately after finishing the word to practice stuttering on it with less abnormality. For in-depth information about teaching these techniques, see Van Riper (1973).

Relaxation. One fact about stuttering on which there is almost universal agreement is that those who have the disorder evince excessive muscle tension in their speech mechanism immediately before and during moments of stuttering. There is also almost universal agreement that this excessive tension is responsible for at least some of the abnormality present during moments of stuttering. Consequently, any intervention strategy that causes a client to be more relaxed while speaking should reduce his or her stuttering severity, at least a little (see Gilman & Yaruss, 2000).

Two types of strategies for reducing tension when speaking have been used with persons who stutter: direct and indirect. Direct strategies are specifically intended either to cause clients to be more relaxed than usual when entering speaking situations or to train them to relax parts of their speech musculature when they feel tension in them. One such strategy that has been used with persons who stutter is progressive relaxation (Jacobson, 1938). Clients are taught to relax differentially various muscle groups, including those that make up the speech mechanism. Unfortunately, many have been unable to learn to use this technique well enough to reduce stuttering significantly in situations in which they tend to stutter a great deal (Bloodstein, 1987).

Another direct approach that has been utilized for this purpose involves the use of *suggestion* in either the waking or hypnotic state (Ham, 1990b; Macfarlane, 1990; Van Riper, 1973). Suggestion can be communicated by the clinician ("live" or on tape) or by the client to himself or herself—autosuggestion. (See Boome & Richardson, 1931, for information about the use of autosuggestion in treating stuttering.) A number of intervention strategies involving suggestion have been used with persons who stutter to bring about a more relaxed state while speaking. (See Van Riper, 1973 for an in-depth discussion.) Stutterers have, for example, been put into a relatively deep hypnotic state and given the posthypnotic suggestion that they will be relaxed when entering speaking situations and not stutter. Unfortunately, this type of posthypnotic suggestion, if effective, is usually so for only a short period of time (Ingham, 1984). While hypnosis by itself is regarded as being of questionable value in the treatment of stuttering (Ham, 1990b), it appears to have gained some acceptance when used to produce the relaxed state required for strategies such as systematic desensitization (Macfarlane, 1990; Wolpe, 1958).

A third direct approach that has been used for reducing tension uses electromyographic biofeedback instrumentation (Ingham, 1993a). Surface electrodes are attached to the skin over a muscle that tends to tense during moments of stuttering (such as the masseter muscle), and the subject uses variations in the visual or auditory signal generated by the instrument both to monitor the level of tension in the muscle and to learn to relax it.

Indirect approaches that use suggestion for reducing tension while speaking usually do not involve the use of hypnosis. An example of such an approach would be the use of suggestion to modify aspects of clients' belief systems. One belief that clinicians may attempt to modify in their clients through the use of suggestion is that they cannot learn to reduce the severity of their stuttering. A client who regards previous therapy as having been unsuccessful is likely to have such a belief.

The suggestion that a client's severity of stuttering *can* be reduced would be communicated to him or her while in the "waking" state. However, the client may not be fully aware on a conscious level that the suggestion is being communicated because it may not be conveyed (or communicated completely) by what the clinician *says*. It may be communicated, in part, by the clinician behaving in a manner that *suggests* to the client that the prognosis for improvement is good. Or this idea may be communicated, in part, by the client meeting other stutterers who have improved—the fact that others have improved *suggests* to the client that he or she can also. The suggestion may also be communicated, in part, by the clinician having the client read research reports and other material that *suggest* persons who stutter can improve. Finally, it may be communicated, in part, by the client changing some aspect of his or her behavior that he or she did not believe could be changed (autosuggestion).

This type of suggestion is responsible for the placebo effect (Shapiro, 1964). An intervention strategy can be effective, at least in part, because the client is led to believe through suggestion that it will be effective. Perhaps this is one reason why many seemingly different intervention strategies have been effective with persons who stutter.

Slow, prolonged speech. Most persons who stutter do so less severely while speaking under the condition of delayed auditory feedback (DAF) in which there is a 250 millisecond delay (see chapter 2). While doing so, their speaking rate tends to be slower than usual and they tend to prolong sounds and syllables. Based on the assumption that it is these changes in speaking behavior rather than DAF, per se, that are responsible for the reduction in stuttering severity, a number of clinicians have attempted to teach delayed-auditory-feedback-type (slow, prolonged) speech to persons who stutter (Ingham, 1993a). Some have recommended using a delayed auditory feedback unit, possibly a portable one, when teaching this form of speech—(see Kalinowski, 2003; Stuart, Xia, Jiang, et al., 2003; Perkins, 1973). Others (e.g., Watts, 1971), however, have reported that it is not necessary to use such a device. They provide data that suggest that the *imitation* of speech produced under DAF is just as effective for reducing stuttering severity as is producing the altered speech pattern with a DAF unit. Those who do recommend using the device, however, gradually wean their clients from it. In some cases this is accomplished by gradually increasing the interval of delay, thereby reducing the impact of the DAF unit on their clients' speech (Perkins, 1973). As this is being done, clients are encouraged to use the slow, prolonged DAF-type speech pattern voluntarily.

When clients use slow, prolonged speech, they are speaking in a nonhabitual manner, which tends to reduce stuttering severity (see chapter 2). Hence, the reduction in stuttering that occurs while using slow, prolonged speech may result, at least in part, from speaking in a nonhabitual manner. If this is the case, then the effect of this strategy on stuttering may only be temporary.

There is an issue to consider before encouraging clients to speak in a manner, like the one just suggested, that listeners are likely to regard as abnormal. Will listeners tend to react more favorably to clients' "new" way of speaking than to their "old" way? There are data suggesting that listeners *may* react more favorably to a client's stuttering than to his or her "new" speech pattern if they regard it as sounding "unnatural" (see Berlin & Berlin, 1964; Franken et al., 1992; Perkins, 1983b; Silverman & Trotter, 1973c). According to Perkins (1983b, p. 157), "Unless use of fluency skills yields speech that sounds reasonably normal, stuttered speech is apt to seem preferable."

Rate reduction.   Some persons who stutter become more fluent, at least temporarily, when they reduce their speaking rate (Ramig, 1984). This has been used alone and in combination with other speech modification strategies to reduce stuttering severity (Perkins, 1973; Schwartz, 1976; Shames & Florance, 1980; Webster, 1980). It has been suggested, in fact, that this is an "active ingredient" in many of the strategies that have been used for this purpose (Ramig, 1984; Wingate, 1976).

Rhythmic (metronome-timed) speech.   Most persons who stutter become more fluent, at least temporarily, when they speak using an artificial rhythm—for example, when pacing their speech with the beats of a metronome (see chapter 2). This phenomenon has been used clinically for several centuries (Eldridge, 1968). Two behavior-modification based approaches that utilize rhythmic speech for reducing stuttering severity were developed during the past twenty-five years. With the first, *metronome-timed speech* (Brady, 1971), clients are encouraged to pace their speech with the beats of a miniature electronic metronome (one word or syllable per beat) that is worn like a behind-the-ear-type or eyeglass-type hearing aid (see figure 2-1). With the second, *syllable-timed speech* (Andrews & Harris, 1964), clients are encouraged to speak rhythmically (one syllable at a time with even stress and timing) without using a device. Both have been reported to be effective in reducing the stuttering of some persons, at least temporarily (Andrews & Harris, 1964; Brady, 1971).

Clients using rhythmic speech—like those using slow, prolonged speech—are speaking in a nonhabitual manner, which by now you know tends to result in reduced stuttering (see chapter 2). Another factor that could partially explain this result is reduced fear of stuttering and desire to avoid it (see Silverman, 1971b).

Do listeners tend to react more favorably to clients' rhythmic speech than to their usual stuttering? There are data (Mallard & Meyer, 1979; Silverman & Trotter, 1973c) suggesting that they may not, particularly if their usual stuttering tends to be relatively mild or if they pace their speech in a staccato, machine-like manner.

Speaking while listening to loud masking noise. Some persons who stutter become more fluent—at least temporarily—when they speak while listening to loud masking noise (see chapter 2). Doing so interferes with their ability to monitor their speech auditorily and, as a consequence, there are changes in their speaking behavior—such as a tendency for their voices to grow louder. This phenomenon has been utilized clinically by having clients use portable masking-noise generators (e.g., Carlisle, 1985; Ingham et al., 1981; Moore & Adams, 1985; Trotter & Lesch, 1967; Trotter & Silverman, 1973). These devices look like binaural body-type hearing aids. Some have a switch that clients can use to turn on the masking noise if they anticipate blocking or begin to block (Trotter & Lesch, 1967; Trotter & Silverman, 1973). Others, such as the *Edinburgh Masker* (Carlisle, 1985; Ingham, 1993a; Ingham et al., 1981; Moore & Adams, 1985), are voice actuated—that is, the masking noise is turned on when the person begins to phonate and turned off when phonation ceases. Some relatively severe stutterers have reported being helped by this type of device (Carlisle, 1985; Trotter & Lesch, 1967). The reduction in stuttering that occurs while using such a device may result, at least in part, from speaking in a nonhabitual manner.

The following comments by STUTT-L participants provide some insight into how a stutterer could benefit from the use of this type of device:

> I have met a certain number of people during the past 25 years who
> did recover from moderate to severe stuttering. Bob is one good

example. If you've ever heard Bob's story about the difficulties he had as a police officer, you'll know that his success has been significant. Bob recovered, in part, because he wore an Edinburgh Masker under his uniform for a dozen years while he was on the job, and this gave him the confidence to move out in the world, interact with the public and with his department, and develop his interpersonal skills.

My own experience has been that using an Edinburgh Masker to talk on the telephone whenever it was an important conversation, such as business related, over the course of three years has led me to the point where I often reach for the masker out of habit and realize I don't need it. I still have some blocks on the phone, but my fear of the phone is totally gone, and I can call people, introduce myself, and speak maybe 90% fluently without thinking about it—and much of this is simply from using the Masker to just nullify that fear response.

Reducing anomalies in laryngeal functioning. Many persons who stutter have anomalies in laryngeal functioning during moments of stuttering (see chapter 3). These include problems with initiating phonation and sustaining it in a relatively relaxed manner with adequate breath support. Several strategies have been proposed that require clients to monitor and attempt to modify one or both of these problems—that is, to have a gentle voice onset target. For example, Schwartz (1976) taught clients to monitor airflow and encouraged them to let some breath flow out passively before initiating phonation for each utterance. Webster (1980), as a part of his Precision Fluency Shaping Program, taught clients to monitor onset of phonation (initially using a biofeedback device) and encouraged them to do it in a manner that is "gentle." While many persons were reported to stutter less severely after learning to use these techniques, some were unable to maintain their post-therapy fluency level for the long term (Andrews & Tanner, 1982b; Pill, 1988).

The improvement in fluency reported by those who used these techniques may have resulted, in at least some cases, from speaking in a non-habitual manner and/or from strong suggestion that the approach would be effective. With regard to the latter, Schwartz (1976) entitled his first book *Stuttering Solved* and his second (1986, with Carter) *Stop Stuttering*.

Reducing abnormalities in breathing. Many stutterers exhibit abnormalities in respiratory functioning during moments of stuttering (see chapter 2). Attempts have been made for hundreds of years to teach stutterers to breathe more normally (Van Riper, 1973). With one such contemporary approach—the *regulated-breathing method*—clients are taught to

> . . . breathe in a smooth manner, to pause at natural juncturing points, to breathe deeply, to plan ahead for the content of speech, and to relax chest and neck muscles. (Azrin, Nunn, & Frantz, 1979)

While Azrin and his associates (1979) reported good results using the technique, Andrews and Tanner (1982a) and Ladouceur, Cote, Leblond, and Bluchard (1982) were unable to replicate them. Consequently, the usefulness of this technique for reducing stuttering is uncertain. Another contemporary approach to treating stuttering through reducing abnormalities in breathing is the *perfectly mastered breathing* (PMB) program (Tonev, 1994).

Punishing stuttering and positively reinforcing fluency.   There have been attempts to reduce stuttering severity by using the operant conditioning methodology developed by B. F. Skinner and his followers (Martin, 1993). If stuttering is the type of behavior that can be manipulated by response-contingent reinforcement, punishment should cause it to occur less frequently. And if speaking "fluently" is such a behavior, positive reinforcement should cause it to occur more frequently.

There have been a number of laboratory studies in which stuttering was reduced *temporarily* following response-contingent presentation of such stimuli as shock, noise, verbal disapproval, response cost, and time-out from speaking that probably would be interpreted by the recipient as punishment (see chapter 2). A few attempts have been reported to use such reinforcement clinically with children who are thought to be beginning to stutter. For example, Martin, Juhl, and Haroldson (1972) reported on the use of a time-out procedure with two preschool children; and Reed and Godden (1977) reported on the use of verbal disapproval (the words "slow down"), also with two preschool children. For all four children, a decrease in stuttering was reported following intervention. (However, see the cautionary note in the following paragraph.) Onslow, Andrews, and Lincoln (1994) reported on its "successful" use with young children in a parent-administered program in which stutter-free utterances were rewarded with praise. In addition, Stocker and Gerstman (1983) have reported positive results from a strategy they refer to as the "probe technique" in which the therapist rewards the child for "reductions in disfluencies with bits of candy or pennies" (p. 336).

Response-contingent punishment should be used with extreme caution with preschool children because there is reason to believe that it can precipitate stuttering. According to the diagnosogenic theory (see chapter 5), communicating to children that their disfluencies (such as sound and syllable repetitions) are undesirable can precipitate the disorder. While the evidence certainly is not conclusive that doing so will always precipitate stuttering or that this is the only way stuttering can begin, it strongly suggests that it is *one* such way (Tudor, 1939; Silverman, 1988b).

Concerns have been expressed about the reliability of perceptual judgments of moments of stuttering. Both interjudge and interclinic disagreements have been reported for relatively experienced judges (Ingham & Cordes, 1992). Consequently, it may not be possible to punish moments of stuttering consistently and immediately after they occur.

Thus far, response-contingent punishment of stuttering has been discussed. A second way that operant conditioning methodology has been used is reinforcement for periods of fluency. Moments of stuttering are ignored and positive reinforcement is given for saying particular words or utterances fluently or for speaking fluently during a particular period of time. Leach (1969), for example, gave a twelve-year-old child one cent for each 15-second period of fluent speech, and Manning, Trutna, and Shaw (1976) gave three children—ages six, nine, and eleven—verbal rewards (such as "Good speech" and "You sounded real nice") for such performances. Some short-term improvement in fluency was reported in both studies.

Positive reinforcement for fluency may be interpreted by clients in the same manner as punishment for stuttering. By equating fluency with speaking well, you indirectly are equating being disfluent with speaking poorly.

Systematic desensitization.   Stuttering severity varies on a situational basis (see chapter 2). One reason a person stutters more than usual in some situations may be that a stimulus associated with those situations elicits higher than usual amounts of anxiety (Wolpe, 1958). If the reaction to this stimulus could be changed, there would likely be some reduction in stuttering severity (Brutten & Shoemaker, 1967). Systematic desensitization (which utilizes the reciprocal inhibition principle) has been used for this purpose (Wolpe, 1958; Brutten & Shoemaker, 1967).

The reciprocal inhibition principle, as formulated by Wolpe (1958), states that each time a person does not become highly anxious in the presence of a stimulus that ordinarily elicits a high level of anxiety, the link between that stimulus and the "old" response is weakened a little. How can it be arranged that a person will be unlikely to respond to such a stimulus with a high level of anxiety? One way is to produce in them an emotional state while they are in the presence of the stimulus that is not compatible with anxiety. One such state is deep relaxation (Wolpe, 1958). A person cannot be deeply relaxed and highly anxious simultaneously!

To desensitize a client to a stimulus using this principle, it is necessary first to get him or her deeply relaxed. A number of techniques can be used for this purpose (Jacobson, 1938; Wolpe, 1958). You would then present the stimulus a number of times in a way that should elicit a relatively low level of anxiety. If, for example, the act of talking on the telephone usually causes a client to become highly anxious, the stimulus could be presented to elicit a relatively low level by having

the client repeatedly enter and leave a room in which there is a telephone, or imagine doing so. Imagining an act is reported to be as effective as actually doing it (Wolpe, 1958). When the client ceased
responding to the stimulus with anxiety when the stimulus was presented in this manner, it next would be presented in a way that would
be expected to elicit a somewhat higher level of anxiety.

For example, the client would be required again and again to say
something on the telephone (or to imagine doing so) to someone with
whom he or she felt comfortable speaking. After the client ceased
responding with anxiety to this version of the stimulus, it would be
presented in a manner that would be expected to elicit a little more
anxiety. This process would be repeated until the client ceased
responding to the stimulus with a high level of anxiety when he or she
encountered it in the "real world." Getting a client to this point can
take many months (Wolpe, 1958).

The application of the reciprocal inhibition principle that was
described in the preceding paragraph is highly structured. This principle also can be utilized in less formal ways. If, for example, a client
were encouraged to discuss a situation that usually causes him or her
to become highly anxious over and over again while he or she was
fairly relaxed, this would tend to weaken the link between this situation and anxiety. This is one reason, incidentally, why psychotherapy
in which clients "talk out their problems" often is beneficial (Wolpe,
1958). It is also the reason why you may feel less anxious after talking
with a friend about what is causing your anxiety.

The reciprocal inhibition principle applied "informally" can be
quite useful when working with persons who stutter. If, for example,
the thought of bringing stuttering out into the open causes a client so
much anxiety that he or she is unwilling to do it, having the client
repeatedly talk about doing so with a person or group with whom he or
she feels comfortable may reduce anxiety sufficiently to enable him or
her to do it. This is one way, incidentally, that a support group, such
as one sponsored by the National Stuttering Association (see Appendix B), can be helpful to persons who stutter.

Emotional flooding (implosive therapy). This, like systematic desensitization, is a behavior therapy method that involves having clients
enter or imagine themselves in disturbing situations (Stampfl & Levis,
1967). While with systematic desensitization these situations are
intended to be initially experienced by the client at a level that is only
slightly disturbing, with emotional flooding they are intended to be experienced by him or her initially at a level that is highly disturbing—one
that should produce an *emotional flood.* The theory is that repeatedly
experiencing situations in this manner can cause the anxiety elicited by
them to dissipate, or *implode* (Stampfl & Levis, 1967). Voluntary stutter-

ing (Van Riper, 1973), which is described elsewhere in this chapter, is an example of a technique that can produce such flooding. For further information about how this method has been used in the treatment of stuttering see Adams (1982) and Van Riper (1973).

Drugs and acupuncture.   There have been a number of attempts to use prescription drugs to reduce stuttering severity (Bloodstein, 1987; Ludlow & Braun, 1993; Van Riper, 1973). Six that have been used with stutterers are bethanechol, carbamazepine, clomipramine, verapamil, and haloperidol. While these drugs appear to make some stutterers more fluent, most of those who become so eventually discontinue their use because of unacceptable side effects such as drowsiness and nausea (Bloodstein, 1987).

Acupuncture also has been reported to be effective as a component of a therapy program for reducing stuttering severity. According to Brauneis (1994, p. 159), "Modern research has shown that acupuncture is able to influence neurophysiological and neurochemical (neurotransmitter) processes as well as relax the patient."

Strategies for modifying listeners' reactions to the client's speech fluency

Most stutterers stutter more severely when talking to some persons than to others (see chapter 2). Almost any older child or adult who has the disorder can name categories of people with whom he or she tends to stutter more severely than usual. An example of such a category for some stutterers is order takers in fast-food restaurants.

According to the interaction-frame model (see figure 7-1) the reactions of listeners to stuttering can influence its severity. Stutterers tend to stutter more severely when with persons whom they expect to react negatively to their stuttering than when with those whom they do not expect to do so. This is because they tend to stutter most when they want to stutter least (Williams, 1982). Consequently, it may be possible to reduce the severity of a client's stuttering in some situations, at least a little, by changing the reactions of certain listeners.

We discussed, in the preceding section, how clinician-administered response-contingent punishment of stuttering and positive reinforcement of fluency can increase stuttering by increasing the desire to avoid it. A person who stutters is likely, at times, to receive both types of feedback from listeners. One who laughs after the person stutters would be administering response-contingent punishment for stuttering. One who complements a stutterer for saying something fluently would be administering response-contingent reinforcement for fluency. Actually, anything a client interprets (rightly or wrongly) as either punishment for stuttering or positive reinforcement for fluency can have this effect.

Strategies for reducing the likelihood that particular listeners will unintentionally deliver response-contingent punishment for stuttering and/or response-contingent reinforcement for fluency are discussed in this section. These are of two types. With one the client attempts to modify these reactions; with the other, somebody else attempts to do so. The "somebody else" is most likely to be a clinician, a parent, or teacher.

Several strategies that a client could utilize for modifying these reactions are now considered. The first involves the use of response-contingent punishment. Immediately after the listener reacts to the client's stuttering or fluency in a way that he or she does not like, the client would do something that the listener would regard as adversive. One of my teenage clients solved the problem of being mocked frequently by a classmate for his stuttering by "beating him up." And one of my adult clients, after being treated in a demeaning way by a store clerk because of his stuttering, asked to see the manager and complained. Both of these resulted in the client feeling more in control and less like a victim. Overtly expressing anger when it is appropriate to do so is also likely to benefit clients in other ways (Rubin, 1969).

Another strategy that a client could use for modifying such reactions is to bring his or her stuttering problem out into the open—to acknowledge it. Listeners are less likely to react to stuttering in ways that clients are likely to regard as objectionable if they do not have to play "The Emperor's New Clothes" game—make believe that they are not aware that the client's speech is abnormal. A client can acknowledge the problem verbally or through a printed message. He or she can do so, for example, by wearing a T-shirt on which is printed "I stutter. So what!" (Silverman, 1988a; Silverman, Gazzolo, & Peterson, 1990). The findings of several studies (ibid.) suggest that listeners tend to react more positively to a stutterer who wears such a shirt than they would otherwise.

A third strategy that clients can use for this purpose is to present themselves as often as possible in a way that suggests they have a good self-concept (Cash & Pruzinsky, 1990). Doing so could involve being clean and well-groomed, being assertive, and not constantly signaling listeners that they are ashamed or embarrassed about stuttering. What clients perceive as reactions to their stuttering may actually be, at least in part, reactions to the feelings of shame and embarrassment about it that they are communicating to listeners, for example, by having poor eye contact during moments of stuttering (see chapter 3). Thus, encouraging clients to try to maintain normal eye contact at these times should help to reduce negative reactions to their disfluency. One strategy for helping clients learn to do this involves the use of response-contingent verbal reinforcement and successive approximations. The client initially would receive such reinforcement for even minimal attempts to improve eye contact during moments of stuttering. As his or her ability to approximate normal eye contact improved, the client would cease receiving reinforcement for minimal attempts. Eventually, only those attempts that resulted in eye contact that was within normal limits would be reinforced.

Another strategy involves modifying clients' feelings of shame and embarrassment about stuttering. While it may not be possible to eliminate these totally, it should be possible to reduce them at least a little (Cash & Pruzinsky, 1990). These feelings are likely to have been caused, at least in part, by certain beliefs (or "certainties"), some of which are listed below:

- "I should be able to talk all the time without stuttering because I can do so some of the time."
- "If I had tried hard enough while in therapy, I would have learned to talk without stuttering."
- "I am weak. If I had been able to exercise a normal amount of self-control (willpower), I would have been able to conquer my problem."
- "The cause of my stuttering is psychological (learned behavior) and, hence, I should have been able to conquer it."
- "People dislike listening to stuttering and, hence, I am making them feel uncomfortable."
- "Since stuttering reduces my speaking rate, I am taking more than my fair share of time while talking."

If it seems likely that a client's feelings of shame and embarrassment about stuttering arise, at least in part, from this source, the first step would be to identify the client's certainties and the second would be to reduce his or her confidence in their accuracy. One way would be to present evidence that does not support them. The evidence could come from research data, the client's (or others') life experiences, and/or arguments developed by the clinician. The client initially is likely to reject such challenges to his or her belief system—or is likely to react in a manner that indicates he or she does not want to be "confused by facts." However, if the clinician is persistent, if the data are compelling, and if the arguments are cogent, the client's belief system is likely to be modified, at least a little. Techniques developed by the general semanticists for modifying erroneous beliefs can be useful here (see Johnson, 1946).

The focus so far has been on strategies that clients can use for modifying listener reactions to their disfluency. We will now consider strategies for clinicians, parents, and teachers.

What strategies can clinicians use? In particular, how can they modify undesirable reactions of a child's parents to his or her disfluency when it appears to be "normal?" Since it seems likely that children can begin to stutter in the manner specified by the diagnosogenic theory (see chapter 5), modifying parents' reactions may be necessary.

It may be possible to modify undesirable reactions of children's parents to their "normal" disfluency by doing one or more of the following:

- providing parents with information about normal childhood disfluency
- providing parents with information about how certain reactions to their child's disfluency could increase it (This can be done in a way that is unlikely to make parents feel guilty if they have already reacted inappropriately to it.)
- identifying the undesirable reactions parents are having to their child's disfluency and increasing their awareness of them
- teaching parents how to react appropriately to their child's speech disfluency

The first task in an intervention program for modifying parents' reactions to their child's disfluency is providing them with information about normal childhood disfluency (see chapter 4). If their child's disfluency is found to be within normal limits, merely providing them with this information may be sufficient to eliminate undesirable reactions to it. That is, if they no longer regard the behavior as abnormal, they probably will cease reacting to it in undesirable ways, particularly if they are made aware that continuing to do so could cause it to become abnormal.

Several problems can be encountered when trying to convince parents that their child's fluency is within normal limits. The first is particularly likely to occur if a child's disfluency level is at the *upper end* of normal limits—that is, if he or she repeats sounds and syllables more often than most other children of the same age. Parents may have a difficult time accepting that it is normal because they are aware of other children their child's age who are not as disfluent. It can be pointed out to them that there are *individual differences* in all aspects of childhood behavior, including disfluency, and that their child just tends to be more disfluent than many others of the same age.

Another problem that can be encountered when trying to convince parents that their child's fluency is within normal limits is their having a mind-set to perceive their child's disfluency as stuttering because of a history of it in the family. They are particularly likely to have such a mind-set if they remember a stutterer in the family being disfluent in a similar way during childhood. They can be made aware that most children born into families in which there is a history of stuttering do not stutter, even if one or both parents do so.

Parents probably should be given information about normal childhood disfluency even if their child exhibits abnormal disfluency behavior. There are at least two reasons. First, it is important for them to be aware that not all the disfluency in their child's speech is abnormal. Their child may not be stuttering, therefore, as severely as they think he or she is. Second, they have to learn to discriminate between normal disfluency and stuttering if they are being asked to inform the clinician about the child's stuttering at home.

After the child's parents have been given information about normal speech disfluency, the clinician's next task is to provide them with information about how certain reactions to their child's disfluency could increase it, and to present the information in a way that is unlikely to make them feel guilty if they have already reacted to it in these ways. If this is not done, they are likely to interpret this information to mean that the reason for their child stuttering is poor parenting. This interpretation could cause them to feel guilty, to reject the clinician's recommendations, or both. To reduce the likelihood of such an interpretation, one or more of the following can be mentioned:

- They were reacting to the child's disfluencies in a way that would seem to be appropriate, based on "common sense." Unfortunately, this is one of those rare instances when common sense can lead you astray.

- They obviously reacted to their child's disfluency as they did because they loved and wanted to help him or her.

- Since there is a history of stuttering in their family and they heard that the disorder can be transmitted genetically, it is understandable that they perceived their child's repetitions as abnormal.

- Since the child's disfluency level appears to be at the upper end of normal limits, it is understandable that they perceived it as being abnormal.

- The fact that they brought their child in for an evaluation is evidence that they love the child and are willing to do whatever is necessary to help him or her.

After the parents appear to accept (perhaps with minor reservations) that certain of their reactions to their child's disfluency and/or demands they are placing on their child for fluency may be increasing his or her disfluency, the clinician should increase their awareness of their occurrence. There are two approaches that can be used, singly or in combination. The first is telling parents, in a "face-saving" way, what they are doing that they need to change. The second is having them watch videotapes of the interaction between themselves and their child while the clinician points out both the desirable and undesirable ways they are reacting to his or her disfluency. Hopefully, there will be some of the former so that the experience will not be totally negative. Film the scene, if possible, so that they can see their child's face immediately after they react to the disfluency. This may help to increase their awareness of the effect their reactions are having on their child.

After the parents are made aware of which aspects of their behavior need to be changed, they are taught how to react appropriately to their child's disfluency. Doing so may involve training them to stop saying things that indicate to the child that he or she is doing something "bad" by being disfluent (such as "Take a deep breath before you talk.") and/or to stop doing the things (such as looking away) that communicate a negative message. This could involve teaching them *things to do* when their child is being disfluent, such as listening to and concentrating on the "message" he or she is attempting to communicate and giving the child positive reinforcement for communicating it successfully, regardless of disfluency (Yovetich, 1984). It also could involve teaching them ways to manipulate unobtrusively their child's spontaneous communicative behaviors that are likely to result in increased fluency. One approach that has been used for teaching parents to react appropriately to their child's disfluency is having them watch videotapes of the clinician interacting with their child and then trying to imitate what they see (Daly, 1987).

Another group whose reactions may have to be changed is classroom teachers. How they react to a child's disfluency can strongly influence how his or her peers are likely to do so. If they react to it in undesirable ways, the child's classmates will be likely to react similarly. Examples of such a reaction would be refusing to allow the child to contribute to class discussions when he or she volunteers, or having the child give oral presentations to the teacher privately rather than to the class. The clinician, therefore, may have to counsel the child's classroom teacher in much the same way he or she would the child's parents. Such counseling, of course, should be done in a manner that is unlikely to make the teacher feel guilty or lose face. Otherwise, it could cause the situation in the classroom to deteriorate rather than improve.

There is another reason why it may be desirable to work with the classroom teacher. He or she could provide the child an opportunity to bring the problem out into the open. The child could be encouraged to give an informal talk about it to classmates. The teacher may want to set the stage by providing information about stuttering, including the names of famous people who had the disorder (for example, Moses). The children probably should be given an opportunity to ask questions. It may be desirable for the child's speech-language pathologist to be present.

The approaches considered thus far for modifying parents' and teachers' reactions to children's speech disfluency attempt to do so directly—that is, by increasing their awareness of reactions that are desirable and undesirable. Many young children who stutter or appear to be at risk for developing the disorder have articulation, auditory processing, language formulation, and/or oral motor problems (Riley & Riley, 1979). An indirect approach (that may be used alone or in combination with the others) is switching the focus of attention and concern from fluency to another aspect of speech, language, and/or communication behavior. Riley and Riley (1979) have described a program for treating young children who stutter that features this component.

Strategies to modify clients' reactions to their stuttering and the reactions of others

We have established that the more clients are disturbed by their stuttering and others' reactions to it, the stronger their desire to avoid stuttering will probably be and, hence, the more severely they are apt to stutter (see figure 7-1). This section focuses on strategies for modifying the reactions of clients to their stuttering as well as the reactions of others, or for *desensitizing* the client to these reactions. The reciprocal inhibition principle (Wolpe, 1958) can be used to explain how such strategies work. This principle, discussed earlier in the chapter, states that each time a person does not experience anxiety (or as much anxiety as usual) while in the presence of a stimulus that usually elicits it, the link between that stimulus and the old, anxiety-type response is weakened. Hence, if clients can be kept a number of times from reacting to their stuttering and to their anticipation of it with the usual amount of anxiety, there should be a reduction in the amount of anxiety these stimuli tend to elicit. Consequently, there should be some reduction in the severity of their stuttering. The same should be true for anticipated undesired listener reactions to their stuttering.

Is it possible to desensitize clients completely or almost completely to their stuttering and the negative reactions of listeners? While clinical experience suggests that this is not an attainable goal for many clients, *reducing* the amount of anxiety with which they tend to react to these occurrences should be possible for almost all of them (Wolpe, 1958). Even if this amount were only reduced 15 or 20 percent, it would contribute to the overall goal of reducing stuttering severity.

While any strategy that can cause clients to respond to stuttering or negative listener reactions with less than the usual amount of anxiety is worth considering, some methods are less acceptable and/or practical than others. For example, voluntary stuttering outside of the clinic environment can be effective, but many stutterers are unwilling to do so. Using systematic desensitization with hypnotic relaxation (Wolpe, 1958) can be effective, but very few speech-language pathologists have been trained to use hypnosis.

The strategies described below can be used (singly or in combination) for desensitizing clients to their stuttering and/or negative reactions to it.

Voluntary stuttering. This strategy, which is described in this chapter, can be effective for desensitizing clients if they are willing to use it and can remain relatively relaxed while doing so. Voluntary stuttering can be used in several ways. One is for the client to stutter voluntarily for a period of time in all (or almost all) situations. Another is for the client to use it as a tool to reduce his or her anxiety temporarily in specific situations. Clients who are extremely anxious about the possibility of stuttering—or stuttering severely—in a particular situation may be able to reduce their anxiety by voluntarily stuttering. The second of these methods is likely to be more acceptable to clients than the first because it does not require them to do as much voluntary stuttering and gives them *control* over when they will do so. Feeling in control, in and of itself, may reduce a client's anxiety level (Van Riper, 1973).

Systematic desensitization. In this strategy (described earlier in the chapter), after a client is relaxed, he or she is made to experience a stimulus that is related either to stuttering or to others' reactions to it, the client is asked to imagine doing so a number of times. An example of such a stimulus is stuttering while talking on the telephone. If the client can remain fairly relaxed while doing this, the strength of the link between this stimulus and anxiety should be reduced, at least a little.

Paradoxical intention. This is a technique in which the client is encouraged to *intend*, or wish, something to occur that he or she fears. According to Frankl (1985, p. 147), "This procedure consists of a reversal of the patient's attitude, inasmuch as his fear is replaced by a paradoxical wish. By the treatment the wind is taken out of the sails of the anxiety." Paradoxical intention has been used for treating a number of conditions in which there is anticipatory anxiety (Frankl, 1985).

How might paradoxical intention be used for desensitizing clients to their stuttering? They could be told that when they anticipate stuttering or begin to stutter they should resolve deliberately to show people how severely they can stutter. That is, rather than desiring to avoid stuttering, they should have the paradoxical intention: desiring to stutter as much as possible. If they are successful in doing this for a period of time, the amount of anxiety that the anticipation of stuttering tends to elicit should be reduced.

The effect of paradoxical intention on anxiety can be explained by the reciprocal inhibition principle (Wolpe, 1958). By desiring to stutter, clients experience less anxiety than usual when they do stutter or anticipate doing so. Consequently, there is a weakening in the link between stuttering and anxiety.

Training clients to control (modify) their moments of stuttering. To learn to do this, clients have to practice, and they cannot practice if they do not stutter. Hence, stuttering becomes desirable behavior and consequently is less likely than before to elicit high levels of anxiety. This strategy may be usable for encouraging clients to adopt the mindset required for using paradoxical intention (the strategy discussed prior to this one). It is easier for some to adopt this mind-set (decide that they want to stutter) if they are doing so for a purpose.

Assertiveness training. This technique for enhancing interpersonal skills can facilitate the development of a state which, like relaxation, is not compatible with anxiety (Wolpe, 1969). Hence, if stutterers behave in an assertive manner in situations in which they usually tend to stutter relatively severely, they are likely to become less anxious in them than usual and consequently are likely to stutter less severely than they usually do (Schloss, Freeman, Smith, & Espin, 1987). Based on the reciprocal inhibition principle (Wolpe, 1958), being assertive in the presence of stimuli that ordinarily elicit relatively high levels of anxiety should cause them to elicit less of it, thereby weakening the link (at least a little) between these stimuli and anxiety.

Talking with a clinician or a support group. Having clients talk with a clinician or a support group about their stuttering and their reactions to it can reduce the related anxiety, provided that the clients are not highly anxious while doing so (Moore & Rigo, 1983). Here, again, the mechanism is the reciprocal inhibition principle. Because clients are talking about these problems without becoming as upset as they usually do, the strength of the link between them and their anxiety is weakened a little.

The ameliorating effect of such talking explains, in part, why some stutterers benefit from attending meetings of a support group, such as those sponsored by the National Stuttering Association (Diggs, 1990; Paul-Brown, 1990). Most persons who participate on a regular basis probably enjoy doing so (experience "positive" emotion). Hence, when they talk with group members about their stuttering and negative reactions to it, they are unlikely to become as upset about these issues as they usually do.

In addition to local support group meetings, there are national and international conventions for stutterers at which there are activities that can desensitize them (a little) to their stuttering. The following accounts by STUTT-L participants illustrate one such activity—a group of attendees going to a restaurant:

> At a European stuttering convention, we went as a group to a restaurant where all these flower salespeople never let you eat in peace. They were at our table all the time. So when we got tired of them, we all started to perform our best (or worst) stutter, all of us in our native languages (English, German, Icelandic and Swedish). Can you imagine the look on their faces? I can still feel my stomach ache . . . :-)

One of the things I enjoy about National Stuttering Association conventions is going out to a restaurant with a group of people and watching the server's reaction when the first person stutters while ordering food, and the second person stutters, and so on. If we feel charitable we may tell the server that we're from a stuttering convention, but sometimes it's fun just to let them wonder.

Reducing the tendency to overvalue fluency.   Our focus thus far in this section has been on strategies for reducing clients' desire to avoid stuttering by desensitizing them to it. A second approach can be used for this purpose: reducing their tendency to use fluency as the primary measure of how well they speak. Many clients tend to overvalue fluency (Perkins, 1983b). This approach can be implemented by encouraging them to redirect their attention from how they are speaking to what they are saying (Yovetich, 1984). The less frequently they judge how well they speak by how much they stutter rather than by how well they communicate, the weaker should be their desire to avoid stuttering. Yovetich (1984) has described a strategy, which he refers to as message therapy, for doing this with children. Shklovskii, Krol, and Mikhailova (1988) have described a group psychotherapy program for adults that attempts, in part, to make participants more aware of verbal and nonverbal aspects of their communication and to try to "normalize" them. If the program is successful, the result should be their considering these aspects more and stuttering less when judging how well they spoke in a particular situation.

Maintenance of Fluency Following Treatment

Fewer than 50 percent of older children and adults who acquire a degree of "normal fluency" during treatment are able to maintain it permanently. According to Perkins (1983b):

> Judging from published and unpublished reports of fluency shaping programs, reports that accord with our experiences, the most predictable outcome is relapse of varying amounts and durations. Not that all progress is lost or that other forms of treatment yield better or more permanent results. Quite the contrary. But the expectation of permanent fluency is an expectation rarely realized. (p. 158)

The relapse rates that have been reported for young children, particularly of preschool age, are considerably less (Starkweather, Gottwald, & Halfond, 1990).

A program for post-treatment maintenance of fluency can minimize or even prevent relapse. It could include periodic clinic contacts to check on status and/or periodic participation in "refresher programs" (Boberg, 1981) or self-help groups for former clients (Howie, Tanner, & Andrews, 1981). For children it could include training parents to administer a fluency maintenance program (Schwartz,

1994). It may be desirable to encourage clients to participate in such programs regardless of whether they appear to be experiencing relapse. It is quite possible that to maintain treatment gains they will have to continue to work on their speech for the rest of their lives (Ingham, 1993b).

Several things can be done while clients are in treatment that reportedly reduce the likelihood of their relapsing after treatment ceases, either permanently or for a relatively long period. One is training them to be their own clinician—to do self-therapy. Another is modifying their self-concepts and their attitudes toward speaking, with the goal of making them both more similar to those of "normal speakers" (DiLollo, Neimeyer, & Manning, 2002) A third is to "normalize" their speech fluency fully before permanently terminating therapy. If this is done while they exhibit "tenuous fluency"—that is, while they continue to exhibit behaviors in rate, rhythm, or vocal characteristics that would enable listeners to differentiate their speech from that of normal speakers (Adams & Runyan, 1981)—they may have a greater potential for relapse. The fluent speech of some stutterers who were regarded by their clinicians as having been "successfully therapeutized" has been shown to be perceptually different from that of normal speakers (Onslow & Ingham, 1987). However, there is a little evidence that providing clients with feedback about this can enable them to make their speech sound more normal (Ingham, Martin, Haroldson, Onslow, & Leney, 1985). A fourth is to prepare them for and train them to cope with relapse, to "cease pretending that the majority of stutterers will be able to maintain fluent or stutter-free speech on a long-term basis" (Kamhi, 1982, p. 460). A fifth is to desensitize them to feeling pressured to speak faster, if the strategy they are using to reduce stuttering severity results in a reduction in speaking rate (Craig & Calver, 1991).

One issue relevant to maintaining fluency is assessing whether a relapse is occurring. Ordinarily, the sooner it can be detected, the better the prognosis for the client successfully coping with it. While casual observation often is adequate for detecting a relapse—particularly one of relatively large magnitude—after it has occurred, it may not be adequate for detecting its beginning stages. Clinicians have used both overt and covert procedures for observing their clients' post-therapy fluency, and there are some data suggesting that, for individuals (as opposed to groups), some overt ones may lead to underestimates of amount of disfluency (Ingham, 1990b).

Strategies for Reducing the Degree to which Clients Are Handicapped by Stuttering

Our primary focus thus far has been on reducing stuttering severity. For most adults who stutter, this is unlikely to be the only important goal.

The set of behaviors that defines their stuttering problem will include some that are not aspects of speaking behavior. They result from living with the disorder and can significantly increase clients' handicaps.

The degree to which clients are handicapped by stuttering (or another fluency disorder) is determined by how much it keeps them from doing what they want to do. The severity of the handicap is not necessarily related to the amount of disfluency. Some persons who stutter very little are more handicapped because of their attitude toward stuttering than some whose stuttering is severe.

The severity of their handicap will be determined, in part, by their beliefs about the impact the disorder has on them. Some such beliefs, or "certainties," can cause them to limit their activities and thereby increase the degree to which they are handicapped. Persons who have other fluency disorders also can be handicapped by these certainties. One or more of their certainties may not be true. Modifying these should cause them to place fewer limitations on themselves and, as a consequence, to be less handicapped than previously. Strategies for working toward this goal are discussed later in this section.

Following are examples of certainties that can cause clients to limit their activities:

A person who stutters cannot be successful in a field that requires a great deal of talking, such as teaching, acting, law, politics, public relations, the clergy, sales, speech-language pathology, and medicine. While a person who stutters may have difficulty getting hired in such a field (Silverman & Paynter, 1990), the fact is that persons who stutter have been successful in all of them. The memberships of the National Stuttering Project and the National Council on Stuttering, for example, include persons who have been employed in these fields for a number of years.

A person who stutters must conquer the disorder before getting on with his or her life. Persons who have this belief tend to put their lives "on hold." While clients certainly should be encouraged to try to reduce the severity of their stuttering (assuming that this would be an attainable goal for them), it probably is unnecessary for them to put their lives on hold until they do so. Many persons who stutter relatively severely appear to have had satisfying lives, professionally and otherwise.

A person who stutters is unworthy. Persons who have this belief tend to withdraw from people—they may almost become hermits. An extreme example would be an attorney with whom I worked briefly who stuttered. He lived for a number of years on a small island in the Pacific because he did not feel he was sufficiently worthy to live on the mainland. Those who view themselves in this way obviously have a poor self-concept and may benefit from psychotherapy.

A person who has normal speech will not want to date someone who stutters. Clients who have this belief will rarely, if ever, try to get a date because they anticipate rejection. While there probably are persons who would refuse to date someone for this reason, the fact that many persons who stutter are married to nonstutterers suggests that this is not true in general. While a person who stutters may attribute his or her lack of success in dating to stuttering, the real reason may be a poor self-concept. He or she may not dress attractively, be well-groomed, have a good sense of humor, and/or in other ways be the kind of positive, self-confident person with whom people enjoy spending time.

If I talk in a particular situation, people will react to my stuttering in ways I'll find upsetting. Clients are likely to avoid talking in certain situations at least some of the time because of bad experiences they have had in the past. For example, a child may avoid asking questions in class or contributing to class discussions because classmates have laughed at his stuttering. Clients assume that because their stuttering was reacted to negatively in the past, it is likely to be treated this way in the future. This may or may not be true. If it is not true, then they are unnecessarily handicapping themselves by not talking. If it is true, they may be losing more than they gain by doing so. For example, while children can reduce negative reactions to their stuttering by not participating in class discussions, doing so can also contribute to their doing less well academically than they would have done otherwise (Williams, Melrose, & Woods, 1969).

Because I stutter I can't participate in a particular activity I think I'd enjoy. Over the years I have met persons who stutter who have participated in a wide variety of activities, many of which involve speaking. They have been debaters, actors, singers, telephone answerers on suicide "hot lines," members of volunteer fire departments, leaders of religious services, and advocates for political candidates and causes. They have even run for and been elected to political office. Hence, clients who have this certainty may be handicapping themselves unnecessarily.

Intervention for reducing the degree to which clients are handicapped by their beliefs is a two-step process (Johnson, 1946). The first involves questioning clients in a way that will reveal the limitations they are placing on themselves. Answers to the following questions can provide useful information: If your stuttering were to disappear tomorrow, what effects would it have on your life? What would you do that you do not do now? Would you change jobs? If you think that you might do so, what field would you enter? Do you think you would do better in school? Why? Would you engage in activities in which you do not participate now? With what people, if any, would you talk more often? Would you date more often? Would you feel better about yourself—more "worthy?" Would you further your education? Would you have more friends?

After at least some of a client's certainties have been identified, the second step is to make an attempt to modify them. This usually involves providing the client with information and/or experiences that hopefully will cause him or her to question the accuracy of such certainties. This information can be provided in several ways. The clinician can do so orally, can encourage the client to read informative material, or can encourage the client to talk to stutterers who do not have these certainties.

The process used for encouraging clients to modify their certainties is similar to hypothesis testing in research (Silverman, 1998). Certainties can be looked upon as hypotheses that may or may not be valid. To assess their validity, clients would be encouraged to make the observations necessary to consider them as objectively as they can. If, for example, one of a client's certainties pertains to how specific listeners will react to his or her stuttering (e.g., how classmates will react if he or she stutters while asking questions in class), the client would be encouraged to stutter while talking to them and observe how they react. If they do react negatively, this would suggest that the certainty is accurate. On the other hand, if they do not do so, this should make the client at least a little less confident in its accuracy. Since a single observation is not adequate for testing any hypothesis, clients should be encouraged to test their certainties more than once.

What if this process indicates that such a certainty probably is accurate—that, for example, stuttering decreases employability in some occupations even if it does not interfere with job performance? (Hurst & Cooper, 1983a, 1983b) Should the client be encouraged to accept the limitations it imposes? If the client is highly unlikely to be able to overcome certain obstacles, it probably would be best for his or her mental health that they be accepted. On the other hand, if there is a good chance they can be overcome and the client is willing "to pay a price" for trying, whether he or she should be encouraged to do so would depend on whether the potential benefits from trying exceed the potential losses from doing so.

Counseling the Client's Family

There may be a need to counsel members of the client's family for reasons other than advising them on how to facilitate his or her therapy. They may need help in coping with situations they themselves encounter because they live with a person who has a fluency disorder. Perhaps the persons most likely to be in need of such help are the parents of children and the spouses of adults who have such a disorder. For descriptions of coping strategies for parents, see Conture and Fraser (1989) and Zebrowski and Schum (1993); and for spouses, see Boberg and Boberg (1990), and Boberg and Kully (1997).

What Constitutes Recovery?

Recovery from stuttering isn't easy to define from a stutterer's perspective. The following comments by STUTT-L participants shed a little light on why this is so:

There are people who do not consider what they do to be stuttering. I have two friends like that. One I know from a church I used to go to, and one is married to a friend of mine. They are mild stutterers, but they are definitely not covert. They have obvious blocks and stammers. They know me pretty well. I have asked them both about their stuttering, and they both gave me the same answer: "I used to stutter but I don't anymore." Uh, excuse me, but what do you call that not being able to say a word? Yodeling? I didn't say that, I just thought it. I figured if they don't consider it something that needs to be dealt with, then that's their business. And apparently neither of them feels it's a problem for them. One of them is a middle-school history teacher who used to be a guard at a prison (same job, right?). The other is one of the biggest talkers I know. I'm in awe of him because he'll walk up to anybody and talk to them about anything.

Personally, I believe recovery from stuttering is not full until we're able to speak to our family members about it without shame and guilt.

My definition of recovery is your stuttering no longer limiting your ability to lead the life YOU WANT to lead.

To me using the word "recovery" does NOT necessarily mean your stuttering is gone—it means you've been able to maintain a level of managing your own stuttering to where YOU are comfortable.

Ironically, what hurts us persons who stutter more is avoidance of speaking, not the disfluencies per se. If a person is taking as much a part in speaking activities as the next person, fluency is just a cosmetic thing.

SELECTING AND IMPLEMENTING INTERVENTION STRATEGIES FOR CLUTTERING

Authorities agree that persons who clutter are abnormally disfluent because they do not monitor their speech adequately (e.g., Daly, 1986, 1993b; Luchinger & Arnold, 1965; Weiss, 1964). This may also be the reason for their language and articulation disorders (Myers, 1992). Consequently, they usually aren't aware of their disfluency and other speech-language disorders (Daly, 1986). Although they usually do not monitor their speech adequately, they apparently can do so judging by the fact that they tend to be more fluent when performing a task that requires them to pay attention to how they talk—as in reading unfamiliar material or speaking a foreign language (see table 2-2). Therefore, to reduce their disfluency it is necessary to get them to monitor their speech more carefully.

Their lack of self-monitoring affects aspects of their speaking behavior other than fluency. Their rate of speaking tends to be excessive, and they make frequent errors related to language formulation and expression. The general disturbance in speech-language functioning of many persons who have this disorder caused Weiss (1964) to hypothesize that cluttering is one manifestation (symptom) of a central language imbalance in the area of verbal utterances. This underlying condition (portion of the "iceberg below the surface"), according to Weiss (1964), also produces disorders that are not directly related to speech and language functioning. Clients who have this disorder, therefore, are also likely to have others that require treatment.

One problem likely to be encountered (at least at first) when working with clients who clutter is lack of motivation. Most are seen by speech-language pathologists because they are told by someone (usually a parent, teacher, or employer) that they need therapy. Their attitude upon being told so is likely to be negative. According to Daly (1986):

> . . . cluttering children are frequently confused by a listener's inability to understand their speech. Clutterers accept no blame for the communication breakdown, thinking instead that the listener should pay closer attention. Adolescent and adult clutterers are annoyed and often angered by the persistent attempts of teachers or speech-language pathologists to find a problem, when in the clutterers' minds none exists. (The author has treated a number of salespersons who clutter. Their sales managers insisted that treatment be obtained because customers had complained that the salespersons were difficult to understand. Even when therapy was mandatory to maintain employment, some adult clutterers would not take their speech treatment seriously. They preferred to believe that their boss was being "hard-nosed" or unreasonable.) (pp. 159–160)

It may be possible to motivate clutterers to invest in therapy by making them more aware of the effect that improved self-monitoring has on their speech and by having them receive positive reinforcement for attempting to improve it, particularly from those who previously complained about it. The first can be accomplished by having clutterers listen to tape recordings made both while they *are* and *are not* adequately monitoring their speech (Daly, 1987). The second can be done by informing persons concerned about clutterers' speech of the importance of providing such reinforcement (Daly, 1986).

Lack of motivation isn't the only problem encountered when working with clutterers. Because their fluency tends to increase significantly when they speak more slowly than usual, one goal of therapy is to encourage them to do so. However, many clutterers cannot tolerate speaking at a slower rate unless they are desensitized to doing so. Van Riper (1982) has suggested several strategies for desensitizing a clutterer to a slower speaking rate:

At first don't ask him to speak slowly even though, when he does so, his communication will markedly improve. You'll find that he cannot tolerate the slower rate. Instead, find other ways of slowing him down until that tolerance is increased. Try reading in unison and begin by using a very fast rate yourself, then gradually returning to a more normal rate. Have him learn to shadow your speech and then the speech of others. Have him repeat phrases and sentences that you utter with different tempos. Have him write down the words he wants to say before saying them. Have him tap the words of his forthcoming utterance before he speaks them or hums them. Record samples of his rapid, confused speech, desensitize him to them, then have him translate. Have him teach you how to speak clutteringly. Using recorded speech samples, jointly analyze the omissions, repetitions, slurrings, and other cluttering features. With prepared written material teach him how to clutter on purpose before trying to say it better. Have him echo both your deliberately cluttered speech and then your normal version. Using more prepared sentences, have him read them faster and faster until complete breakdown occurs, then listen to the recording.

A most valuable technique is to teach him to pause and to tolerate that pause for increasing lengths of time. For this you will have to use modeling and various signals to indicate when to stop and when to get going again. Adequate pausing will slow down his speech more than any amount of exhortation to talk slowly. The clutterer's speech is highly disorganized and he needs some training in this area. . . . Have him paraphrase things he reads or what you tell him. . . . Do some role playing of situations in which he must speak coherently such as applying for a job or asking for a date or giving directions to a stranger hunting for a store. (p. viii)

Other authors also have suggested strategies for encouraging clutterers to monitor their speech more closely and to develop tolerance for a slower speaking rate. They include:

- having clients use a miniature masking noise generator, such as the Edinburgh Masker, while speaking (Dewar, Dewar, & Anthony, 1976). The resulting disturbance in auditory feedback causes them to concentrate more than usual on how they are speaking.

- having clients pace their speech with a metronome (Tiger, Irvine, & Reis, 1980). Doing so would cause them to concentrate more on how they are speaking and thus reduce their speaking rate.

- using a delayed auditory feedback (DAF) device to desensitize clients to speaking more slowly (Daly, 1992). If they can learn to tolerate slow, distorted DAF speech, they will almost certainly be better able to tolerate a slower speaking rate.

- telling clients to pronounce each syllable slowly, giving each syllable equal stress (Weiss, 1964). The resultant speech sounds similar to that produced by using a delayed auditory feedback machine. This exercise tends to heighten their awareness of tactile and kinesthetic feedback (Daly, 1986).

- having the client practice reading material aloud, in which the words are exposed one at a time through a hole (a "window" in a sheet of paper) at a relatively slow rate. This exercise can be used to desensitize a client to slower speech. (See Daly, 1988, for structured therapy materials and evaluations forms for this task.)

- having clients count backward by a specific amount (ones, twos, threes, or fours) to increase their concentration (Weiss, 1964).

- having clients speak in unison with or "shadow" (see chapter 2) tape-recordings made by the clinician in which the rate/prosody are appropriate. Ham (1988) has described in detail a program that can be used for this purpose.

- having clients visualize themselves speaking fluently in as many situations and with as many people as possible, including those who have reacted negatively to their speech (Daly, 1988; Daly, Thompson, & Simon, 1985).

- encouraging clients to watch videotapes of themselves, filmed both while they are and are not adequately monitoring their speech (see Daly, 1987).

- using Shames and Florance's (1980) Stutter-Free Speech Program. Daly (1986) has reported some success using a modified version of the program with clutterers. He concluded that this program was beneficial because "Their emphasis on slow, smooth speech initiations and continuous phonation, first with delayed feedback and later without it, provides the clutterer with concrete, verifiable components of the speech act that can also be monitored." (Daly, 1986, p. 181)

How likely is a person who has this disorder to be completely cured? The prognosis for a cure is poor, but better for children than for adults (Daly, 1986, 1993b; Luchinger & Arnold, 1965; Myers & St. Louis, 1992; Weiss, 1964).

For further information about the management of cluttering, as well as its symptomatology and etiology, see the special 1996 issue of the *Journal of Fluency Disorders* devoted to the disorder.

SELECTING AND IMPLEMENTING INTERVENTION STRATEGIES FOR NEUROGENIC ACQUIRED STUTTERING

Several strategies that have been suggested for reducing the abnormal disfluency associated with this disorder are described here.

Word-retrieval deficits appear to be at least partially responsible for the abnormal disfluency exhibited by some persons who have this disorder (Brown & Cullinan, 1981). It has been suggested that teaching a delay strategy to provide more time for word retrieval may be one way to reduce such disfluency (Linebaugh, 1984). One such strategy is self-monitoring.

Whitney and Goldstein (1989) described a self-monitoring program they found successful in reducing the disfluency of three mild aphasics. Three disfluency types were used as target behaviors: repetition (part-word, word, and phrase), interjection, and revision (see chapter 1). Target behaviors are treated one at a time. The program consists of the following four steps:

1. Clients listen to tape recordings of their speech while their clinician points out instances of the target behavior to them. The purpose is to begin to make them aware of the behavior they are to self-monitor.

2. Clients listen to other tape recordings of their speech and signal (for example, activate a counter) each time they hear the target behavior. If they do not signal an instance within three seconds after it occurs, the clinician stops the tape and points it out to them. If they accurately identify most instances, this would suggest that they understand what their clinician wants them to self-monitor.

3. Clients self-monitor while performing a speaking task (such as describing a picture). They are told to signal each time they produce the target behavior, in the same way they did in step 2. If they do not signal an instance within three seconds, the clinician stops them and points out the target behavior, using a recording.

4. Clients self-monitor while performing the speaking task used in step 3 without the clinician providing feedback and reinforcement. Their performance is recorded and the amount of the target behavior they evince is compared to that in a recording they made before beginning the training program. If there is less of the target behavior in the post- than in the pre-intervention recording, this would suggest that self-monitoring could be helpful for decreasing their disfluency. They would then be encouraged and trained to use it outside the clinic environment.

Whitney and Goldstein (1989) used this program for more than 10 sessions with each client. It probably would take considerable practice before most clients would be able to self-monitor successfully during nonstructured conversational speech.

This strategy may also be worth trying with clients who are excessively disfluent for other reasons—such as a relatively mild dysarthria—because it reduces their speaking rate. To determine whether a client would be likely to benefit from the use of this strategy, have him or her speak at a very slow rate. If doing so results in increased fluency, it is likely that he or she would be helped by self-monitoring.

Several other strategies have also been suggested for reducing the speaking rates of clients who exhibit this type of disfluency. These include having them pace their speech in a syllable-by-syllable manner, auditorily with the beats of a metronome or tactually with a pacing board (Helm-Estabrooks, 1986). With the latter, the client taps his or her finger from square to square while speaking in this manner (see Helm-Estabrooks, 1986, for an illustration of this board and further information about tactile pacing). Other strategies that have been suggested for this purpose include speaking under the condition of delayed auditory feedback (Helm-Estabrooks, 1986). Fluency-enhancing strategies used for treating stuttering—including utilizing a slow rate, learning to initiate phonation with an easy onset, and systematic desensitization—have also been used with such clients (Market et al., 1990).

Thus far, the discussion has been on treating clients with neurogenic acquired stuttering by encouraging them to speak in a manner that will cause the abnormal disfluency to occur less frequently. Since the disorder results from the abnormal functioning of one or more structures in the central nervous system, if it were possible to reduce the extent to which they malfunction, it also would be possible to reduce the resulting disfluency. There is some evidence that it may be possible to treat the disorder in this manner.

Bhatnagar and Andy (1989), for example, have described a person with this disorder who had a thalamic stimulation electrode implanted because of chronic pain. Within the first three weeks of daily self-stimulation, a noticeable reduction was reported in the client's disfluency. After two months, the client was reported to have become almost normally fluent. A two-and-a-half-year post-therapy follow-up indicated that he had not relapsed. (In another paper [Andy & Bhatnagar, 1991], incidentally, they reported that electrical stimulation at the same thalamic site in a normal speaker during surgery resulted in abnormal disfluency.) Also, Manders and Bastijns (1988) described a child with this disorder who recovered after an epileptic attack—a condition that by causing further damage may have normalized the functioning of some structure in the central nervous system.

Others (Van Riper, 1982) have reported similar outcomes. Perhaps, sometime in the future, it will be possible to normalize the functioning of such structures through the use of pharmacological agents (Helm-Estabrooks, 1986).

If a person who has neurogenic acquired stuttering fears being disfluent and desires to avoid it, he or she can develop stuttering as an overlay on the disorder. The mechanism by which this overlay can develop is essentially the same as that which both the diagnosogenic and expectancy neurosis theories (discussed elsewhere in the book) posit as being responsible for a child developing stuttering. That is, the person tries to avoid being disfluent and by so doing becomes even more disfluent.

Few persons who have neurogenic acquired stuttering are likely to develop a stuttering overlay. However, it is important to be cognizant of this possibility whenever you treat a client who has neurogenic acquired stuttering and to treat the overlay if a client appears to be developing one. The approach you would use for doing so would be essentially the same as you would use to reduce a stutterer's desire to avoid stuttering. Stressing the fact that the disfluency associated with neurogenic acquired stuttering has an organic etiology and, consequently, cannot be avoided may help to discourage the person from trying to avoid being disfluent. Getting the client to the "acceptance" stage in the grieving process (for normal speech) can also help to get his or her focus off of disfluency.

SELECTING AND IMPLEMENTING INTERVENTION STRATEGIES FOR PSYCHOGENIC ACQUIRED STUTTERING

The treatment of clients who have this disorder may require a combination of psychotherapy and speech therapy (Roth et al., 1989). With regard to the speech therapy component of management, clients are,

> . . . as a group, receptive and responsive to speech therapy, if the same techniques used in the treatment of adult stuttering that originates in childhood are applied. . . . When patients are persuaded that they have greater-than-expected capacity for fluent speech and are shown how to decrease the severity of stuttering blocks through the use of such traditional techniques as easy onset of voicing, light touch, or bounce during phonatory or articulatory blocking or struggle, their stuttering can diminish or disappear. A strong attitude of clinician encouragement and optimism seemed to be an indispensable component of such therapy. (Roth et al., 1989, p. 64)

If there is any doubt about the client's emotional health, he or she should be referred to a psychologist or psychiatrist for evaluation (Roth et al., 1989).

SELF-HELP FOR STUTTERING AND OTHER FLUENCY DISORDERS

The self-help movement has come a long way since its beginnings in 1935 with the founding of Alcoholics Anonymous. In 1990, it was estimated that 12,000,000 people "get help from helping" in approximately 500,000 such groups (Diggs, 1990). The largest self-help organization for persons who stutter or have another fluency disorder in the United States is the National Stuttering Association (NSA). (See Bradberry, 1997; Gregory, 1997; Reardon & Reeves, 2002; and Yaruss, Quesal, & Murphy, 2002.)

There are local self-help groups for persons who stutter, some of which are affiliated with national organizations (see Appendix B). Those who participate in them may or may not be receiving therapy concurrently. In some a speech-language pathologist attends meetings on a regular basis.

Through participating in meetings sponsored by local and national groups, reading their newsletters, and visiting their Web sites, stutterers are likely to become more aware that the problems they encounter in living with the disorder are not unique and can be coped with. They also may benefit from learning about the experiences others have had with particular approaches to therapy, about speech-language pathologists in their community who are experienced working with persons who have the disorder, and about books that may help them better understand and cope with stuttering (e.g., Carlisle, 1985; Tillis & Wager, 1984). According to Diggs (1989):

> Many self-help organizations encourage discussing how members cope with upsetting events. Problems are shared with other people who care. As one consumer said, "I'm not singled out. Somebody else is in the same boat." Members listen without judgment and learn together, recognizing others rights to their own beliefs.
>
> Through such experiences, many self-helpers decide for the first time that they don't have to hide their problem. A sense of normalization grows from being with people who share a problem, and often a social support system emerges. This socialization process seems to be quite important in the generic self-help movement, but may be even more critical to people with communication disorders where often the problems themselves promote social isolation. (p. 33)

Speech-language pathologists should refer clients to such groups if they feel they could benefit from participating in them. Those who have chronic perseverative stuttering syndrome are particularly likely to do so (Cooper, 1993). Some speech-language pathologists resist making such referrals (Pill & St. Louis, 1994). According to Cooper (1986):

> Many factors might be cited to explain the typical professional's lack of enthusiasm for self-help groups. I suspect that one of those factors is the professional's failure to accept the fact . . . that some individuals will continue to stutter no matter what they may do or have done to them and that even some successfully controlled stutterers need such continuing support to maintain their control. Clinicians may be uncomfortable with the existence of groups of individuals who may or may not continue to experience disfluencies but appear to benefit from the association with others with similar experiences. Perhaps professionals experience discomfort believing that they or their colleagues have failed if former clients seek such support. (p. 325)

Such resistance also can result from misconceptions clinicians have about these groups. They may think, for example, that group members just talk about depressing experiences and feel sorry for themselves. I agree with Diggs (1990, p. 33) that "Consumers are becoming more interested in taking charge of their own lives. Professionals need to recognize this trend and acknowledge the potential benefits of self-help." The families of persons who stutter—particularly the parents of young children who do so—may also benefit from participating in self-help groups (Aguirrebengoa, 1994).

Self-help groups for persons who stutter or have another fluency disorder exist in many countries. Information about them can be obtained from the European League of Stuttering Associations (ELSA) and the International Stuttering Association (ISA), a worldwide network of national self-help organizations (Pill & St. Louis, 1994). According to Pill and St. Louis:

> Around the world, support groups are variously termed self-help groups, therapy groups, and maintenance groups among other labels. Some groups dissociate themselves from speech professionals, some are autonomous organizations which communicate and closely cooperate with clinicians, and others function primarily as proponents of particular treatment methods or programs. (p. 201)

While members of self-help groups usually interact face-to-face, other options are possible. Starkweather (1994), for example, has reported on an electronic self-help group in which stutterers interact through e-mail.

In addition to self-help groups, there are self-help books. The Speech Foundation of America has published some that are co-authored by speech-language pathologists regarded as authorities on stuttering. These books are usable for parent counseling and for communicating to teenage and adult clients that their experiences with and feelings about stuttering are not unique and that they can cope with the disorder.

ASSESSING/DOCUMENTING THERAPY OUTCOME

The philosophy of management throughout this chapter (and, indeed, throughout this book) is based on the assumption that management of stuttering usually has two aspects: reduction (or elimination) of abnormal disfluency and reduction of the extent to which the disorder (assuming that it is not cured) interferes with the client's life. Consequently, when assessing/documenting therapy outcome, both aspects should be considered.

What strategies are likely to yield data possessing adequate levels of validity, reliability, and generality for this purpose? Pros and cons of a number of strategies are discussed in the "Proceedings of the NIDCD Workshop on Treatment Efficacy Research in Stuttering," published in 1993 in the *Journal of Fluency Disorders* (pp. 121–361), and in papers by Hillis (1993) and Franken, Boves, Peters, and Webster (1995).

In my own clinical practice, the strategy I have found most useful for gathering such data is questioning the client and possibly members of his or her family as well as others (such as teachers) who spend a significant amount of time with the client. I ask if aspects of the client's stuttering problem have changed and, if so, how. For gathering such data from the client, the *Stuttering Problem Profile* (see Appendix C) can be helpful: The client, who completed the profile prior to therapeutic intervention, is asked for each statement circled whether he or she is any closer to being successful now than prior to therapy.

My decision to evaluate therapy outcome clinically, primarily by questioning clients and those with whom they interact, was based on the results of a large-scale study of approaches for evaluating stuttering therapy that was summarized in a report by Drs. Wendell Johnson and William Trotter of the University of Iowa to the federal agency that funded it. The study was done in the late 1940s or early 1950s and, to my knowledge, was never published. One conclusion was that skillfully questioning a client about how he or she has changed yields data that are as reliable as those yielded by the 20 or more "objective" measures they evaluated. If a client has changed in any meaningful ways outside the therapy room, the client and/or members of his or her family are likely to be aware of it. The findings of a study by Finn and Ingham (1994), incidentally, in which stutterers were shown to be able to reliably rate an attribute of their "speech quality," tends to support this conclusion.

ASSIGNMENTS

Behavior Modification

Select an aspect of your behavior that you would like to modify and attempt to do so for a period of at least two months. Changes that my students have attempted to make include exercising more frequently, studying on a more regular schedule, losing weight, eating less junk food, keeping their apartments cleaner, biting their fingernails less frequently, being on time more often, watching less TV, and being less "negative" when talking with people. Keep a weekly journal in which you describe your successes and failures as honestly and objectively as you can. What problems did you encounter while doing this assignment? How did your motivation level vary during the months you were "in therapy?" What insights did you gain that hopefully will result in your functioning as a more effective clinician? This assignment is quite similar to one used by Leahy (1994).

Fluency-Facilitating Speech Strategy

A number of fluency-facilitating speech strategies are described in this chapter. Use one in all communication situations for at least a day. An example of a strategy you could use for this assignment is "a lengthening of vowels beyond that perceived . . . [by you] as being normal, short utterance lengths, and the use of frequent pauses" (McKeehan, 1994, p. 114). How did people react while you were using the strategy? How did their reactions affect you? What did you learn while doing this assignment that will affect your use of such strategies with clients? (This assignment is based on one described by McKeehan in her 1994 paper.)

Badge Wearing

One strategy for bringing stuttering out into the open is wearing a badge or a shirt on which a message is printed acknowledging the disorder. There is a store or kiosk in some shopping malls at which you can have such a badge printed. Make a badge, or have one made, that says "I stutter. So what!" and wear it for a day. Did you feel self-conscious at first while wearing it? It you did, were you less self-conscious at the end of the day than you were at the beginning? What reactions, if any, did you get while wearing it? In what situations do you think a stutterer might benefit from doing so?

Certainty Testing

We discussed in this chapter how people are handicapped by their "certainties." Identify one certainty you have that may be handicapping you. If possible, test it and describe what happened when you did so.

Support Group

There are support/self-help groups for persons who stutter in many communities. If there is one in your community, attend a meeting. In what ways are stutterers likely to benefit from participating in such a group? Should speech-language pathologists refer clients to them? Why?

Telecommunication Relay Service

Telecommunication relay services (TRSs) enable a speech-impaired person to communicate by telephone without having to speak (Silverman, 1997b, 1999b). They do so by typing what they want to "say," using either a personal computer with a modem attached or a telecommunication device for the deaf (TDD). For many stutterers, the telephone situation is one in which they stutter very severely (see chapter 2). Make at least two calls using your state's TRS. Under what circumstances might a stutterer benefit from using one?

8

Preventing Stuttering

> ### INSTRUCTIONAL OBJECTIVES
>
> By the end of this chapter, you should be able to:
>
> ▸ Specify two cultural factors that can prevent the onset of stuttering in children and the precipitation of stuttering overlays on other types of fluency disorders.
>
> ▸ Describe a strategy for preventing stuttering in young children.
>
> ▸ Describe a strategy for preventing stuttering from becoming a disability and/or a handicap.
>
> ▸ Describe a strategy for preventing overlays of stuttering on other fluency disorders.

Stuttering is a preventable disorder in the same sense that diabetes is a preventable disorder. While having a history of diabetes in your family places you at greater risk for developing the disorder than would be the case if there were no such history, there are things you can do—like not allowing yourself to become overweight—that can greatly reduce the likelihood of your developing diabetes, even though you may have a genetic predisposition to do so. Likewise, even though you have a genetic or other predisposition to develop stuttering, there are things that can be done that can greatly reduce the likelihood of your developing the disorder—to prevent the disorder from being precipitated. Our focus in this chapter will be on strategies for reducing the likelihood that stuttering will be precipitated, either by itself or as a psychological overlay on other fluency disorders (i.e., cluttering, neurogenic acquired stuttering, or psychogenic acquired stuttering).

CULTURAL CONSIDERATIONS

The cultural factors discussed in chapters 6 and 7 that can affect the clinical relationship when evaluating and treating clients who stutter can also affect it when attempting to prevent children from stuttering and both children and adults from developing stuttering overlays on their existing cluttering, neurogenic acquired stuttering, or psychogenic acquired stuttering

Two cultural factors are discussed in this section that can very adversely affect the prognosis for preventing stuttering and stuttering overlays. The first of these factors is what people in the culture believe to be the cause of stuttering. If it is believed to be a punishment for sin, or simply God's will, then it may not be considered appropriate to try to prevent it. Attempts to prevent stuttering and stuttering overlays are highly unlikely to be successful if it isn't possible to get clients and families who hold these beliefs to change them. A clergy member or a community cultural leader whom they respect may be able to facilitate their doing so.

The second of these factors is the value placed in the culture on not "losing face." The approach advocated here for preventing stuttering in young children is likely to require parents to change how they react to their child's syllable repetitions and other disfluencies, because their current reactions increase the likelihood of their child developing stuttering. That is, it requires parents to acknowledge (at least to themselves) that what they are doing is making it more, not less, likely that their child will stutter. By acknowledging this situation and changing how he or she reacts to the child's disfluencies, that parent could lose face with his or her spouse or with other family members. There is a script elsewhere in the chapter that may be helpful for dealing with this issue.

PREVENTING STUTTERING IN YOUNG CHILDREN

The goal on which I'll focus in this section is reducing the likelihood that a preschool-age child whose parents are concerned about his or her syllable repetitions and/or other disfluencies will develop stuttering. These disfluencies may result from a genetic predisposition to stutter. However, just like keeping weight down can reduce the likelihood that someone with a genetic predisposition for type-two diabetes will develop the disorder, the advice given here can reduce the likelihood that someone with a genetic predisposition to stutter will stutter.

The advice given in this chapter, even if conscientiously followed, is unlikely to prevent all cases of stuttering. One reason is that the disorder may have more than one cause (see chapter 5). The situation for conscientiously following advice for preventing stuttering, therefore, is similar to that for doing so to prevent type-two diabetes. That is, a person who tries to keep from becoming diabetic by being thin may still become diabetic, but he or she is considerably less likely to develop diabetes than someone who is fat.

Assumptions

The recommendations I'll be making are based on a slightly modified version of Wendell Johnson's diagnosogenic theory (see chapter 5). While Johnson appeared to believe that his theory, by itself, could explain the onset of stuttering, this may not be true. It may only specify a series of events that can precipitate the disorder in children who have a genetic predisposition to develop it. Regardless of whether or not a genetic predisposition is a necessary condition for a child to begin to stutter, the recommendations in this section should help to reduce the likelihood of the disorder being precipitated.

These recommendations are intended primarily for preschool-age children who are not exhibiting secondary symptoms and who do not appear to be aware of and concerned about their disfluency. Some of these children may, in fact, have begun to stutter. The overlap between Bloodstein's Phase I stuttering and the normal syllable repetition of preschoolers is considerable. For children who are exhibiting secondary symptoms and/or appear to be aware of and concerned about their disfluency, these recommendations, by themselves, are not adequate for managing their impairment. A more direct approach is necessary.

Recommendations

The child's parents and others in the child's environment must cease making the child conscious of and cease reacting negatively to his or her syllable repetitions and other disfluencies. The more the child attempts to avoid repeating syllables and being disfluent in other ways, the more frequently he or she is likely to repeat syllables and otherwise be disfluent, regardless of whether or not the child has already begun to stutter. This is likely to involve getting parents and others to cease saying things to the child like "talk more slowly," "stop and start over again," "think of what you're going to say before you say it," and/or "take a deep breath before you talk." It may also involve getting them to cease reacting nonverbally to the child' disfluency in ways that signal to the child that being disfluent is bad (e.g., having a disapproving-type facial expression while the child is being disfluent).

If the parents and others haven't been concerned about the child's disfluency for very long and/or haven't reacted to it very much in the ways indicated in the previous paragraph, merely telling them to avoid making the child self-conscious about his or her disfluency is likely to be sufficient. However, if the parents and/or others have been reacting to it in negative ways for a period of time, more counseling will probably be needed. One reason is that they're likely to reject this recommendation because accepting it would make them feel guilty—that is, it would either make them feel responsible for their child's stuttering or for placing the child at risk for doing so. Such feelings of guilt must be addressed for at least two reasons. First, failure to alleviate them would be doing the parents (or others) harm, which would be a violation of the ASHA ethical injunction "to hold paramount the welfare of persons served professionally." Second, the parents (or others) would probably resist modifying the reactions that make the child self-conscious about being disfluent and, hence, he or she would be likely to become increasingly more disfluent. The script reproduced below can be used by the clinician to enable those who are making a child feel self-conscious about being disfluent to save face and feel less guilty:

> I know that you love your child and that you were trying to help your child. You were doing what by "common sense" seemed to be the appropriate thing to do to help him (or her) talk better. Common sense usually works. This is one of those rare occasions when it doesn't. Indicating to your child that he (or she) should try to be more fluent is like telling yourself that you have to get a good night's sleep. The harder you try to make yourself sleep, the less likely you are to do so. The syllable repetitions and other hesitations in your child's speech work the same way. Consequently, what we have to do is to get your child to stop trying to avoid them and just concentrate on what he (or she) has to say. You should do everything that you can to encourage your child to talk and ignore his (or her) repetitions and other hesitations. Hopefully, your ignoring them will encourage your child to do so also. I hope that you won't feel too guilty about this. You did what was the common-sense thing to do to help your child. Furthermore, you sought an evaluation for your child, which tells me that you love and really want to help him (or her).

This script is not intended to be read aloud. Paraphrase and modify it in any way necessary to make it appropriate for a particular person.

A second objective is to make the child feel good about himself or herself as a communicator. Parents and others should be encouraged to focus more on what the child is saying than on how he or she is saying it. Communicating effectively and communicating fluently are not the same. Many stutterers now and in the past (e.g., Moses) have been very effective as communicators. The amount of positive reinforcement that a child receives for talking should be based on how well he or she communicates, not on how disfluency-free he or she talks. Having a child feel good about himself or herself as a communicator should reduce the likelihood that the child will stutter if he or she isn't already doing so. Furthermore, if the child is already stuttering and it isn't possible to ameliorate the disorder, feeling adequate as a communicator can help to prevent his or her impairment from becoming a disability, a handicap or both.

PREVENTING STUTTERING FROM BECOMING A DISABILITY AND/OR A HANDICAP

Stuttering is an impairment that rarely causes a preschooler who has it to be disabled or handicapped. Both tend to develop later. Their development can, in part, be accounted for by the impairment (i.e., the moments of stuttering) becoming more severe. However, the relationship between severity of stuttering and degree of disability and handicap is far from perfect. Many moderately severe stutterers are only minimally disabled and handicapped because of stuttering, and many mild stutterers are severely disabled or handicapped because of it. It would seem reasonable to conclude, therefore, that at least some of the disability and handicap associated with stuttering can be prevented.

Once it has been determined that a child has begun to stutter, one of the goals for managing it should be to prevent (or at least minimize) the emergence of disabilities and handicaps. Helping the child develop strategies for stuttering less severely should help to prevent their development, at least a little. However, these efforts may not be as effective as you'd expect. Almost any amount of residual stuttering can disable and/or handicap someone. If this weren't the case, very mild stutterers would rarely, if ever, be disabled or handicapped by their disorder.

One of the best ways to prevent stuttering from becoming a disability or a handicap is to do whatever you can to help children who have the disorder to feel good about themselves, particularly as communicators. A number of things you can do to help them are listed below.

- Base your comments to children on how well they *communicate* while speaking, rather than on how *fluent* they are.

- Encourage parents, teachers, and others who interact with children who stutter to base their comments to them on how well they communicate, rather than on how fluent they are.

- Encourage children who stutter to become involved with speech-related extracurricular activities (such as debating) in which success is determined by how well one communicates.

- Encourage children who stutter to read biographies of persons who were high achievers in spite of stuttering and to adopt such persons as role models.
- Discourage children who stutter from viewing their future as that of "a giant in chains."
- Encourage children who stutter to view living with stuttering as a *challenge*, which, if met, can possibly yield a more fulfilling life than otherwise.
- Encourage children who stutter to bring their stuttering out into the open.
- Encourage children who stutter to view their disfluency as a genetically-based individual difference (like being left-handed) rather than as a disorder.
- Encourage children who stutter to participate in an online or "live" self-help/support group for children with the disorder.
- Encourage their parents to get them some psychotherapy if they appear to be developing a poor self-concept.
- Encourage children who stutter to pursue interests and strengthen skills (e.g., in sports, art, or music) that are likely to cause them to be respected by their peers.

PREVENTING OVERLAYS OF STUTTERING ON OTHER FLUENCY DISORDERS

A person can develop stuttering as an overlay on cluttering, neurogenic acquired stuttering, and possibly even on psychogenic acquired stuttering. The development of such an overlay, fortunately, can sometimes be prevented. Some strategies you can use to reduce the likelihood of developing a stuttering overlay appear in this section.

Assumption

The assumption being made here is that the more strongly a person who evinces cluttering, neurogenic acquired stuttering, or psychogenic acquired stuttering fears being disfluent and desires to avoid being so, the more at risk he or she is for developing a stuttering overlay. (For a rationale for this assumption, see the discussion of stuttering as anticipatory-struggle behavior in chapter 5.)

Recommendation

Do whatever you can to keep the client from fearing disfluency. Some of the ways it might be possible to accomplish this goal are to:

- base your comments to the client on how well he or she communicates, rather than on how fluent he or she is.

- encourage the client to focus more on communication effectiveness, and less on disfluency, when judging how well he or she spoke in a situation.

- discourage the client from attempting to conceal being disfluent by avoiding talking.

- encourage the client to bring the fluency disorder out into the open—to be willing to acknowledge having it.

- do whatever you can to minimize the degree to which a fluency impairment disables or handicaps a client.

- do whatever you can to minimize the client's feelings of guilt, shame, and embarrassment about speaking disfluently.

- do whatever you can to facilitate the client accepting the fluency impairment and getting on with his or her life.

CAN CLUTTERING, NEUROGENIC ACQUIRED STUTTERING, AND PSYCHOGENIC ACQUIRED STUTTERING BE PREVENTED?

Based on the assumptions currently being made about the etiology of these disorders, they do not appear to be preventable. The consensus appears to be that cluttering is precipitated by a type of cerebral dysfunction that probably has a genetic etiology; neurogenic acquired stuttering is thought to be precipitated by damage to the brain; and psychogenic acquired stuttering is thought to be precipitated by a traumatic experience. Consequently, it's difficult to see how a speech-language pathologist could make a meaningful contribution toward preventing any of these disorders, except possibly by offering counseling to families in which there is a history of cluttering. Few persons, however, would be likely to consider cluttering sufficiently handicapping to warrant such counseling.

APPENDIX A

Wordings and Structures for Paragraphs and Sections in Fluency Disorder Evaluation Reports

A number of paragraphs and sections from evaluation reports of children and adults who have fluency disorders are reproduced in this appendix to be used as "boilerplate" for evaluation reports. These were abstracted from reports submitted to me by the following speech-language pathologists who have national and international reputations as authorities on the treatment of stuttering: Dr. Martin R. Adams, University of Houston; Dr. Oliver Bloodstein, Brooklyn College; Dr. Edward Conture, Syracuse University; Dr. Steven B. Hood, University of South Alabama; Dr. William H. Perkins, University of Southern California; Dr. Richard Shine, East Carolina University; and Dr. Ehud Yahri, University of Illinois at Urbana–Champaign. They are intended to suggest wordings and structures for communicating some types of information in such reports about the fluency disorder. All of the reports, incidentally, contained other types of information (e.g., birth and developmental histories and statements of the results of hearing and language tests). Family names were replaced with *Smith* to maintain confidentiality.

IDENTIFYING INFORMATION

Name:	Date Seen:
File Number:	Examiner:
Birthdate:	Parents:
Age:	Informant:
Address:	Referral:
Telephone:	Report Sent To:

Name:	Date of Evaluation:
Birthdate:	Informant for History:
Age:	Clinic File Number:
Sex:	Diagnostic Code Number:
Address:	Statement of Diagnosis:
Telephone::	

STATEMENT OF THE PROBLEM

This young boy, accompanied by his father and mother, appeared at the Speech, Hearing, and Language Clinic for a differential diagnosis of a suspected incipient stuttering problem.

℘   ℞

Stanley Smith, age eight years-eight months, was seen at this center for a speech and language evaluation. History information was provided by Stanley and his mother. Mrs. Smith indicated that she felt Stanley was becoming concerned about his speech and stated that Stanley has requested finding someone who could "help him with his speech." Of paramount concern to both Stanley and his mother was the increasingly frequent repetitions exhibited in Stanley's speech and his mounting concern over them.

℘   ℞

John, a four-year, nine-month-old male, was referred to the Speech and Hearing Clinic for a stuttering evaluation by his parents. His mother expressed concern about his stuttering and indicated it has worsened during the past year.

℘   ℞

Mr. Smith is a personable young man who appeared immediately open, confident, and relaxed in the relationship he established with me. He did almost no stuttering during the interview and could offer no explanation for his fluency in speaking with me. He reports that at times he stutters severely, however.

When he tried to imitate his stuttering it seemed to consist of hard contacts of the articulators. He says he feels marked muscular tension when he stutters, especially in the throat area. He is concerned about the fact that his stuttering has been getting worse lately; he feels it is unrealistic to hope for a complete cure but wants to "contain" the problem and if possible to ameliorate it. Another reason he has for desiring therapy at this time is that he is hoping for advancement in his job. He works for the phone company as a repairman and aspires to a management position in the company. He does not believe that his stuttering would hinder such advancement but feels it would be more appropriate if he stuttered less.

HISTORY OF THE DEVELOPMENT OF THE DISORDER

In regard to speech development, Jim's parents reported that he produced his first words before the age of 12 months and was speaking in sentences prior to the age of two years. At approximately two years, five months, Mr. and Mrs. Smith began to be concerned about their son's speech development. Mrs. Smith stated that Jim was repeating words and syllables at the beginning of sentences. Recently, he had also begun to experience difficulty with other words within his utterances. This behavior was particularly evident when Jim was excited or under stress. His parents further reported that Jim's fluency appeared to break down when he was engaged in competitive conversations with his brother and when Jim took his turn speaking to his father on the telephone while Mr. Smith was out of town on business.

$\wp$ ϖ

Joe could not report exactly when he began stuttering but stated that he was aware of it by age 10. He did not believe that there was any medical or traumatic experience at that time which precipitated his stuttering. During his high school years, when stress was intensified as a result of increased academic responsibility, Joe's stuttering became more severe. In college, familiar speaking situations and speaking with friends were thought by him to be relatively easy whereas speaking to professors and in front of classes have posed more difficulties.

$\wp$ ϖ

ℬ   ℭ

Mike's mother could not recall when he spoke his first word or when he started producing sentences. However, she did report that his stuttering behavior was first noticed at approximately two and a half years of age. His mother reported that "at one time his stuttering became better but then he went back to the speech problem." During the last six to eight months, his nursery school reported that during "circle time" the children were having trouble understanding Mike, and that this has caused him to become upset.

The patient is aware of his stuttering and dislikes slowing down or starting over when instructed by a parent. He reportedly is frustrated by his stuttering and dislikes his peers "making fun" of his speech.

The parents view Mike's stuttering as significant and stated that his stuttering has worsened during the past year. His mother is concerned about his self-esteem and aggressive behavior due to constant ridiculing from his peers at school. Initially, their attempts to "help" him overcome stuttering by having him "slow down" or stop and start over again were helpful, but during the past year his attempts to change his speaking behavior have been unsuccessful. At times he gets upset when asked to slow down or change his speaking pattern. According to his mother, his stuttering becomes worse when another person is present, especially his older sister. His mother feels he competes for attention and conversation with his sister, which results in his increased stuttering.

ℬ   ℭ

During a thirty-minute interview, Sam provided information about the onset and development of his fluency disorder. Sam reported that he began stuttering around the age of eight, and in second grade he was enrolled in speech therapy for remediation of his disfluencies. He explained that when his family moved to Greenfield, speech therapy was no longer available. He further explained that the period of time during which he did *not* receive any speech therapy at school was from the beginning of third grade until last spring (2003). Susan Jones, speech/language clinician at Greenfield High School, has reportedly provided fluency therapy services to Sam since the spring of 2003.

Sam recalled that his speech disfluencies during elementary school were mostly sound/syllable repetitions. He stated that "at first I wouldn't do it that much," and that since elementary school his speech disfluencies have "gotten worse." Sam reported that there were instances when he was unable to "get the word out."

Sam said that he became the most "conscious" of his speech in junior high. He stated that currently his disfluencies "come and go," and that he is the most disfluent during "one on one" situations. Sam explained that the aspect of his speech fluency which concerns him the most is its effect on his education. He gave the following example: "If

I've got to do a speech, I won't do it: then I get a bad grade." Sam reported that he is sometimes "embarrassed" by his speech disfluencies and expressed the hope that the problem will change so that he "will be able to talk clearer."

EVALUATION RESULTS—
SPEECH SAMPLE ANALYSES

An analysis of a 566-word sample of Tim's conversational speech revealed a total of 133 disfluencies, or 23.5 stuttered words per 100 words spoken. The breakdown of this figure according to specific disfluency types was as follows:

Part-word repetitions	7.95
Whole-word repetitions	4.77
Phrase repetitions	1.06
Interjections	9.01
Incomplete phrases	0.71
TOTAL	23.50

As can be seen, the predominant types of disfluencies in Tim's speech were interjections and part-word repetitions. The clinician estimated the average repetition to be three or four times. Although Tim indicated no specific phonemes on which he had more disfluencies, it was noted that the disfluencies occurred most consistently on words or syllables beginning with the vowel /I/. Tim exhibited quite fluent reading ability when he was asked to read both "The Rainbow Passage" and "My Grandfather." Analysis of these two reading samples revealed only one repetition and one prolongation throughout the total 463 words read. Tim's conversational speech was timed. His average rate of speaking of 169.5 words per minute was within the normal range.

Physical behaviors that typically accompany stuttering were observable as Tim spoke. Eye blinking, poor eye contact, and neck and facial muscle tension occurred quite consistently during moments of disfluency. Tim was often observed wringing his hands while he held the rest of his body rather still. Avoidance behaviors observed consisted primarily of interjections used as "starters."

On a seven-point scale for rating severity of stuttering, with one being very mild stuttering and seven being very severe stuttering, Tim's speech was rated by the clinician at five, although moments of more severe stuttering did occur.

$\wp$ $\wp$

Joseph engaged in a number of different speaking tasks. He was totally fluent during rote, automatic tasks such as counting, saying the days of the week and months of the year, and reciting the "Pledge of Allegiance." He was normally fluent when repeating sentences and reading a passage written for readers at the third-grade level.

Analysis of a 145-word spontaneous speech sample during dialogue yielded 54 disfluent moments (37%). Within these 54 disfluencies there were five instances of vocalized pauses and interjections which were "normal" disfluencies. Of particular concern, however, was the fact that syllable repetitions were noted to occur 34 times. For the most part repetitions were disrhythmic and accompanied by mild signs of tension. Most of the syllable repetitions were accompanied by increases in either pitch and/or loudness, and the schwa vowel was often substituted for the correct vowel. For most of the syllable repetitions the number of units ranged from three to five (i.e., *bo-bo-bo-boating, ba-ba-ba-ba-ba-badly*). During 21 of the 34 part-word repetitions, there was some degree of vowel prolongation during the final unit of repetition (row-row-*roooo*wing). There were 12 instances of vocalized sound prolongations (*wwwww*indow), nine of which were also accompanied by increases in either pitch and/or loudness. The remaining two disfluencies were single-unit whole-word repetitions. Moments of stuttering were usually between one and two seconds in duration. Avoidance behaviors were not observed.

Joseph's rate of speech was inconsistent. Because of the frequency and duration of disfluencies, his rate of speech in terms of meaningful words spoken was only 84 words per minute. However, this is misleading. Analysis of his articulation rate during fluent utterances yielded a typical range of between seven and nine syllables per second. Therefore, while his speech rate was slow, his fluent articulation rate was very fast.

ℰᴏ   ℛℯ

Martin was seen on July 8, 2003 for a speech evaluation. The assessment included obtaining a sample of his speech on videotape during a face-to-face conversation with a stranger and while reading.

The clinician observed that Martin's speech was marked by a high degree of disfluency. During the face-to-face conversation he stuttered on 18% of the syllables he uttered and spoke at an average rate of 153 syllables per minute. While reading, Martin averaged a speech rate of 162 syllables per minute with disfluency on 11% of his uttered syllables (above 7% disfluency is typically considered abnormal; 150 syllables spoken per minute is considered the low end of the normal speech rate range with the average speaker speaking about 225 syllables per minute). Martin's speech rate fell at the lower end of the normal range, in part because of numerous stops resulting from blocks while stuttering.

Martin's speech was characterized by prolongation and repetition of sounds, whole words, and phrases: it was also observed that he would sometimes run out of air at the ends of phrases. Accompanying his stuttering struggle were head jerks, general upper body movement, eye blinks, and facial tension. Though Martin related that he typically does not maintain eye contact during a moment of stuttering, during the evaluation his eye contact was excellent.

ℛ   ℛ

The *Stuttering Severity Instrument* (Riley, 1972) was administered to assess the severity of stuttering based on percentage of stuttered words, duration of the longest instance of stuttering, and physical concomitants.

During a 200-word spontaneous speech sample, Adam stuttered on 14% of the words spoken. The longest instance of stuttering was three seconds. Physical concomitants included lip pressing, tense jaw muscles, poor eye contact, and constant looking around. He obtained an overall score of 23, which placed him at the 77th percentile and resulted in the highest moderate rating of stuttering severity. A score of 24 would have placed him in the lowest level of the severe range. Based on reports by his parents that his stuttering is often more severe than it was during the evaluation, it would appear that Adam's stuttering severity sometimes falls at the low end of the severe range.

ℛ   ℛ

Administration of the *Stocker Probe Technique* (Stocker, 1980), which associates the level of communicative responsibility with the frequency of speech disfluencies, resulted in Dan producing a *total* of 19 speech disfluencies in response to 50 questions asked in reference to common objects. Dan's typical level of breakdown (the level at which speech disfluencies were *most* frequent) was level IV (8 speech disfluencies per 10 questions asked at this level). His typical level of recovery (the level at which speech disfluencies were *least* frequent) was level I (0 speech disfluencies per 10 questions asked at this level).

EVALUATION RESULTS—AVOIDANCES, ATTITUDES, AND BELIEFS

Harold was asked to list the people, situations, words, and sounds that he associates with the presence of at least mild stuttering. In response, the patient cited: (1) talking to his mother, grandmother, and grandfather; (2) talking with friends; (3) talking with professors; (4) talking on the phone; (5) answering questions or having to give a report in class; (6) introducing himself; and (7) saying words that begin with /w/ or /a/. Harold was quite candid in admitting that he routinely practices situational and word avoidance. That is, he will consciously seek to evade speaking in certain situations and using certain words. If he has no alternative but to speak, the patient indicated that he would say as little as possible.

Continuing the interview, the patient was asked to identify the behaviors that he uses to avoid an expected stuttering or to escape from a stuttering that is in progress. As regards avoidances, Harold replied with: (1) slowing down and breaking words into syllables; (2) taking a deep breath; (3) making word substitutions; (4) interjections; and (5) throat clearings. To escape from a stutter that is in progress, the client said that he might: (1) change to another word; (2) skip over the stuttered word; (3) interrupt the stutter and (a) take a deep breath before re-trying the word; (b) repeat the phrase leading up to the stuttered word; or (c) interject a sound before again attempting the stuttered word. All of these behaviors were observed by the clinician during the evaluation.

ℬ   ℭ

Jerry feels that some situations increase the severity of his stuttering. He has a harder time speaking to a group than to individuals. It is more difficult for him to speak to strangers than to people with whom he is familiar. Jerry did state, however, that he feels most people generally ignore his stuttering, although some of his students have expressed difficulty in listening to and understanding him at times. Some of the anxiety-producing situations Jerry mentioned were: speaking with people in authority, particularly professors; addressing his class; having to talk after arriving late to a meeting; and some phone conversations.

ℬ   ℭ

Michael reported that he has distinct anticipations of stuttering and often "looks ahead" as he speaks and chooses circumlocutions to avoid stuttering. Yet he deliberately avoids using word substitutions and believes he always has, by choice. He rarely avoids speaking situations. His most frequent emotional reaction when he stutters is frustration. Fear is a reaction he has only occasionally. He does not seem to be strongly driven to hiding his stuttering. Most of his close associates know he stutters and he is not excessively troubled by their reactions, although he finds it irritating when listeners supply words for him.

ℬ   ℭ

Results from responses to the Situational Reaction Questionnaire, Fluency Attitude Scale, and general background questions revealed that Kevin feels as though his stuttering holds him back in daily-life communication interactions as well as to some degree in communicative situations at work. Kevin reported that he is seeking help now because he wants to express himself "more freely."

Kevin seems to be very strongly motivated to improve his communication ability in order to experience greater personal satisfaction—to say what he wants to say and participate in speaking situations in which he would like to be involved with greater confidence and ease of speaking.

SUMMARY AND RECOMMENDATIONS

The general picture is that of a typical case of adult stuttering that has fallen somewhat short of its potential development as a serious personal problem. There is an absence of continual fear and shame, and systematic avoidance. Andrew's greatest fear is that the problem will continue to become more severe.

I outlined for Andrew the two major philosophies of stuttering therapy, the "talk differently" and the "stutter differently" approaches, emphasizing the advantages and disadvantages of each as objectively as possible, on the assumption that the choice should always lie with the stutterer. Without hesitation he expressed his preference for the stutter-differently method. He expressed a strong aversion to any approach that attempted to train him to speak in an unnatural manner. He was also emphatic in stating that his goal was not normal speech but a reduction in the severity of his stuttering. He expressed considerable enthusiasm about the idea of learning to stutter with less effort and tension. Accordingly, I suggested that we try the Van Riper techniques of cancellation and pull-outs.

80   03

Throughout the diagnostic session, Jerry exhibited moderate to severe stuttering. Although the speech therapy he received two-and-a-half years ago had been successful, it is apparent that he needs additional therapy. Jerry's stuttering clearly interferes with his personal and academic life, and his professional aspirations. Because he is a teaching assistant at present, it seems apparent that there is a need for him to obtain help for his stuttering. Jerry has expressed a desire to begin speech therapy and stated that his main goal to accomplish is to be able to go before a class "without stuttering much" and to be able "to handle it better." It is recommended, therefore, that he be enrolled in speech therapy.

80   03

This young man is presently exhibiting a stuttering problem of no worse than moderate severity. The problem seems weakly associated with anxiety, but closely connected to problems with the prompt, easy initiation and maintenance of voicing. Roy's clinical picture is further complicated by his extensive use of word and situational avoidance, and by his employment of other "tricks" that are designed to minimize or altogether mask the stuttering.

It was recommended to the client that he place himself on our clinic's waiting list for therapy this coming fall. Roy was agreeable to this suggestion.

When therapy is undertaken, it should involve two procedures that are utilized simultaneously. These procedures are training in breathstream management and conscious suppression of all escape/ avoidance behaviors. Treatment should be instituted on as intensive a basis as possible, certainly no less frequently than two, one-hour clinic visits per week.

APPENDIX B

Organizations and Web Sites for Persons Interested in Stuttering and Other Fluency Disorders

SELF-HELP ORGANIZATIONS

These organizations from the United States and Canada desire participation by speech-language pathologists as well as stutterers. There are comparable organizations in other countries. For further information about self-help organizations for stutterers worldwide, go to the Stuttering Home Page (www.stutteringhomepage.com) and click on "Support Organizations for PWS."

Friends
1220 Rosita Road
Pacifica, CA 94044-4223

Friends is a self-help organization for children who stutter and their parents. It sponsors an annual convention, a newsletter, and a Web site (www.friendswhostutter.org).

National Stuttering Association
5100 East LaPalma Avenue, Suite 208
Anaheim Hills, CA 92807

The NSA (which began in 1977 as the National Stuttering Project) is the largest of the self-help groups for persons who stutter in the United States. It has many local chapters for teenagers and adults. About 20 percent of its members are speech-language pathologists. It sponsors an annual convention, a newsletter, and a Web site (www.nsastutter.org).

Speak Easy Inc. of Canada
(speakez@NBNET.NB.CA)

Speak Easy Inc. of Canada is a self-help organization for Canadian persons who stutter. It provides information and support to both adults who stutter and the parents of children who stutter. It sponsors an online newsletter (send a blank e-mail to *speakeasycanada-subscribe@yahoogroups.com* to subscribe).

Stuttering Foundation of America
(www.stutteringhelp.org)

The Stuttering Foundation of America (formally known as the Speech Foundation of America) publishes low-cost books on stuttering for stutterers, their parents, and speech-language pathologists.

PROFESSIONAL ORGANIZATIONS

American Speech-Language-Hearing Association (ASHA)
10801 Rockville Pike
Rockville, MD 20852

ASHA is the major professional organization in the United States for speech-language pathologists and audiologists. It accredits clinical training programs in these fields and offers a Certificate of Clinical Competence in each of them. Its members treat and research all types of communicative disorders, including stuttering and other fluency disorders. ASHA has a Special Interest Division on Fluency and Fluency Disorders that offers advanced training and voluntary specialty certification for practitioners who specialize in managing these disorders. Information about fluency disorders is published in its journals and presented at its annual convention. For further information about ASHA and its involvement with fluency disorders, visit its Web site (www.asha.org).

Canadian Association of Speech-Language Pathologists and Audiologists (CASLPA) (www.caslpa.ca)

CASLPA performs much the same functions in Canada for regulating the practice of speech-language pathology and audiology that ASHA does in the United States.

International Fluency Association (IFA) (www.ruhr-uni-bochum.de/ifa/index.html)

IFA is an interdisciplinary, international organization for clinicians and researchers who specialize in fluency disorders as well as for persons who have them. Its publication is the *Journal of Fluency Disorders*. It usually sponsors an international congress on fluency disorders every three years.

State and Provincial Speech, Language, and Hearing Associations

Most of the states in the United States and provinces of Canada have a professional association for speech-language pathologists and audiologists. They almost always have an annual convention, the program of which is likely to include at least one session on stuttering or one of the other fluency disorders. The U.S. state associations can be accessed through the ASHA Web site and the Canadian provincial ones through the CASLPA Web site.

WEB SITES

Stuttering Homepage (www.stutteringhomepage.com)

This Web site, maintained by Dr. Judy Kuster at Minnesota State University at Mankato and updated frequently, provides links to many (perhaps most) of the Web sites that contain information about stuttering, cluttering, neurogenic acquired stuttering, and/or psychogenic acquired stuttering. A great place to begin any fluency-disorder-related Web site search.

STUTT-L

This listserv functions almost like an online self-help group. Contributors include speech-language pathologists, students training to become speech-language pathologists, and persons who stutter or have another fluency disorder. Students are encouraged to subscribe. Messages provide considerable insight about how persons who stutter (or have another fluency disorder) feel about their lives, their disorders, various approaches to therapy, and speech-language pathologists. To subscribe: Send an e-mail message to: *listserv@vm.temple.edu*. Type "Subscribe Stutt-l yourfirstname yourlastname" in the body of the message and send.

APPENDIX C

Evaluation Forms
and Tasks

1. The Rainbow Passage
2. Arthur the Young Rat
3. Sentence Repetition Task
4. The S-Scale
5. Stutterers Self-Ratings of Reactions to Speech Situations
6. Stuttering Problem Profile
7. Inventory of Communication Attitudes
8. Problem Profile for Elementary-School-Age Children Who Stutter about Talking
9. Physician's Screening Procedure for Children Who May Stutter
10. Stuttering Severity Instrument
11. Iowa Scale of Severity of Stuttering
12. Checklist of Stuttering Behavior
13. Perceptions of Self Semantic Differential Task
14. Southern Illinois University Speech Situation Checklist
15. Disfluency Descriptor Digest
16. Children's Attitudes about Talking—Revised (CAT-R)
17. The Cooper Chronicity Prediction Checklist
18. Daly's Checklist for Possible Cluttering—Experimental Edition

The Rainbow Passage

When the sunlight strikes raindrops in the air, they act like a prism and form a rainbow. A rainbow is a division of white light into many beautiful colors. These take the shape of a long round arch, with its path high above, and its two ends apparently beyond the horizon. There is, according to legend, a boiling pot of gold at one end. People look, but no one ever finds it. When a man looks for something beyond his reach, his friends say he is looking for the pot of gold at the end of the rainbow.

Throughout the centuries men have explained the rainbow in various ways. Some have accepted it as a miracle without physical explanation. To the Hebrews it was a token that there would be no more universal floods. The Greeks used to imagine that it was a sign from the gods to foretell war or heavy rain. The Norsemen considered the rainbow as a bridge over which the gods passed from earth to their home in the sky. Other men have tried to explain the phenomenon physically. Aristotle thought that the rainbow was caused by reflection of the sun's rays by the rain. Since then physicists have found that it is not reflection, but refraction of the raindrops which causes the rainbow. Many complicated ideas about the rainbow have been formed. The difference in the rainbow depends considerably upon the size of the water drops, and the width of the color band increases as the size of the drops increases. The actual primary rainbow observed is said to be the effect of superposition of a number of bows. If the red of the second bow falls upon the green of the first, the result is to give a bow with an abnormally wide yellow band, since red and green light when mixed form yellow. This is a very common type of bow, one showing mainly red and yellow, with little or no green or blue.

Reproduced with permission from Fairbanks, 1960, p. 127.

Arthur The Young Rat

Once, a long time ago, there was a young rat named Arthur who could never make up his flighty mind. Whenever his swell friends used to ask him to go out and play with them, he would only answer airily, "I don't know." He wouldn't try to say yes or no either. He would always shrink from making a specific choice.

His proud Aunt Helen scolded him: "Now look here," she stated, "no one is going to aid or care for you if you carry on like this. You have no more mind than a stray blade of grass."

That very night there was a big thundering crash and in the foggy morning some zealous men—with twenty boys and girls—rode up and looked at the fallen barn. One of them slipped back a broken board and saw a squashed young rat, quite dead, half in and half out of his hole. Thus, in the end the poor shirker got his just dues. Oddly enough his Aunt Helen was glad. "I hate such oozy, oily sneaks," said she.

Reproduced with permission from Darley & Spriestersbach, 1978, p. 276.

SENTENCE REPETITION TASK

The child is instructed to repeat each of the following sentences after the examiner.

1. Mother is cooking dinner.
2. Grandmother likes to receive letters.
3. Father's swimming suit has black and white stripes.
4. My sister really likes painting pictures.
5. Please give me the yellow balloon.
6. It was chilly at the football game.
7. Peter picked some green peppers.
8. Bring the broom and sweep the floor.
9. The wind blew briskly.
10. Frank likes to read sports magazines.
11. The baby carriage has been painted white.
12. David rode his bicycle to school.
13. On Sundays Christians go to church.
14. The bell on the fire engine rings loudly.
15. We had fresh bread for lunch on Tuesday and Wednesday.
16. The sun shone brightly today.

THE S-SCALE

The response for each statement that indicates an "undesirable" attitude is printed in brackets following it.

1. I usually feel that I am making a favorable impression when I talk. [F]
2. It is easy for me to talk to important people. [F]
3. More than anything else I would like to be able to talk better. [T]
4. You can't gain much by arguing. [T]
5. I find it easy to talk with almost anyone. [F]
6. I find it very easy to look at my audience while speaking to a group. [F]
7. I have felt self-conscious when reciting in class. [T]

continued →

8. A person who is my teacher or my boss is hard to talk to. [T]
9. I am often in places where I need to introduce one person to another. [F]
10. I would like to introduce the speaker at a meeting. [F]
11. I never did volunteer much to recite in class. [T]
12. Even the idea of giving a talk in public makes me afraid. [T]
13. Some words are harder than others for me to say. [T]
14. I would rather not introduce myself to a stranger. [T]
15. I forget all about myself shortly after I begin to give a speech. [F]
16. I am a good mixer. [F]
17. People sometimes feel uncomfortable when I am talking to them. [T]
18. I dislike introducing one person to another. [T]
19. I often ask questions in group discussions. [F]
20. I find it easy to keep control of my voice when speaking. [F]
21. I become suddenly afraid when called upon to speak. [T]
22. I do not mind speaking before a group. [F]
23. I find it easier to talk with persons younger than me. [T]
24. I do not talk well enough to do the kind of work I'd really like to do. [T]
25. My speaking voice is rather pleasant and easy to listen to. [F]
26. I am sometimes embarrassed by the way I talk. [T]
27. I face most speaking situations with complete confidence. [F]
28. There are few people I can talk with easily. [T]
29. I talk better than I write. [F]
30. My speech is the same as always. [F]
31. I wish it did not bother me to talk to people. [T]
32. It is easier to answer questions in class than to ask them. [T]
33. I often feel nervous while talking. [T]
34. In school I found it very hard to talk before the class. [T]
35. I find it hard to make talk when I meet new people. [T]
36. I often have to search for the words I want. [T]
37. I feel pretty confident about my speaking ability. [F]
38. I wish I could say things as clearly as others do. [T]
39. Even though I knew the right answer I often failed to give it because I was afraid to speak out. [T]

STUTTERER'S SELF-RATINGS OF REACTIONS TO SPEECH SITUATIONS

The four five-point scales used for rating speaking situations are defined as follows:

A. *Avoidance:*

1. I never try to avoid this situation and have no desire to avoid it.
2. I don't try to avoid this situation, but sometimes I would like to.
3. More often than not I do not try to avoid this situation, but sometimes I do try to avoid it.
4. More often than not I do try to avoid this situation.
5. I avoid this situation every time I possibly can.

B. *Reaction* [enjoyment of speaking in the situation]

1. I definitely enjoy speaking in this situation.
2. I would rather speak in this situation than not.
3. It's hard to say whether I'd rather speak in this situation than not.
4. I'd rather not speak in this situation.
5. I very much dislike speaking in this situation.

C. *Stuttering* [or substitute another type of abnormal disfluency behavior]:

1. I don't stutter at all (or only rarely) in this situation.
2. I stutter mildly (for me) in this situation.
3. I stutter with average severity (for me) in this situation.
4. I stutter more than average (for me) in this situation.
5. I stutter severely (for me) in this situation.

D. *Frequency:*

1. This is a situation I meet very often, two or three times a day, or even more, on the average.
2. I meet this situation at least once a day with rare exceptions (except Sunday perhaps).
3. I meet this situation from three to five times a week on the average.
4. I meet this situation once a week, with few exceptions, and occasionally I meet it twice a week.
5. I rarely meet this situation, certainly not as often as once a week.

Reproduced from Darley & Spriestersbach, 1978, pp. 317–318.

The speaking situations rated include the following:

1. Ordering in a restaurant
2. Introducing myself (face to face)
3. Telephoning to ask the price, train fare, etc.
4. Buying a plane, train, or bus ticket
5. Short class recitation (ten words or less)
6. Telephoning for a taxi
7. Introducing one person to another
8. Buying something from a store clerk
9. Conversation with a good friend
10. Talking with an instructor after class or in his or her office
11. Long distance telephone call to someone I know
12. Conversation with my father
13. Asking a person for a date (or talking to a person who asks me for a date)
14. Making a short speech
15. Giving my name over the telephone
16. Conversation with my mother
17. Asking a secretary if I can see her employer
18. Going to a house and asking for someone
19. Making a speech to an unfamiliar audience
20. Participating in a committee meeting
21. Asking an instructor a question in class
22. Saying hello to a friend going by
23. Asking for a job
24. Telling a person a message from someone else
25. Telling a funny story with one stranger in the crowd
26. Playing games requiring speech
27. Reading aloud to friends
28. Participating in a bull session
29. Dinner conversation with strangers
30. Talking with my barber (or beauty operator)
31. Telephoning to make an appointment, or arrange a meeting place with someone
32. Answering roll call in class
33. Asking at a desk for a book, or card to be filled out, etc.

continued →

34. Talking with someone I don't know well while waiting for a bus or class, etc.
35. Talking with other players during a playground game
36. Taking leave of a hostess
37. Conversation with a friend while walking along the street
38. Buying stamps at a post office
39. Giving directions or information to strangers
40. Taking leave of a girl (boy) after a date

Reproduced from Darley & Spriestersbach, 1978, pp. 318–319.

Means for adult male stutterers in terms of the twenty-fifth, fiftieth, and seventy-fifth percentile values for each of the four modes of response.

Response Mode of	Twenty-fifth Percentile	Fiftieth Percentile	Seventy-fifth Percentile
Avoidance	1.82	2.20	2.80
Reaction	2.10	2.56	2.97
Stuttering	2.08	2.53	2.98
Frequency	3.48	3.88	4.11

Adapted from Shumak, 1955, p. 356.

STUTTERING PROBLEM PROFILE

Name: _____ **Age:** _____ **Date:** _____

Address: _____

Instructions:

On the following pages are a list of statements made by stutterers about their stuttering problem following a period of therapy. In order to help you and your clinician to define goals for therapy, please circle the numbers of those statements that you would like to be able to make at the termination of therapy that you don't feel you could make now. If there are statements you would like to be able to make that aren't included in the list, write them on the last page.

1. I am usually willing to stutter openly.
2. I have learned to speak on exhalation rather than on inhalation.
3. I don't usually have trouble with the first sounds of words.
4. I no longer have a great deal of difficulty speaking in school.

continued →

5. I am able to give myself assignments and carry them out to my own satisfaction.

6. I am usually willing to use the telephone.

7. I am as cheerful as most people.

8. I don't usually experience a great mounting of tension and feeling of panic before speaking engagements.

9. I repeat sounds, syllables, and words infrequently.

10. I have a strong desire to do something about my stuttering problem.

11. I used to be quiet and shy. Now I tend to be outgoing.

12. My attitude toward my stuttering is no longer one of embarrassment.

13. I am not in a rush to respond when talking with people.

14. I don't usually experience emotional depression after stuttering in front of other people.

15. I can usually control the level of tensing when involved in speaking situations.

16. I can read relatively fluently.

17. I have learned to live with my problem.

18. I have learned not to be afraid of people.

19. I no longer have the feeling that stuttering is a miserable abnormality.

20. I am putting more emphasis on communicating well than on not stuttering.

21. I have learned how to stutter in a way that is more acceptable to the listener.

22. I have gained a better overall understanding of the problem.

23. I am confident that if I work at it, I can do something about my stuttering.

24. I understand how fluent speakers react to stutterers and why.

25. I usually don't hold myself back from talking when with a group of people.

26. I am not as ashamed as I used to be because of my stuttering.

27. I usually don't stutter much when giving a formal report to a group of people.

28. I have gained increased courage to participate in conversations, answer phone calls, and talk to strangers.

29. I am reasonably tolerant of nonfluency in general.

30. I usually don't avoid feared words and situations.

31. I no longer have a feeling of hopelessness about my stuttering.

32. My mental attitude toward my stuttering has changed. The gist of my present attitude is "true acceptance of the fact that I *am* a stutterer."

33. I talk as much as most people.

34. When around other people, I usually don't hold back my feelings because of fear of stuttering.

35. I usually am not preoccupied with myself.

36. I am usually willing to discuss my problem with other people.

37. I no longer object to my therapy program.

38. I have expanded my activities, both social and business.

39. I usually don't have strong feelings of shame and embarrassment when I block.

40. I now feel I could change what I do when I stutter if I would wake up and do it.

continued →

41. I no longer anticipate stuttering on certain sounds.
42. I am convinced that I can talk without having to struggle.
43. I don't usually become very anxious when I have to initiate a phone call.
44. My breathing while speaking usually isn't irregular.
45. When I stutter, related movements such as hand jerks and eye blinkings rarely occur.
46. I no longer speak at an excessive rate.
47. I usually am not afraid of public speaking.
48. I find it relatively easy to ask a clerk for something in a store.
49. I can purposely speak the way I want in the majority of situations.
50. I would be willing to become an officer in a club where I would have to give speeches.
51. I have learned that speaking can be an enjoyable experience.
52. I don't usually worry about entering speaking situations.
53. I don't usually become extremely depressed when in a period of "regression" in my speech.
54. I no longer consider myself an oddity because I stutter.
55. I usually am willing to say what I feel like saying.
56. I usually am not afraid to stutter in front of people.
57. My self-confidence has increased considerably.
58. It doesn't bother me to hear other stutterers speak.
59. I try to avoid changing words I think I will stutter on.
60. Words that I used to use as "starters" have all but completely disappeared.
61. I am getting involved in many speaking situations.
62. I believe I can overcome my problem to the extent I can live comfortably with it.
63. I look upon my stuttering as something that can be changed or modified.
64. I have as many friends as most people.
65. I have learned to modify some of the overt behavior, e.g., facial grimaces.
66. I am relatively relaxed in speaking situations.
67. I am sure I can completely conquer the problem.
68. I recognize the worth of experimenting and playing around with my stuttering.
69. I don't usually experience feelings of failure when in a period of "regression" in my speech.
70. I no longer try to avoid looking at the person with whom I am talking when I am stuttering.
71. I now rarely anticipate stuttering.
72. I feel that I have learned to accept the fact that I stutter.
73. I have quit being a lone wolf.
74. I do not react violently to my nonfluencies.
75. I feel fairly confident I can do something about my stuttering.
76. I have finally accepted the fact I am a stutterer. Before I never felt like I was one and always tried to "hide" it.

continued →

77. I push myself to enter situations in which I know I will stutter instead of avoiding them.
78. I probably talk to as many people as most persons.
79. I am usually willing to modify my stuttering blocks outside the therapy situation in the manner recommended by my therapist.
80. I usually don't worry very much about the reactions of others when I have a speech block.
81. I am paying more attention to my strengths than my weaknesses.
82. I tend to be relatively relaxed when giving a formal report to a group of people.
83. I usually am not afraid to approach people and talk to them.
84. I realize that improving my speech must be a day-to-day affair with specific goals and assignments set up.
85. I have accepted a certain amount of nonfluency as normal speech behavior.
86. I recite in the classroom as much as most students.

Additional Statements

INVENTORY OF COMMUNICATION ATTITUDES

Response Scales of the Inventory of Communication Attitudes

Affective Scale 1

1 __ I definitely enjoy speaking in this situation.

2 __

3 __

4 __

5 __

6 __

7 __ I hate speaking in this situation.

continued →

Behavioral Scale 2

1 __ My speech skills are excellent in this situation.

2 __

3 __

4 __

5 __

6 __

7 __ My speech skills are poor in this situation.

Cognitive-A Scale 3

1 __ Most speakers definitely enjoy speaking in this situation.

2 __

3 __

4 __

5 __

6 __

7 __ Most speakers hate speaking in this situation.

Cognitive-B Scale 4

1 __ Most speakers' speech skills are excellent in this situation.

2 __

3 __

4 __

5 __

6 __

7 __ Most speakers' speech skills are poor in this situation.

Frequency Scale 5

1 __ I meet this situation 2 or 3 times a day, or more, on the average.

2 __

3 __

4 __

5 __

6 __

7 __ I never meet this situation.

Thirteen Situational Subscales and Associated Items of the Inventory of Communication Attitudes

Subscale 1: Telephone Conversations
Item 01 Telephoning to ask a price, train fare, etc.
Item 02 Telephoning to make an appointment with a stranger.
Item 03 Talking with a salesperson on the telephone.

Subscale 2: Argument/Conflict with a Friend
Item 04 Refusing a friend a favor
Item 05 Confronting a friend who has failed to fulfill an agreement.
Item 06 Criticizing a friend for a mistake he or she has made.

Subscale 3: Argument/Conflict with a Stranger
Item 07 Arguing with a salesperson about an overcharge.
Item 08 Arguing with a service person to provide additional service or to lower the cost of service.
Item 09 Complaining to a waiter/waitress about poor service.

Subscale 4: One-to-One Conversation with a Family Member
Item 10 Talking with my father.
Item 11 Talking with my mother.
Item 12 Talking with a family member while riding in a car.

Subscale 5: One-to-One Conversation with an Authority Figure
Item 13 Telling my doctor what is ailing me.
Item 14 Talking with a lawyer.
Item 15 Talking with a store manager.

Subscale 6: Group Conversation with Known Group (Informal)
Item 16 Telling a funny story to a group of 2 to 8 friends.
Item 17 Talking with a group of 2 to 8 friends at a party.
Item 18 Carrying on a conversation with 2 to 8 friends during a card, golf, or other game.

Subscale 7: Group Conversations with Unknown Group (Informal)
Item 19 Talking with 2 to 8 strangers during dinner.
Item 20 Taking part in a discussion group of 2 to 8 strangers.
Item 21 Starting off a discussion in a group of 2 to 8 strangers.

Subscale 8: Formal Presentations
Item 22 Making a short speech (1 or 2 minutes) at work or in a class.
Item 23 Making a 5- to 10-minute speech at work or in a class.
Item 24 Acting as a spokesperson or representative of a group in a meeting at work or in a class.

continued →

Subscale 9: *Questioning a Friend or Family Member to Obtain Information or to Elicit Action*

Item 25 Asking a friend for a ride.

Item 26 Asking a family member for money (a small loan).

Item 27 Asking a family member for advice.

Subscale 10: *Questioning a Stranger to Obtain Information or to Elicit Action*

Item 28 Asking a stranger for the time of a movie or other event.

Item 29 Asking for stamps at the post office.

Item 30 Asking a waiter/waitress for help.

Subscale 11: *Questioning an Authority Figure to Obtain Information or to Elicit Action*

Item 31 Asking a police officer for directions or information.

Item 32 Asking a question of a boss at work or an instructor in class.

Item 33 Asking a question of an authority at a forum or a meeting.

Subscale 12: *Situations Involving Time Constraints*

Item 34 Asking a secretary to see his or her employer when I am late for an appointment.

Item 35 Asking for flight or bus information when I am late for that plane or bus.

Item 36 Talking to a store clerk when a number of other customers are waiting for help.

Subscale 13: *Situations Involving Memorized Content or Unchangeable Content*

Item 37 Telling someone my address.

Item 38 Telling someone my telephone number.

Item 39 Telling someone my name.

Reproduced from Watson, Gregory, & Kistler, 1987, pp. 449–450.

PROBLEM PROFILE FOR ELEMENTARY-SCHOOL-AGE CHILDREN WHO STUTTER ABOUT TALKING

Below are the aspects of talking sampled and some examples of questions that would be asked about each:

"Whom Do You Like to Talk to?" Questions   Whom do you like to talk to at home; at school? Whom don't you like to talk to at home; at school? Whom do you think likes to talk with you at home; at school? Whom do you think doesn't like to talk with you at home; at school? Questions of this kind can also be asked in terms of a 3-point scale, such as, "Who likes to talk to you best at home, the next best, the least best?" After each answer you can obtain additional information by asking questions such as "Why do you think this is so?"

"Who Talks the Most?" Questions   Who talks the most (the least) at home? Whom do you talk to the most (the least) at home; at school? Whom does your father, mother, brother, . . . talk to the most (the least) at home? Again, these questions can be put on a scale whereby the child ranks the relative amount each member of the family talks. The same scale can be used to find the relative amount the child talks in comparison with other children at home or at school. Where appropriate, follow his or her answer with "Why?"

"Who Interrupts?" Questions   Who interrupts the most at home, school, play? Who interrupts the least? This question can be pursued by asking who interrupts father, mother, brother, the most? Who interrupts you the most (the least)? Whom do you interrupt the most (the least) at home; at school? An answer obtained to any question can [and probably should] be pursued by asking "why" questions.

"Who Are Good Talkers?" Questions   Who's the best talker at home? Who's the next best talker? Who's the poorest talker at home? Why do you consider him or her to be a good talker? Why do you consider (the ones named toward the bottom of the list) not to be very good talkers? If the child does not include her- or himself, you can ask directly about where he puts her- or himself on the scale of "good talker" or "poor talker." The same question can be asked about his or her school environment.

"When Do You Want to Talk Well?" Questions   Are there times when you want to talk extra well? Where? Why? Are there times when you don't care particularly how you talk? Where? Why? Do you think this is true about other people who talk?

"Where Do You Want to Talk More than You Do?" Questions   In school, on the playground, at parties, when company comes, do you talk more than, less than, or about the same amount as other children in your class? Are there times when you wish you could talk more but aren't permitted to? Why do you think this is so? Does this happen with other children? Why?

"Who Listens?" Questions   Who pays the most (the least) attention to you when you talk at home; at school? What do you like listeners to do when you talk to them? How do you want them to listen? For example, do you want them to look down; to look at you; to smile; to frown; to interrupt you; to talk for you? Who does the most and the least of those things that you (like) (don't like) at home; at school? Why do you think they do it?

Reproduced with permission from Williams, 1978, pp. 68–70.

PHYSICIAN'S SCREENING PROCEDURE FOR CHILDREN WHO MAY STUTTER

Child's Name _____   File _____

Date of Birth _____   Age _____

Exam Date _____

	Normal	Borderline	Abnormal	Very Abnormal
Area A *Types of disfluencies*	1. Repeats phrases or whole words. 2. Interjects "uh" while thinking.	3. Repeats the first sound of a word 2 or 3 times without tension.	4. Repeats sound 4 or more times before getting the word out.	5. Child has tense voice during the repetitions. 6. Child has "hard" blocks. Gets stuck on words.
Area B *Other behaviors during abnormal disfluencies*				1. Tries to change words for fear of stuttering. 2. Child struggles to get word out as seen in facial grimaces and/or hand, arm or foot movements.
Area C *Frequency of abnormal disfluencies*		1. Infrequent (less than 2%).	2. Frequent (one in every 2–3 sentences).	3. Very frequent (one or more per sentence).
Area D *Child's reactions to the abnormal disfluencies*	1. None. Seems unaware of them.		2. Child just keeps on trying.	3. Child gives up trying to say the sentence or asks, "Why can't I talk right?"

continued →

	Normal	Borderline	Abnormal	Very Abnormal
Area E *Other people's reactions to the abnormal disfluencies.*	1. No one is bothered by the disfluencies.		2. Parents are afraid he/she will not outgrow the stuttering.	3. Child is very upset by teasing or other listener reactions.
Area F *How long since the abnormal disfluencies were first noticed?*		1. They began less than four months ago.	2. They began 4 to 12 months ago.	3. They began more than 12 months ago.

Examiner's Comments: _____

Note the number of "Abnormal" and "Very abnormal" symptoms on the right-hand half of the page.

1 or 2 symptoms?___ (Monitor)   3 or more symptoms?___ (Refer)

Examiner: _____

Reproduced with permission from Riley & Riley, 1989, p. 64.

STUTTERING SEVERITY INSTRUMENT (SSI)

Frequency (Use A or B, not both)

A. For readers. Use 1 and 2				B. For nonreaders		
1. Job Task		*2. Reading Task*		*Picture Task*		
Per-centage	Task Score	Per-centage	Task Score	Per-centage	Task Score	
1	2	1	2	1	4	
2–3	3	2–3	2	2–3	6	
4	4	4–5	5	4	8	
5–6	5	6–9	6	5–6	10	*Total*
7–9	6	10–16	7	7–9	12	*Frequency*
10–14	7	17–26	8	10–14	14	*A (1 & 2)*
15–28	8	27 and up	9	15–28	16	*or*
29 and up	9			29 and up	18	*B*

Duration

Estimated Length of Three Longest Blocks	Task Score	
Fleeting	1	
One half second	2	
One full second	3	
2 to 9 seconds	4	
10 to 30 seconds (by second hand)	5	*Total*
30 to 60 seconds	6	*Duration*
More than 60 seconds	7	*Score*

Physical Concomitants

Evaluating Scale   0 = *none;* **1** = *not noticeable unless looking for it;* **2** = *barely noticeable to casual observer;* **3** = *distracting;* **4** = *very distracting;* **5** = *severe and painful looking.*

1. Distracting sounds. Noisy breathing, whistling, sniffing, blowing, clicking sounds	0 1 2 3 4 5	
2. Facial grimaces. Jaw jerking, tongue protruding, lip pressing, jaw muscles tense	0 1 2 3 4 5	
3. Head movement. Back, forward, turning away, poor eye contact, constant looking around	0 1 2 3 4 5	*Total*
4. Extremities movement. Arm and hand movement, hands about face, torso movement, leg movements, foot tapping or swinging	0 1 2 3 4 5	*Physical Concomitant Score*

IOWA SCALE OF SEVERITY OF STUTTERING

Speaker _____   **Age** ___ **Sex** ___ **Date** _____

Rater _____   **Identification** _____

Instructions:

Indicate your identification by some such term as "speaker's clinician," "clinical observer," "clinical student," or "friend," "mother," "classmate," et cetera. Rate the severity of the speaker's stuttering on a scale from 0 to 7, as follows:

0   No stuttering

1   *Very mild*—stuttering on less than 1 percent of words; very little relevant tension; disfluencies generally less than one second in duration; patterns of disfluency simple; no apparent associated movements of body, arms, legs, or head.

2   *Mild*—stuttering on 1 to 2 percent of words; tension scarcely perceptible; very few, if any, disfluencies last as long as a full second; patterns of disfluency simple; no conspicuous associated movements of body, arms, legs, or head.

3   *Mild to moderate*—stuttering on about 2 to 5 percent of words; tension noticeable but not very distracting; most disfluencies do not last longer than a full second; patterns of disfluency mostly simple; no distracting associated movements.

4   *Moderate*—stuttering on about 5 to 8 percent of words; tension occasionally distracting; disfluencies average about one second in duration; disfluency patterns characterized by an occasional complicating sound or facial grimace; an occasional distracting associated movement.

5   *Moderate to severe*—stuttering on about 8 to 12 percent of words; consistently noticeable tension; disfluencies average about 2 seconds in duration; a few distracting sounds and facial grimaces; a few distracting associated movements.

6   *Severe*—stuttering on about 12 to 25 percent of words; conspicuous tension; disfluencies average 3 to 4 seconds in duration; conspicuous distracting sounds and facial grimaces; conspicuous distracting associated movements.

7   *Very severe*—stuttering on more than 25 percent of words; very conspicuous tension; disfluencies average more than 4 seconds in duration; very conspicuous distracting sounds and facial grimaces; very conspicuous distracting associated movements.

Reproduced from Sherman, 1952.

Checklist of Stuttering Behavior

Name_____   Age ____   Sex ____

Observer_____   Date _____

Instruction to Observer:

Observe the stutterer as he or she speaks or reads aloud. Focus your attention on such disfluencies and related reactions as you would classify as stuttering. Observe these reactions as they are associated with the speaking of specific words. Write each such word at the top of a column and make a checkmark in the appropriate space to indicate each type of disfluency or other reaction observed. Note by the use of 1, 2, 3, et cetera, the sequencing of behaviors. Under "Supplementary Observations" add descriptive details concerning any of the numbered items checked, and comment on apparent emotionality of the speaker, general degree of tension, relevant remarks made by the speaker, and so on.

Types of Reaction	Word 1	Word 2	Word 3	Word 4	Word 5	Word 6
1. Repeating part of word	—	—	—	—	—	—
2. Repeating whole monosyllabic word	—	—	—	—	—	—
3. Repeating this and other word(s)	—	—	—	—	—	—
4. Saying "uh—uh" or the like	—	—	—	—	—	—
5. Prolonging sound(s)	—	—	—	—	—	—
6. Pausing in the middle of word	—	—	—	—	—	—
7. Failing to complete the word	—	—	—	—	—	—
8. Holding breath	—	—	—	—	—	—
9. Gasping	—	—	—	—	—	—
10. Inhaling irregularly	—	—	—	—	—	—
11. Exhaling irregularly	—	—	—	—	—	—
12. Speaking on exhausted breath	—	—	—	—	—	—
13. Delay in starting word	—	—	—	—	—	—
14. Pressing lips together	—	—	—	—	—	—
15. Pressing tongue against teeth or palate	—	—	—	—	—	—
16. Closing eyes	—	—	—	—	—	—
17. Protruding tongue	—	—	—	—	—	—
18. Enlarging eyes	—	—	—	—	—	—
19. Opening mouth irrelevantly	—	—	—	—	—	—
20. Dilating nostrils	—	—	—	—	—	—

continued →

Types of Reaction	Word 1	Word 2	Word 3	Word 4	Word 5	Word 6
21. Turning head sideways	—	—	—	—	—	—
22. Bending head downward	—	—	—	—	—	—
23. Moving head up or back	—	—	—	—	—	—
24. Moving hands or fingers	—	—	—	—	—	—
25. Moving legs or feet	—	—	—	—	—	—
26. Moving body	—	—	—	—	—	—
27. Other (specify)	—	—	—	—	—	—
28. _____	—	—	—	—	—	—
29. _____	—	—	—	—	—	—
30. _____	—	—	—	—	—	—

Supplementary Observations:

Reproduced with permission from Darley & Spriestersbach, 1978, pp. 307–308.

PERCEPTIONS OF SELF SEMANTIC DIFFERENTIAL TASK

Below are some rating scales each with nine points. I would like you to evaluate YOURSELF, as you typically are, on each of these scales. Please circle the number on the scale that best describes yourself, on each scale.

	1	2	3	4	5	6	7	8	9
1.	Open								Guarded
	1	2	3	4	5	6	7	8	9
2.	Nervous								Calm
	1	2	3	4	5	6	7	8	9
3.	Cooperative								Uncooperative
	1	2	3	4	5	6	7	8	9
4.	Shy								Bold
	1	2	3	4	5	6	7	8	9
5.	Friendly								Unfriendly
	1	2	3	4	5	6	7	8	9
6.	Self-conscious								Self-assured
	1	2	3	4	5	6	7	8	9
7.	Tense								Relaxed
	1	2	3	4	5	6	7	8	9
8.	Sensitive								Insensitive
	1	2	3	4	5	6	7	8	9
9.	Anxious								Composed
	1	2	3	4	5	6	7	8	9
10.	Pleasant								Unpleasant
	1	2	3	4	5	6	7	8	9
11.	Withdrawn								Outgoing
	1	2	3	4	5	6	7	8	9
12.	Quiet								Loud
	1	2	3	4	5	6	7	8	9
13.	Intelligent								Dull
	1	2	3	4	5	6	7	8	9
14.	Talkative								Reticent
	1	2	3	4	5	6	7	8	9
15.	Avoiding								Approaching

continued →

	1	2	3	4	5	6	7	8	9
16.	Fearful								Fearless
	1	2	3	4	5	6	7	8	9
17.	Aggressive								Passive
	1	2	3	4	5	6	7	8	9
	Afraid								Content
	1	2	3	4	5	6	7	8	9
19.	Introverted								Extroverted
	1	2	3	4	5	6	7	8	9
	Daring								Hesitant
	1	2	3	4	5	6	7	8	9
21.	Secure								Insecure
	1	2	3	4	5	6	7	8	9
22.	Emotional								Bland
	1	2	3	4	5	6	7	8	9
23.	Perfectionistic								Careless
	1	2	3	4	5	6	7	8	9
24.	Bragging								Self-derogatory
	1	2	3	4	5	6	7	8	9
25.	Inflexible								Flexible

Reproduced with permission from Kalinowski et al., 1987, pp. 329–331.

SOUTHERN ILLINOIS UNIVERSITY SPEECH SITUATION CHECKLIST

Instructions:

The items in this checklist refer to speech situations, situations where you are involved in talking. Talking in these situations may or may not currently cause you some negative emotion, e.g., fear, tension, anxiety, or other unpleasant feelings. In the column as indicated put the number that best describes how much each of these speech situations disturbs you nowadays.

0 = not relevant
1 = not at all
2 = a little
3 = a fair amount
4 = much
5 = very much

continued →

Rating	Speech Situation
1.	Talking on the telephone
2.	Talking to a stranger
3.	Giving your name
4.	Talking with a young child
5.	Saying a sound or word that has been troublesome in the past
6.	Placing an order in a restaurant
7.	Talking to an animal
8.	Placing a person-to-person telephone call
9.	Talking with a close friend
10.	Arguing with parents
11.	Talking with a sales clerk
12.	Talking in a rap or bull session
13.	Being criticized
14.	Meeting someone for the first time
15.	Talking after being teased about your speech
16.	Saying hello
17.	Reading an unchangeable passage aloud
18.	Being misunderstood
19.	Answering a specific question
20.	Asking for information
21.	Being interviewed for a job
22.	Trying to get across your own point of view
23.	Introducing yourself
24.	Giving directions
25.	Talking when "high"
26.	Talking to hairdresser
27.	Talking when trying to make a good impression
28.	Talking when generally happy
29.	Talking with teachers
30.	Making an appointment with a secretary
31.	Asking the teacher a question
32.	Answering questions about your speech
33.	Being asked to repeat your answer
34.	Being asked to give your name
35.	Making introductions
36.	Being asked to give personal information
37.	Asking if someone is at home
38.	Buying a plane, bus, or train ticket to a specific place

continued →

Rating	Speech Situation
39.	Telling a taxicab driver where to take you
40.	Asking a gas station attendant for a specific amount of gas
41.	Speaking before a group
42.	Making an appointment
43.	Giving a prepared speech
44.	Being rushed when speaking
45.	Apologizing
46.	Being with a member of the opposite sex
47.	Refuting a criticism
48.	Giving a telephone number
49.	Giving an ad lib report
50.	Returning a call
51.	Selling a product

Reproduced with permission from Hanson, Gronhovd, & Rice, 1981, pp. 354–355.

DISFLUENCY DESCRIPTOR DIGEST

The University of Alabama
Department of Communicative Disorders

Personalized Fluency Control Therapy
Disfluency Descriptor Digest,
For the Identification of
Appropriate Fluency Initiating Gestures

Client _____   File No. _____
Clinician _____   Date _____

Directions:

Below are statements describing behavior frequently observed in the disfluent speech of stutterers. Place a check (✓) in the box preceding the statement if the behavior is present in the client's stuttering pattern even if the behavior occurs only occasionally.

☐   1. Disfluencies are characterized by obvious "struggle behavior" in the laryngeal area prior to speech onset.

continued →

☐ 2. Frequently the disfluency is characterized by obvious articulatory posturings of the jaw, lips, or tongue prior to the initiation of sound.

☐ 3. Speech appears monotone with abnormally little variation in intensity and pitch.

☐ 4. The onset and the termination of speech sounds in continued speech appears abnormally abrupt.

☐ 5. The breathing pattern for speech appears to be more "clavicular" or "thoracic" than abdominal.

☐ 6. Articulatory movements appear abnormally rapid.

☐ 7. The habitual pitch level appears too high or low for the individual's age, sex, and size.

☐ 8. The voice quality appears "harsh," "husky," or "hoarse."

☐ 9. In general, the rate of speech appears rapid.

☐ 10. Disfluencies frequently are characterized by rapid and repetitious articulatory movements of the jaw, lips, or tongue.

☐ 11. During periods of disfluency, the breathing pattern appears asynchronous and disruptive to fluent speech.

☐ 12. Disfluencies frequently are characterized by fixed articulatory placements of the jaw, lips, or tongue resulting in a complete closure of the vocal tract.

☐ 13. Disfluencies frequently appear to originate at the level of the larynx with an inability to initiate phonation.

☐ 14. Inhalation prior to the speech attempt appears abnormally rapid.

☐ 15. Inhalation prior to the speech attempt appears insufficient.

☐ 16. Inhalation prior to the speech attempt appears abnormally prolonged.

☐ 17. Speech appears abnormally soft with respect to loudness.

☐ 18. Disfluencies appear to occur at the end of an exhalation—client appears "out-of-breath."

☐ 19. Pauses are observed between the cessation of inhalation and the initiation of phonation.

☐ 20. Speech appears abnormally loud.

continued →

Directions:

Now place a check (✓) before those numbers in the box below that correspond to the statement numbers that you checked above. When finished you might be able to identify more clearly which FIG or FIGs will be most helpful for your client.

FIG Fluency Initiating Gesture	Numbers of statements above describing behavior modified by the FIG						
Slow Speech	☐6	☐9	☐10				
Smooth Speech	☐4	☐8	☐12				
Easy Onset	☐1	☐2	☐7	☐12	☐13	☐19	
Deep Breath	☐5	☐7	☐11	☐14	☐15	☐16	☐18
Syllable Stress	☐3	☐11	☐12				
Loudness Control	☐3	☐8	☐17	☐20			

Reproduced with permission from Cooper, 1982, p. 357.

CHILDREN'S ATTITUDES ABOUT TALKING—REVISED (CAT-R)

Read each sentence carefully so you can say if it is true or false for you. The sentences are about your talking. If you feel that the sentence is right, circle "True." If you think the sentence about your talking is not right, circle "False." Remember, circle "False" if you think the sentence is wrong and "True" if you think it is right.

1.	I don't talk right.	**True**	False
2.	I don't mind asking the teacher a question in class	True	**False**
3.	Sometimes words will stick in my mouth when I talk.	**True**	False
4.	People worry about the way I talk.	**True**	False
5.	It is harder for me to give a report in class than it is for most of the other kids.	**True**	False
6.	My classmates don't think I talk funny.	True	**False**
7.	I like the way I talk.	True	**False**
8.	People sometimes finish my words for me.	**True**	False
9.	My parents like the way I talk.	True	**False**
10.	I find it easy to talk to most everyone.	True	**False**
11.	I talk well most of the time.	True	**False**
12.	It is hard for me to talk to people.	**True**	False
13.	I don't talk like other kids.	**True**	False
14.	I don't worry about the way I talk.	True	**False**
15.	I don't find it easy to talk.	**True**	False

continued →

16.	My words come out easily.	True	**False**
17.	It is hard for me to talk to strangers.	**True**	False
18.	The other kids wish they could talk like me.	True	**False**
19.	Some kids make fun of the way I talk.	**True**	False
20.	Talking is easy for me.	True	**False**
21.	Telling someone my name is hard for me.	**True**	False
22.	Words are hard for me to say.	**True**	False
23.	I talk well with most everyone.	True	**False**
24.	Sometimes I have trouble talking.	**True**	False
25.	I would rather talk than write.	True	**False**
26.	I like to talk.	True	**False**
27.	I wish I could talk like other kids.	**True**	False
28.	I am afraid the words won't come out when I talk.	**True**	False
29.	I don't worry about talking on the phone.	True	**False**
30.	People don't seem to like the way I talk.	**True**	False
31.	I let others talk for me.	**True**	False
32.	Reading out loud in class is easy for me.	True	**False**

(The answers in "bold" indicate a negative attitude toward talking.)

Reproduced with permission from De Nil & Brutten, 1991a, pp. 65–66.

THE COOPER CHRONICITY PREDICTION CHECKLIST

Instructions:

To be completed for children ages three to eight. Answers to questions require the assistance of the child's parents. Each item should be explained and discussed with the parents. Place a check (✓) on the appropriate blank.

	Yes	No	Unknown

I. Historical Indicators of Chronicity

1. Is there a history of chronic stuttering in the family? ___ ___ ___

2. Is the severity (frequency, duration, consistency) of the disfluencies increasing? ___ ___ ___

3. Did the disfluencies begin with blockings rather than with easy repetitions? ___ ___ ___

4. Have the child's disfluencies persisted since being observed (as opposed to being episodic with long periods of normal fluency)? ___ ___ ___

5. Has the child been disfluent for two or more years? ___ ___ ___

continued →

	Yes	No	Unknown

II. Attitudinal Indicators of Chronicity

   1. Does the child perceive himself or herself to be disfluent? ___ ___ ___

   2. Does the child experience communicative fear because of the disfluencies? ___ ___ ___

   3. Does the child believe the disfluency problem to be getting worse? ___ ___ ___

   4. Does the child avoid speaking situations? ___ ___ ___

   5. Does the child express anger or frustration because of the disfluencies? ___ ___ ___

III. Behavioral Indicators of Chronicity

   1. Do sound prolongations or hesitations occur among the disfluencies? ___ ___ ___

   2. Are the repetitions more frequently whole-word or phrase repetitions rather than part-word repetitions? ___ ___ ___

   3. Are the part-word repetitions accompanied by visible tension or stress? ___ ___ ___

   4. Do the part-word repetitions occur more than three times on the same word? ___ ___ ___

   5. Is the rapidity of the syllable repetitions faster than normal? ___ ___ ___

   6. Is the schwa vowel inappropriately inserted in the syllable repetition? ___ ___ ___

   7. Is the air flow during the repetitions often interrupted? ___ ___ ___

   8. Do prolongations last longer than one second? ___ ___ ___

   9. Do prolongations occur on more than one word in a hundred during periods of disfluency? ___ ___ ___

   10. Are the prolongations uneven or interrupted as opposed to being smooth? ___ ___ ___

   11. Is there observable tension during the prolongation? ___ ___ ___

   12. Are the terminations of the prolongations sudden as opposed to being gradual? ___ ___ ___

   13. During prolongations of voiced sounds is the airflow interrupted? ___ ___ ___

   14. Are the silent pauses prior to the speech attempt unusually long? ___ ___ ___

   15. Are the inflection patterns restricted and monotone? ___ ___ ___

   16. Is there loss of eye contact during the moment of disfluency? ___ ___ ___

   17. Are there observable and/or distracting extraneous facial or body movements during the moment of disfluency? ___ ___ ___

                             Total 'Yes' Responses ___ ___ ___

continued →

Instructions:

Place a check (✓) on the appropriate blank.

Predictive of Recovery:	0–6	—
Requiring Vigilance:	7–15	—
Predictive of Chronicity:	16–27	—

Caution: The categorization of scores used on this checklist is based on an interpretation of data reported by McClelland and Cooper (*Journal of Fluency Disorders*, 1978) and on clinical observation. It is not based on longitudinal studies. Judgments as to probable stuttering chronicity should not be based solely on the scoring of this checklist.

From: Cooper, E. B., & Cooper, C. S. (1985). *Cooper personalized fluency therapy handbook* (rev.). Allen, TX: DLM Teaching Resources. Used with permission from DLM Teaching Resources.

Reproduced with permission from Gordon & Luper, 1992.

DALY'S CHECKLIST FOR POSSIBLE CLUTTERING—EXPERIMENTAL EDITION

Client's Name _____   Date_____

Instructions:

Please respond to each descriptive statement below. Your answers should reflect how well you believe the statement describes the child/adult:

Statement True for Client	Not at all 0	Just a little 1	Pretty much 2	Very much 3
1. Repeats syllables, words, phrases	0	1	2	3
2. Started talking late; onset of words and sentences delayed	0	1	2	3
3. Fluency disruptions started early; no remissions; never very fluent	0	1	2	3
4. Speech very disorganized; confused wording	0	1	2	3
5. Silent gaps or hesitations common; interjections; many "filler" words	0	1	2	3
6. Stops before saying initial vowel; no tension; drawn out vowels	0	1	2	3
7. Rapid rate (speaks too fast); tachylalia; speaks in spurts	0	1	2	3
8. Extrovert; high verbal output; compulsive talker	0	1	2	3

continued →

Statement	Not True for Client	Just a at all 0	Pretty little 1	Very much 2	much 3
9.	Jerky breathing pattern, respiratory dysrhythmia	0	1	2	3
10.	Slurred articulation (omits sounds or unstressed syllables)	0	1	2	3
11.	Mispronounciation of /r/, /l/, and sibilants	0	1	2	3
12.	Speech better under pressure; e.g., during short periods of heightened attention	0	1	2	3
13.	Difficulty following directions; impatient/ uninterested listener	0	1	2	3
14.	Distractible; attention span problems; poor concentration	0	1	2	3
15.	Story-telling difficulty (trouble sequencing events)	0	1	2	3
16.	Demonstrates word-finding difficulties resembling anomia	0	1	2	3
17.	Inappropriate reference by pronouns is common	0	1	2	3
18.	Improper language structure; poor grammar and syntax	0	1	2	3
19.	Clumsy and uncoordinated; motor activities accelerated (or hasty)	0	1	2	3
20.	Reading disorder is a prominent disability	0	1	2	3
21.	Disintegrated and fractionated writing; poor motor control	0	1	2	3
22.	Writing shows transposition of letters and words (omits letters and syllables)	0	1	2	3
23.	Left-right confusion; delayed hand preference	0	1	2	3
24.	Initial loud voice; trails off to a murmer; mumbles	0	1	2	3
25.	Seems to think faster than he can talk or write	0	1	2	3
26.	Above average in mathematical and abstract reasoning abilities	0	1	2	3
27.	Poor rhythm, timing, or musical ability (may dislike singing)	0	1	2	3
28.	Improper stress patterns of speech; poor melodic accenting of syllables	0	1	2	3
29.	Appears younger than age; small and/or immature	0	1	2	3
30.	Other family member with same/similar problem; heredity	0	1	2	3
31.	Untidy; careless, hasty; impulsive or forgetful	0	1	2	3
32.	Impatient, superficial, and/or short-tempered	0	1	2	3
33.	Lack of self-awareness; unconcerned attitude over inappropriateness of many behaviors and responses	0	1	2	3

Total Score _____

Diagnosis _____

continued →

Other Relevant Information Determined by Interviewer. (Circle correct answer)

Identified in school as
learning disabled.   Yes   No   Recommended for testing   Don't know

Currently receiving speech/
language therapy   Yes   No   Recommended   Don't know

Comments: _____

_____

_____

Clinician _____

Experimental Edition by
David A. Daly, 1991

Reproduced with permission from Daly, 1993a.

References

Adamczyk, B. (1994). Stuttering therapy with the "Echo Method." *Journal of Fluency Disorders*, 19, 147.

Adams, M. R. (1982). A case report on the use of flooding in stuttering therapy. *Journal of Fluency Disorders*, 7, 343–353.

Adams, M. R. (1992). Childhood stuttering under "positive" conditions. *American Journal of Speech-Language Pathology*, 1(3), 5–6.

Adams, M. R., & Runyan, C. M. (1981). Stuttering and fluency: Exclusive events or points on a continuum? *Journal of Fluency Disorders*, 6, 197–218.

Adams, M. R., Sears, R. L., & Ramig, P. R. (1982). Vocal changes in stutterers and nonstutterers during monotoned speech. *Journal of Fluency Disorders*, 7, 21–35.

Aguirrebengoa, L. (1994). Prevention of stuttering: Parents of stuttering children. *Journal of Fluency Disorders*, 19, 148–149.

Ainsworth, S., & Fraser-Gruss, J. (1981). *If Your Child Stutters: A Guide for Parents*. Memphis, TN: Speech Foundation of America.

Ambrose, N. G., & Yairi, E. (1994). The development of awareness of stuttering in preschool children. *Journal of Fluency Disorders*, 19, 229–245.

Ambrose, N. G., Yairi, E., & Cox, N. (1993). Genetic aspects of early childhood stuttering. *Journal of Speech and Hearing Research*, 36, 701–706.

Amman, J. O. C. (1700). *A Dissertation on Speech*. Reprinted 1965, New York: Stechert-Hafner.

Amster, B. (1994). Perfectionism and stuttering. *Journal of Fluency Disorders*, 9, 150.

Anderson, D. (1994). He stammers! That's a pity!: Historical perceptions of stuttering as reflected in the arts. *Journal of Fluency Disorders*, 19, 150.

Andrews, G. (1984). The epidemiology of stuttering. In R. F. Curlee & W. H. Perkins (Eds.), *The Nature and Treatment of Stuttering: New Directions*. San Diego, CA: College-Hill.

Andrews, G., Craig, A., Feyer, A.-M., Hoddinott, S., Howie, P., & Neilson, M. (1983). Stuttering: A review of research findings and theories circa 1982. *Journal of Speech and Hearing Disorders*, 48, 226–246.

Andrews, G., & Harris, M. (1964). *The Syndrome of Stuttering*. London: William Heinemann Medical Books.

Andrews, G., & Tanner, S. (1982a). Stuttering treatment: An attempt to replicate the regulated-breathing method. *Journal of Speech and Hearing Disorders*, 47, 138–140.

Andrews, G., & Tanner, S. (1982b). Stuttering: the results of 5 days treatment with an airflow technique. *Journal of Speech and Hearing Disorders*, 47, 427–429.

Andy, O. J., & Bhatnagar, S. C. (1991). Thalamic-induced stuttering (Surgical observations). *Journal of Speech and Hearing Research*, 34, 796–800.

Appelt, A. (1911). *Stammering and its Permanent Cure*. London: Methuen.

Arnold, G. E. (1959). Spastic dysphonia: I. Changing interpretations of a persistent affliction. *Logos*, 2, 3–14

Arnott, N. (1828). *Elements of Physics*. Edinburgh: Adams.

Aronson, A. E. (1973). *Psychogenic Voice Disorders; An Interdisciplinary Approach to Detection, Diagnosis, and Therapy*. New York: W. B. Saunders.

Atkins, C. P. (1988). Perceptions of speakers with minimal eye contact: Implications for stutterers. *Journal of Fluency Disorders*, 13, 429–436.

Attanasio, J. S. (1987). A case of late-onset or acquired stuttering in adult life. *Journal of Fluency Disorders*, 12, 287–290.

Azrin, N. H., Nunn, R. G., & Frantz, S. E. (1979). Comparison of regulated breathing vs. abbreviated desensitization on reported stuttering episodes. *Journal of Speech and Hearing Disorders*, 44, 331–339.

Barbara, D. A. (1982). *The Psychodynamics of Stuttering*. Springfield, IL: Charles C. Thomas.

Barber, V. (1939). Studies in the psychology of stuttering: XV. Chorus reading as a distraction in stuttering. *Journal of Speech Disorders*, 4, 371–383.

Baumgartner, J. M. (1999). Acquired psychogenic stuttering. In R. F. Curlee (Ed.), *Stuttering and Related Disorders of Fluency*. New York: Thieme, 269–288.

Baungartner, J. M., & Brutten, G. J. (1983). Expectancy and heart rate as predictors of the speech performance of stutterers. *Journal of Speech and Hearing Research*, 26, 383–388.

Bebout, L., & Arthur, B. (1992). Cross-cultural attitudes toward speech disorders. *Journal of Speech and Hearing Research*, 35, 45–52.

Beech, H. R., & Fransella, F. (1968). *Research and Experiment in Stuttering*. New York: Pergamon.

Bell, A. M. (1853). *Observations on Defects of Speech, the Cure of Stammering, and the Principles of Elocution*. London: Hamilton-Adams.

Bellak, L. (1954). *The Thematic Apperception Test and the Children's Apperception Test in Clinical Use*. New York: Grune & Stratton.

Benecken, J. (1994). On the nature and clinical relevance of a stigma: "The stutterer." *Journal of Fluency Disorders*, 19, 154.

Berlin, C. I. (1960). Parents' diagnoses of stuttering. *Journal of Speech and Hearing Research*, 3, 372–379.

Berlin, S., & Berlin, L. (1964). Acceptability of stuttering and control patterns. *Journal of Speech and Hearing Disorders*, 29, 436–441.

Bernstein-Ratner, N., & Benitez, M. (1985). Linguistic analysis of a bilingual stutterer. *Journal of Fluency Disorders*, 10, 211–219

Bhatnagar, S. C., & Andy, O. J. (1989). Alleviation of acquired stuttering with human centremedian thalamic stimulation. *Journal of Neurology, Neurosurgery, and Psychiatry*, 52, 1182–1184.

Blanton, S., & Blanton, M. G. (1936). *For Stutterers.* New York: D. Appleton-Century.

Blood, I. M., Wertz, H., Blood, G. W., Bennett, S., & Simpson, K. C. (1997). The effects of life stresses and daily stresses on stuttering. *Journal of Speech and Hearing Research*, 40(1), 134–143.

Bloodstein, O. (1960). The development of stuttering: II. Developmental phases. *Journal of Speech and Hearing Disorders*, 25, 366–376.

Bloodstein, O. (1961). The development of stuttering: III. Theoretical and clinical implications. *Journal of Speech and Hearing Disorders*, 26, 67–82.

Bloodstein, O. (1984). *Speech Pathology: An Introduction* (2nd Ed.). Boston, MA: Houghton Mifflin Company.

Bloodstein, O. (1987). *A Handbook on Stuttering* (4th Ed.). Chicago: National Easter Seal Society.

Bloodstein, O. (1988). Verification of stuttering in a suspected malingerer. *Journal of Fluency Disorders*, 13, 83–88.

Bloodstein, O. (1990). On pluttering, skivering, and floggering: A commentary. *Journal of Speech and Hearing Disorders*, 55, 392–393.

Bloom, C. M., & Silverman, F. H. (1973). Do all stutterers adapt? *Journal of Speech and Hearing Research*, 16, 518–521.

Bloom, L. (1978). Notes for a history of speech pathology. *Psychoanalytic Review*, 65, 433–463.

Bluemel, C. S. (1957). *The Riddle of Stuttering.* Danville, IL: Interstate Publishing Company.

Boberg, E. (1981). *The Maintenance of Fluency.* New York: Elsevier.

Boberg, E., Howie, P., & Woods, L. (1979). Maintenance of fluency: A review. *Journal of Fluency Disorders*, 4, 93–116.

Boberg, E., Yeudall, L. T., Schopflocher, D., & Bo-Lassen, P. (1983). The effect of an intensive behavioral program on the distribution of EEG alpha power in stutterers during the processing of verbal and visuospatial information. *Journal of Fluency Disorders*, 8, 245–263.

Boberg, J. M., & Boberg, E. (1990). The other side of the block: The stutterer's spouse. *Journal of Fluency Disorders*, 15, 61–75.

Boberg, J., & Kully, D. (1997). Spouses as adjuncts in stuttering therapy. *Seminars in Speech and Language*, 18(4), 357–369.

Bogue, B. N. (1926). *Stammering: Its Cause and Cure.* Indianapolis, IN: Author.

Boome, E. J., & Richardson, M. A. (1931). *The Nature and Treatment of Stammering.* London: Methuen & Co.

Boone, D. R. (1987). *Human Communication and Its Disorders.* Englewood Cliffs, NJ: Prentice-Hall.

Borden, G. L., Baer, T., & Kenney, M. K. (1985). Onset of voicing in stuttered and fluent utterances. *Journal of Speech and Hearing Research*, 28, 363–372.

Boyce, W., Broers, T., & Paterson, J. (2001). CBR and disability indicators. *ASIA Pacific Disability Rehabilitation Journal*, 12(1), 3–21.

Bradberry, A. (1997). The role of support groups and stuttering therapy. *Seminars in Speech and Language*, 18(4), 391–399.

Brady, J. P. (1971). Metronome-conditioned speech retraining for stuttering. *Behavior Therapy*, 2, 129–150.

Brady, J. P. (1998). Drug-induced stuttering: A review of the literature. *Journal of Clinical Psychopharmacology*, 18(1), 50–54.

Brady, W. A., & Hall, D. E. (1976). The prevalence of stuttering among school-age children. *Language, Speech, and Hearing Services in Schools*, 7, 75–81.

Brauneis, E. (1994). The use of acupuncture in a holistic approach to the treatment of stuttering. *Journal of Fluency Disorders*, 19, 158.

Brill, A. A. (1923). Speech disturbances in nervous and mental diseases. *Quarterly Journal of Speech*, 9, 129–135.

Brown, G., & Cullinan, W. L. (1981). Word-retrieval difficulty and disfluent speech in adult anomic speakers. *Journal of Speech and Hearing Research*, 24, 358–365.

Brown, S. F. (1945). The loci of stutterings in the speech sequence. *Journal of Speech Disorders*, 10, 181–192.

Brutten, G. J., & Shoemaker, D. J. (1967). *The Modification of Stuttering*. Englewood Cliffs, NJ: Prentice-Hall.

Brutten, G. J., & Shoemaker, D. J. (1974). *Speech Situation Checklist*. Carbondale: Speech Clinic, Southern Illinois University.

Bryngelson, B. (1952). Suggestions in the theory and treatment of dysphemia and its symptom, stuttering. *The Speech Teacher*, 1, 131–136.

Canter, G. (1971). Observations on neurogenic stuttering: A contribution to differential diagnosis. *British Journal of Disorders of Communication*, 6, 139–143.

Carlisle, J. A. (1985). *Tangled Tongue: Living with a Stutter*. Toronto: University of Toronto Press.

Cash, T. F., & Pruzinsky, T. (Eds.) (1990). *Body Images*. New York: Guilford Press.

Cherry, C., & Sayers, B. (1956). Experiments upon the total inhibition of stammering by external control and some clinical results. *Journal of Psychosomatic Research*, 1, 233–246.

Cicero (1942). *Cicero de Oratore* [Translated by E. W. Sutton]. London: Heinemann.

Collins, C. R., & Blood, G. W. (1990). Acknowledgment and severity of stuttering as factors influencing nonstutterers' perceptions by stutterers. *Journal of Speech and Hearing Disorders*, 55, 75–81.

Commodore, R. W., & Cooper, E. B. (1978). Communicative stress and stuttering frequency during normal, whispered, and articulation-without-phonation speech modes. *Journal of Fluency Disorders*, 3, 1–12.

Conture, E. G., & Fraser, J. (1989). *Stuttering and Your Child: Questions and Answers*. Memphis, TN: Speech Foundation of America.

Conture, E. G., & Guitar, B. E. (1993). Evaluating efficacy of treatment of stuttering: School-age children. *Journal of Fluency Disorders*, 18, 253–287.

Conture, E. G., & Kelly, E. M. (1991). Young stutterers' nonspeech behavior during stuttering. *Journal of Speech and Hearing Research*, 34, 1041–1056.

Conture, E. G., McCall, G. N., & Brewer, D. W. (1977). Laryngeal behavior during stuttering. *Journal of Speech and Hearing Research*, 20, 661–668.

Cooper, E. B. (1978). Facilitating parental participation in preparing the therapy component of the stutterer's Individualized Education Program. *Journal of Fluency Disorders*, 3, 221–228.

Cooper, E. B. (1982). A disfluency descriptor digest for clinical use. *Journal of Fluency Disorders*, 7, 355–358.

Cooper, E. B. (1986). Treatment of Stuttering: Future trends. *Journal of Fluency Disorders*, 11, 317–327.

Cooper, E. B. (1987). The chronic perseverative stuttering syndrome: Incurable stuttering. *Journal of Fluency Disorders*, 12, 381–388.

Cooper, E. B. (1993). Chronic Perseverative Stuttering Syndrome: A harmful or helpful construct? *American Journal of Speech-Language Pathology*, 2(3), 11–15, 21–22.

Cooper, E. B., Cady, B. B., & Robbins, C. J. (1970). The effect of the verbal stimulus words *wrong, right*, and *tree* on the disfluency rates of stutterers and nonstutterers. *Journal of Speech and Hearing Research*, 13, 239–244.

Cooper, E. B., & Cooper, C. S. (1985b). *Cooper Personalized Fluency Control Therapy Handbook*. Allen, TX: DLM Teaching Resources.

Cooper, E. B., & Rustin, L. (1985). Clinician attitudes toward stuttering in the United States and Great Britain: A cross-cultural study. *Journal of Fluency Disorders*, 10, 1–17.

Cordes, A. K., & Ingham, R. J. (1994). The reliability of observational data: II. Issues in the identification and measurement of stuttering events. *Journal of Speech and Hearing Research*, 37, 279–294.

Coriat, I. H. (1931). The nature and analytical treatment of stuttering. *Proceedings of the American Speech Correction Association*, 1, 151–156.

Craig, A. (1998). Relapse following treatment for stuttering: A critical review and correlative data. *Journal of Fluency Disorders*, 23, 1–30.

Craig, A. R., & Calver, P. (1991). Following up on treated stutterers: Studies of perceptions of fluency and job status. *Journal of Speech and Hearing Research*, 34, 279–284.

Craven, D. C., & Ryan, B. P. (1984). The use of a portable delayed auditory feedback unit in stuttering therapy. *Journal of Fluency Disorders*, 9, 237–243.

Cross, D. E., & Luper, H. L. (1983). Relation between finger reaction time and voice reaction time in stuttering and nonstuttering children and adults. *Journal of Speech and Hearing Research*, 26, 356–361.

Culton, G. L. (1986). Speech disorders among college freshmen: A 13-year survey. *Journal of Speech and Hearing Disorders*, 51, 3–7.

Curlee, R. F. (1993). *Stuttering and Related Fluency Disorders*. New York: Thieme Medical Publishers.

Daly, D. A. (1981). Differentiating stuttering subgroups with Van Riper's developmental tracks: A preliminary study. *Journal of the National Student Speech and Hearing Association*, 9, 89–101.

Daly, D. A. (1986). The clutterer. In Kenneth O. St. Louis (Ed.), *The Atypical Stutterer*. Orlando, FL: Academic Press.

Daly, D. A. (1987). Use of the home VCR to facilitate transfer of fluency. *Journal of Fluency Disorders*, 12, 103–106.

Daly, D. A. (1988). *The Freedom of Fluency: A Therapy Program for the Chronic Stutterer*. Moline, IL: LinguiSystems.

Daly, D. A. (1992). Helping the clutterer: Therapy considerations. In F. Myers & K. O. St. Louis (Eds.), *Cluttering: A Clinical Perspective* Leicester, Great Britain: Far Communications, 107–121.

Daly, D. A. (1993a). Cluttering: Another fluency syndrome. In R. Curlee (Ed.), *Stuttering and Related Disorders of Fluency*. New York: Thieme Medical Publishers, 179–204.

Daly, D. A. (1993b). Cluttering: The orphan of speech-language pathology. *American Journal of Speech-Language Pathology*, 2(2), 6–8.

Daly, D. A., & Burnett, M. L. (1999). Cluttering: Traditional views and new perspectives. In R. F. Curlee (Ed.), *Stuttering and Related Disorders of Fluency*. New York: Thieme Medical Publishers, 222–254.

Daly, D. A., Thompson, J. D., & Simon, C. A. (1985). Treatment of cluttering with stutter-free speech and mental imagery. Paper presented at the annual meeting of the American Speech-Language-Hearing Association in Cincinnati.

Darley, F. L. (1955). The relationship of parental attitudes and adjustments to the development of stuttering. In W. Johnson and R. Leutenegger (Eds.), *Stuttering in Children & Adults*. Minneapolis: University of Minnesota Press.

Darley, F. L., & Spriestersbach, D. C. (1978). *Diagnostic Methods in Speech Pathology* (2nd Ed.). New York: Harper & Row.

Darwin, E. (1800). *Zoonomia*. London.

Deal, J. L. (1982). Sudden onset of stuttering: A case report. *Journal of Speech and Hearing Disorders*, 47, 301–304.

Deal, J. L., & Doro, J. M. (1987). Episodic hysterical stuttering. *Journal of Speech and Hearing Disorders*, 52, 299–300.

Dempsey, G. L., & Granich, M. (1978). Hypno-behavioral therapy in the case of a traumatic stutterer: A case report. *International Journal of Clinical and Experimental Hypnosis*. 26, 125–133.

Denhardt, R. (1890). *Das Stottern. Eine Psychose*. Leipzig: Ernst Keil's Nachfolger.

Dewar, A., Dewar, A. D., & Anthony, J. F. K. (1976). The effects of auditory feedback masking on concomitant moments of stuttering. *British Journal of Disorders of Communication*, 11, 95–102.

Dickson, S. (1971). Incipient stuttering and spontaneous remission of stuttered speech. *Journal of Communication Disorders*, 4, 99–110.

Dietrich, S., Jensen, K. H., & Williams, D. E. (2001). Effects of the label "stutterer" on student perceptions. *Journal of Fluency Disorders*, 26, 55–66.

Diggs, C. C. (1990). Self-help for communication disorders. *ASHA*, 32 (1), 32–34.

DiLollo, D., Neimeyer, R. A., & Manning, W. H. (2002). A personal construct psychology view of relapse: Implications of a narrative therapy component to stuttering treatment. *Journal of Fluency Disorders*, 27(1), 19–40.

Drayna, D. T. (1997). Genetic linkage studies of stuttering: Ready for prime time? *Journal of Fluency Disorders*, 22, 237–241.

Duncan, M. H. (1949). Home adjustment of stutterers and non-stutterers. *Journal of Speech Disorders*, 14, 195–198.

Dunlap, K. (1917). The stuttering boy. *Journal of Abnormal Psychology*, 12, 44–48.

Dunlap, K. (1932). *Habits: Their Making and Unmaking*. New York: Liveright.

Eldridge, M. (1968). *The History of the Treatment of Speech Disorders*. Baltimore, MD: Williams & Wilkins.

Erickson, R. L. (1969). Assessing communication attitudes among stutterers. *Journal of Speech and Hearing Research*, 12, 711–724.

Felsenfeld, S. (2002). Finding susceptibility genes for developmental disorders of speech: The long and winding road. *Journal of Communication Disorders*, 35(4), 329–345.

Fenichel, O. (1945). *The Psychoanalytic Theory of Neurosis*. New York: W. W. Norton.

Finn, P., & Ingham, R. J. (1994). Stutterers' self-ratings of how natural speech sounds and feels. *Journal of Speech and Hearing Research*, 37, 326–340.

Flanagan, B., Goldiamond, I., & Azrin, N. (1958). Operant stuttering: The control of stuttering behavior through response-contingent consequences. *Journal of Experimental Analysis of Behavior*, 1, 173–177.

Fletcher, J. M. (1914). An experimental study of stuttering. *Journal of Applied Psychology*, 25, 201–249.

Franken, M. C., Boves, L., Peters, H. F. M., & Webster, R. L. (1992). Perceptual evaluation of the speech before and after fluency shaping stuttering therapy. *Journal of Fluency Disorders*, 17, 223–241.

Frankl, V. E. (1985). *Man's Search for Meaning*. New York: Washington Square Press.

Fransella, F. (1972). *Personal Change and Reconstruction: Research on a Treatment of Stuttering*. New York: Academic Press.

Freeman, F. J., & Rosenfield, D. B. (1982). A research note on "source" in dysfluency. *Journal of Fluency Disorders*, 7, 295–296.

Freeman, F. J., & Ushijima, T. (1978). Laryngeal muscle activity during stuttering. *Journal of Speech and Hearing Research*, 21, 538–562.

Freund, H. (1966). *Psychopathology and the Problems of Stuttering*. Springfield, IL: Charles C. Thomas.

Froeschels, E. (1950). A technique for stutterers—ventriloquism. *Journal of Speech and Hearing Disorders*, 15, 336–337.

Gaines, N. D., Runyan, C. M., & Meyers, S. C. (1991). A comparison of young stutterers' fluent versus stuttered utterances on measures of length and complexity. *Journal of Speech and Hearing Research*, 34, 37–42.

Geschwind, N., & Galaburda, A. M. (1985). Cerebral lateralization: Biological mechanisms, associations, and pathology: I. A hypothesis and a program for research. *Archives of Neurology*, 42, 429–459.

Gilman, M., & Yaruss, J. S. (2000). Stuttering and relaxation: Applications for somatic education in stuttering treatment. *Journal of Fluency Disorders*, 25(1), 59–76.

Glauber, I. P. (1982). *Stuttering: A Psychoanalytic Understanding.* New York: Human Sciences Press.

Goda, S. (1961). Stuttering manifestations following spinal meningitis. *Journal of Speech and Hearing Disorders,* 26, 392–393.

Goldberg, B. (1989). Historic treatment of stuttering: From pebbles to psychoanalysis. *ASHA,* 31 (6/7), 71.

Goldiamond, I. (1965). Stuttering and fluency as manipulable operant response classes. In L. Krasner & L. P. Ullman (Eds.), *Research in Behavior Modification.* New York: Holt, Rinehart, & Winston.

Gootwald, S. R., & Hall, N. E. (2003). Stuttering treatment in schools: Developing family and teacher partnerships. *Seminars in Speech and Language,* 24(1), 41–46.

Gordon, P. A., & Luper, H. L. (1992). The early identification of beginning stuttering I: Protocols. *American Journal of Speech-Language Pathology,* 1(3), 43–53.

Gregory, H. H. (1997). The speech-language pathologist's role in stuttering self-help groups. *Seminars in Speech and Language,* 18(4), 401–409.

Guitar, B. (1975). Reduction of stuttering frequency using analog electromyographic feedback. *Journal of Speech and Hearing Research,* 18, 672–685.

Guitar, B., Schaefer, H. K., Donahue-Kilburg, G., & Bond, L. (1992). Parent verbal interactions and speech rate: A case study in stuttering. *Journal of Speech and Hearing Research,* 35, 742–754.

Gutzmann, H. (1939). Erbbiologische, soziologische und organische Faktoren die Sprachstorungen begunstigen. *Archive fur Stimmheilkunde,* 3, 133–136.

Haefner, R. (1929). *The Educational Significance of Left-Handedness.* New York: Teachers College, Columbia University Press.

Halvorson, J. A. (1971). The effects on stuttering frequency of pairing punishment (response cost) with reinforcement. *Journal of Speech and Hearing Research,* 14, 356–364.

Halvorson, J. A. (1999). *Abandoned.* Hager City, WI: Halvorson Farms of Wisconsin.

Ham, R. E. (1988). Unison speech and rate control therapy. *Journal of Fluency Disorders,* 13, 115–126.

Ham, R. E. (1990a). Clinician preparation: Experiences with pseudostuttering. *Journal of Fluency Disorders,* 15, 305–315.

Ham, R. E. (1990b). *Therapy of Stuttering: Preschool Through Adolescence.* Englewood Cliffs, NJ: Prentice-Hall.

Hammer, C. S. (1994). Working with families of Chamorro and Carolinian cultures. *American Journal of Speech-Language Pathology,* 3(3), 5–12.

Harle, M. (1946). Dynamic interpretation and treatment of acute stuttering in a young child. *American Journal of Orthopsychiatry,* 15, 156–162.

Helm-Estabrooks, N. (1986). Diagnosis and management of neurogenic stuttering in adults. In Kenneth O. St. Louis (Ed.), *The Atypical Stutterer.* Orlando, FL: Academic Press.

Helm-Estabrooks, N. (1999). Stuttering associated with acquired neurological disorders. In R. F. Curlee (Ed.), *Stuttering and Related Disorders of Fluency.* New York: Thieme, 255–268.

Helm-Estabrooks, N., & Hotz, G. (1998). Sudden onset of "stuttering" in an adult: Neurogenic or psychogenic? *Seminar of Speech and Language*, 19(1), 23–29.

Herodotus (1821). *Herodotus II*. London: S. & R. Bentley.

Hillis, J. W. (1993). Ongoing assessment in the management of stuttering: A clinical perspective. *American Journal of Speech-Language Pathology*, 2(1), 24–37.

Hippocrates (1923a). *Aphorisms* [Translated by W. H. S. Jones]. London: Heinemann.

Hippocrates (1923b). *Precepts* [Translated by W. H. S. Jones]. London: Heinemann.

Hippocrates (1923c). *The Sacred Disease* [Translated by W. H. S. Jones]. London: Heinemann.

Howie, P. M. (1981). Concordance for stuttering in monozygotic and dizygotic twin pairs. *Journal of Speech and Hearing Research*, 24, 317–321.

Howie, P. M., Tanner, S., & Andrews, G. (1981). Short- and long-term outcome in an intensive treatment program for adult stutterers. *Journal of Speech and Hearing Disorders*, 46, 104–109.

Hubbard, C. P., & Prins, D. (1994). Word familiarity, syllabic stress pattern, and stuttering. *Journal of Speech and Hearing Research*, 37, 564–571.

Hubbard, C. P., & Yairi, E. (1988). Clustering of disfluencies in the speech of stuttering and nonstuttering preschool children. *Journal of Speech and Hearing Research*, 31, 228–233.

Hugh-Jones, S., & Smith, P. K. (1999). Self-reports of short- and long-term effects of bullying on children who stammer. *British Journal of Educational Psychology*, 69 (2), 141–158.

Hulit, L. M. (1989). A stutterer like me. *Journal of Fluency Disorders*, 14, 209–214.

Hulit, L. M., & Haasler, S. K. (1989). Influence of suggestion on the nonfluencies of normal speakers. *Journal of Fluency Disorders*, 14, 359–369.

Hulit, L. M., & Wirtz, L. (1994). The association of attitudes toward stuttering with selected variables. *Journal of Fluency Disorders*, 19, 247–267.

Hunt, H. (1861). *Stammering and Stuttering, Their Nature and Treatment*. [A facsimile was published in 1967 by Hafner Publishing Company, New York.]

Hurst, M., & Cooper, E. B. (1983a). Employer attitudes toward stuttering. *Journal of Fluency Disorders*, 8, 1–12.

Hurst, M., & Cooper, E. B. (1983b). Vocational rehabilitation counselors' attitudes toward stuttering. *Journal of Fluency Disorders*, 8, 13–27.

Hutchinson, J. M., & Watkin, K. L. (1976). Jaw mechanics during release of the stuttering moment: Some initial observations and interpretations. *Journal of Communication Disorders*, 9, 269–279.

Ingham, J. C., & Riley, G. (1998). Guidelines for documentation of treatment efficacy for young children who stutter. *Journal of Speech and Hearing Research*, 41(4), 753–770.

Ingham, R. J. (1984). *Stuttering and Behavior Therapy: Current Status and Experimental Foundations*. San Diego, CA: College-Hill.

Ingham, R. J. (1990a). Commentary on Perkins (1990) and Moore and Perkins (1990): On the valid role of reliability in identifying "What Is Stuttering?" *Journal of Speech and Hearing Disorders*, 55, 394–397.

Ingham, R. J. (1990b). Research on stuttering treatment for adults and adolescents: A perspective on how to overcome a malaise. *ASHA Reports*, 18, 91–95.

Ingham, R. J. (1993a). Current status of stuttering and behavior modification—II. Principal issues and practices in stuttering therapy. *Journal of Fluency Disorders*, 18, 57–79.

Ingham, R. J. (1993b). Transfer and maintenance of treatment gains of chronic stutterers. In Richard F. Curlee (Ed.), *Stuttering and Related Disorders of Fluency*. New York: Thieme Medical Publishers, 166–178.

Ingham, R. J. (2001). Brain imaging studies of developmental stuttering. *Journal of Communication Disorders*, 34(6), 493-516.

Ingham, R. J., & Cordes, A. K. (1992). Interclinic differences in stuttering-event counts. *Journal of Fluency Disorders*, 17, 171–176.

Ingham, R. J., Martin, R. R., Haroldson, S. K., Onslow, M., & Leney, M. (1985). Modification of listener-judged naturalness in the speech of stutterers. *Journal of Speech and Hearing Research*, 28, 495–504.

Ingham, R. J., Southwood, H., & Horsburgh, G. (1981). Some effects of the Edinburgh masker on stuttering during oral reading and spontaneous speech. *Journal of Fluency Disorders*, 6, 135–154.

Irwin, J., & Duffy, J. K. (1955). *Speech and Hearing Hurdles*. Columbus, OH: School and College Service.

Jacobson, E. (1938). *Progressive Relaxation*. Chicago: University of Chicago Press.

James, S. E., Brumfitt, S. M., & Cudd, P. A. (1999). Communicating by telephone: Views of a group of people with stuttering impairment. *Journal of Fluency Disorders*, 24, 299–317.

Johnson, W. (1930). *Because I Stutter*. New York: Appleton-Century-Crofts.

Johnson, W. (1946). *People in Quandaries*. New York: Harper & Brothers.

Johnson, W. (1958). Introduction: The six men and the stuttering. In Jon Eisenson (Ed.), *Stuttering: A Symposium*. New York: Harper & Brothers, pp. xi–xxiv.

Johnson, W. (1961). Measurement of oral reading and speaking rate and disfluency of adult male and female stutterers and nonstutterers. *Journal of Speech and Hearing Disorders Monograph Supplement No. 7*, 1–20.

Johnson, W., & Associates (1959). *The Onset of Stuttering: Research Findings and Implications*. Minneapolis: University of Minnesota Press.

Johnson, W., & Knott, J. R. (1937). Studies in the psychology of stuttering: I. The distribution of moments of stuttering in successive readings of the same material. *Journal of Speech Disorders*, 2, 17–19.

Johnson, W., & Rosen, B. (1937). Studies in the psychology of stuttering: VII. The effect of certain changes in speech pattern upon frequency of stuttering. *Journal of Speech Disorders*, 2, 105–109.

Johnson, W., & Sinn, A. (1937). Studies in the psychology of stuttering: V. Frequency of stuttering with expectation of stuttering controlled. *Journal of Speech Disorders*, 2, 98–100.

Johnson, W., & Solomon, A. (1937). Studies in the psychology of stuttering: IV. A quantitative study of expectation of stuttering as a process involving a low degree of consciousness. *Journal of Speech Disorders*, 2, 95–97.

Jones, P. K. (1966). Observations on stammering after localized cerebral injury. *Journal of Neurology, Neurosurgery, and Psychiatry*, 29, 192–195.

Kalinowski, J. (2003). Self-reported efficacy of an all in-the-ear-canal pros-
thetic device to inhibit stuttering during one hundred hours of university
teaching: An authbiographical clinical commentary. *Disability and Rehabilitation*, 25(2), 107–111.

Kalinowski, L. S., Lerman, J. W., & Watt, J. (1987). A preliminary examina-
tion of the perception of self and others in stutterers and nonstutterers.
Journal of Fluency Disorders, 12, 317–331.

Kamhi, A. G. (1982). The problem of relapse in stuttering: Some thoughts on
what might cause it and how to deal with it. *Journal of Fluency Disorders*,
7, 459–467.

Kamhi, A. G., & McOsker, T. G. (1982). Attention and stuttering: Do stutterers
think too much about speech? *Journal of Fluency Disorders*, 7, 309–321.

Kent, R. D. (1983). Facts about stuttering: Neurologic perspectives. *Journal of
Speech and Hearing Disorders*, 48, 249–255.

Klencke, H. (1860). *Die Heilung des Stotterns*. Leipsig.

Knott, J., Johnson, W., & Webster, M. (1937). Studies in the psychology of
stuttering: II. A quantitative evaluation of expectation of stuttering in
relation to the occurrence of stuttering. *Journal of Speech Disorders*, 2,
20–22.

Kroll, R. M., & De Nil, L. (1994). Locus of control and client performance variables as predictors of stuttering treatment outcome. *Journal of Fluency
Disorders*, 19, 186–187.

Kushner, H. S. (1981). *When Bad Things Happen to Good People*. New York:
Avon Books.

Ladouceur, R., Cote, C., Leblond, G., & Bluchard, L. (1982). Evaluation of regulated-breathing method and awareness training in the treatment of stuttering. *Journal of Speech and Hearing Disorders*, 47, 422–426.

Lay, T. (1982a). Nonspecific elements in therapy with stutterers. *Journal of
Fluency Disorders*, 7, 479–486.

Lay, T. (1982b). Stuttering: Training the therapist. *Journal of Fluency Disorders*, 7, 63–69.

Leach, E. (1969). Stuttering: Clinical application of response-contingent procedures. In B. B. Gray & G. England (Eds.), *Stuttering and the Conditioning
Therapies*. Monterey, CA: Monterey Institute of Speech and Hearing.

Leahy, M. M. (1994). Attempting to ameliorate student therapists' negative
stereotype of the stutterer. *European Journal of Disorders of Communication*, 29(1), 39–49.

Lebrun, Y. (1997). *From the Brain to the Mouth: Acquired Dysarthria and Disfluency in Adults*. The Netherlands: Kluwer Academic Publishers.

Lebrun, Y., & Bayle, M. (1973). Surgery in the treatment of stuttering. In Y.
Lebrun & R. Hoops (Eds.), *Neurolinguistic Approaches to Stuttering*. The
Hague: Mouton, pp. 82–89.

Lebrun, Y., & Leleux, C. (1985). Acquired stuttering following right brain
damage in dextrals. *Journal of Fluency Disorders*, 10, 137–141.

Lebrun, Y., Leleux, C., Rousseau, J., & Devreux, F. (1983). Acquired stuttering. *Journal of Fluency Disorders*, 8, 323–330.

Lebrun, Y., & Van Borsel, J. (1990). Final sound repetitions. *Journal of Fluency Disorders*, 15, 107–113.

Leith, W. R. (1986). Treating the stutterer with atypical cultural influences. In Kenneth O. St. Louis (Ed.), *The Atypical Stutterer*. Orlando, FL: Academic Press.

Leith, W. R., & Timmons, J. L. (1983). The stutterer's reaction to the telephone as a speaking situation. *Journal of Fluency Disorders*, 8, 233–243.

Liles, B. Z., Lerman, J., Christensen, L., & St. Ledger, J. (1992). A case description of verbal and signed disfluencies of a 10-year-old boy who is retarded. *Language, Speech, and Hearing Services in Schools*, 23, 107–112.

Lindsay, J. S. (1989). Relationship of developmental disfluency and episodes of stuttering to the emergence of cognitive stages in children. *Journal of Fluency Disorders*, 14, 271–284.

Linebaugh, C. W. (1984). Mild aphasia. In Audrey Holland (Ed.), *Language Disorders in Adults*. San Diego, CA: College-Hill Press, pp. 113–131.

Luchinger, R, & Arnold, G. E. (1965). *Voice-Speech-Language*. Belmont, CA: Wadsworth Publishing Company.

Ludlow, C. L., & Braun, A. (1993). Research evaluating the use of neuropharmacological agents for treating stuttering: Possibilities and problems. *Journal of Fluency Disorders*, 18, 169–182.

Macfarlane, F. K. (1990). The use of hypnosis in speech therapy: A questionnaire study. *British Journal of Disorders of Communication*, 25, 227–246.

Maestas, A. G., & Erickson, J. G. (1992). Mexican immigrant mothers' beliefs about disabilities. *American Journal of Speech-Language Pathology*, 1(4), 5–10.

Maier, S. F., & Seligman, M. E. P. (1976). Learned helplessness: Theory and evidence. *Journal of Experimental Psychology: General*, 105, 3–46.

Mallard, A. R., & Meyer, L. A. (1979). Listener preferences for stuttered and syllable-timed speech production. *Journal of Fluency Disorders*, 4, 117–121.

Manders, E., & Bastijns, P. (1988). Sudden recovery from stuttering after an epileptic attack: A case report. *Journal of Fluency Disorders*, 13, 421–425.

Manning, W. H., Burlison, A. E., & Thaxton, D. (1999). Listener response to stuttering modification techniques. *Journal of Fluency Disorders*, 24, 267–280.

Manning, W. H., Dailey, D., & Wallace, S. (1984). Attitude and personality characteristics of older stutterers. *Journal of Fluency Disorders*, 9, 207–215.

Manning, W. H., Trutna, P. A., & Shaw, C. K. (1976). Verbal versus tangible reward for children who stutter. *Journal of Speech and Hearing Disorders*, 41, 52–62.

Market, K. W., Montague Jr., J. C., Buffalo, M. D., & Drummond, S. S. (1990). Acquired stuttering: Descriptive data and treatment outcome. *Journal of Fluency Disorders*, 15, 21–33.

Martin, R. R. (1993). The future of behavior modification of stuttering: What goes around comes around. *Journal of Fluency Disorders*, 18, 81–108.

Martin, R. R., Juhl, P., & Haroldson, S. (1972). An experimental treatment with two preschool stuttering children. *Journal of Speech and Hearing Research*, 15, 743–752.

Martin, R. R., & Siegel, G. M. (1966a). The effects of response contingent shock on stuttering. *Journal of Speech and Hearing Research*, 9, 340–352.

Martin, R. R., & Siegel, G. M. (1966b). The effects of simultaneously punishing stuttering and rewarding fluency. *Journal of Speech and Hearing Research*, 9, 466–475.

Matsuda, M. (1989). Working with Asian parents: Some communication strategies. *Topics in Language Disorders*, 9(3), 45–53.

McClean, M. D. (1990). Neuromotor aspects of stuttering: Levels of impairment and disability. *ASHA Reports*, 18, 64–71.

McDonough, A., Quesal, R. W. (1988). Locus of control orientation of stutterers and nonstutterers. *Journal of Fluency Disorders*, 13, 97–106.

McKeehan, A. B. (1994). Student experiences with fluency facilitating speech strategies. *Journal of Fluency Disorders*, 19, 113–123

Meltzer, A. (1992). Horn stuttering. *Journal of Fluency Disorders*, 17, 257–264.

Meyers, S. C. (1986). Qualitative and quantitative differences and patterns of variability in disfluencies emitted by preschool stutterers and nonstutterers during dyadic conversations. *Journal of Fluency Disorders*, 11, 293–306.

Miller, D. T., & Turnbill, W. (1986). Expectancies and interpersonal processes. *Annual Review of Psychology*, 37, 233–257.

Miller, S., & Watson, B. C. (1992). The relationship between communication attitude, anxiety, and depression in stutterers and nonstutterers. *Journal of Speech and Hearing Research*, 35, 789–798.

Moeller, D. (1975). *Speech Pathology and Audiology: Iowa Origins of a Discipline.* Iowa City: University of Iowa Press.

Montgomery, B. M., & Fitch, J. L. (1988). The prevalence of stuttering in the hearing-impaired school age population. *Journal of Speech and Hearing Disorders*, 53, 131–135.

Moore, J. C., & Rigo, T. G. (1983). An awareness approach to the covert symptoms of stuttering. *Journal of Fluency Disorders*, 8, 133–145.

Moore, M. A. S., & Adams, M. R. (1985). The Edinburgh Masker: A clinical analog study. *Journal of Fluency Disorders*, 10, 281–290.

Moore, W. H. Jr., (1986). Hemispheric alpha asymmetries of stutterers and nonstutterers for the recall and recognition of words and connected reading passages: Some relationships to severity of stuttering. *Journal of Fluency Disorders*, 11, 71–89.

Morgenstern, J. J. (1956). Socio-economic factors in stuttering. *Journal of Speech and Hearing Disorders*, 21, 25–33.

Muellerleile, S. (1981). Portable delayed auditory feedback device: A preliminary report. *Journal of Fluency Disorders*, 6, 361–363.

Murphy, W. P., & Quesal, R. W. (2002). Strategies for addressing bullying with the school-age child who stutters. *Seminars in Speech and Language*, 23(3), 205–212.

Murray, F. P., & Edwards, S. G. (1980). *A Stutterer's Story.* Danville, IL: Interstate Printers and Publishers.

Myers, F. (1992). Cluttering: A synergistic framework. In F. Myers & K. O. St. Louis (Eds.), *Cluttering: A Clinical Perspective.* Leicester, Great Britain: Far Communications, 71–84.

Myers, F., & St. Louis, K. O. (Eds.) (1992). *Cluttering: A Clinical Perspective.* Leicester, Great Britain: Far Communications.

Mygind, H. (1898). Uber die Ursachen des Stotterns. *Archive fur Laryngologie und Rhinologie,* 8, 294–307.

Nadoleczny, M. (1926). *Kurzes Lehrbuch der Sprach- und Stimmheilkunde mit Besonderer Berucksichtigung des Kindesalters.* Leipzig: Verlag Von F. C. W. Vogel.

Nagel, R., & van Eupen, A-K. (1994). Presentation of a cognitive training program for stuttering children: "Think-Wise!" *Journal of Fluency Disorders,* 19, 196.

Newman, L. L. (1987). The effects of punishment of repetitions and the acquisition of "stutter-like" behaviors in normal speakers. *Journal of Fluency Disorders,* 12, 51–62.

Nowack, W. J., & Stone, R. E. (1987). Acquired stuttering and bilateral cerebral disease. *Journal of Fluency Disorders,* 12, 141–146.

Oates, D. W. (1929). Left-handedness in relation to speech defects, intelligence, and achievement. *Forum of Education,* 7, 91–105.

Ojemann, R. H. (1931). Studies in sidedness, III. Relation of handedness to speech. *Journal of Educational Psychology,* 22, 120–126.

Onslow, M. (1992). Choosing a treatment procedure for early stuttering: Issues and future directions. *Journal of Speech and Hearing Research,* 35, 983–993.

Onslow, M., Andrews, G., & Lincoln, M. (1994). A control/experimental trial of an operant treatment for early stuttering. *Journal of Speech and Hearing Research,* 37, 1244–1259.

Onslow, M., & Ingham, R. J. (1987). Speech quality measurement and the management of stuttering. *Journal of Speech and Hearing Disorders,* 52, 2–17.

Otsuki, H. (1958). Study on stuttering: Statistical observations. *Otorhinolaryngology Clinic,* 5, 1150–1151.

Packman, A., & Onslow, M. (1999). Fluency disruption in speech and in wind instrument playing. *Journal of Fluency Disorders,* 24(4), 293–298.

Paden, E. P. (1970). *A History of the American Speech and Hearing Association 1925–1958.* Washington, DC: American Speech and Hearing Association.

Paul-Brown, D. (1990). National Stuttering Project. *Asha,* 32 (1), 35.

Penfield, W., & Roberts, L. (1959). *Speech and Brain Mechanisms.* Princeton, NJ: Princeton University Press.

Perkins, W. H. (1973). Replacement of stuttering with normal speech: II. Clinical procedures. *Journal of Speech and Hearing Disorders,* 38, 295–303.

Perkins, W. H. (1983a). The problem of definition: Commentary on stuttering. *Journal of Speech and Hearing Disorders,* 48, 246–249.

Perkins, W. H. (1983b). Learning from negative outcomes in stuttering therapy: II. An epiphany of failures. *Journal of Fluency Disorders,* 8, 155–160.

Perkins, W. H. (1990a). What is stuttering? *Journal of Speech and Hearing Disorders,* 55, 370–382.

Perkins, W. H. (1990b). Gratitude, good intentions, and red herrings: A response to commentaries. *Journal of Speech and Hearing Disorders,* 55, 402–404.

Perkins, W. H. (1991). So near and yet so far: A response to Siegel. *Journal of Speech and Hearing Research*, 34, 1083–1086.

Perkins, W. H. (1993). The early history of behavior modification of stuttering: A view from the trenches. *Journal of Fluency Disorders*, 18, 1–11.

Perkins, W. H. (1994). Solving unsolvable stuttering. *American Journal of Speech-Language Pathology*, 3(3), 32–33

Perkins, W. H., Kent, R., & Curlee, R. (1991). A theory of neuropsycholinguistic function in stuttering. *Journal of Speech and Hearing Research*, 34, 734–735.

Perkins, W. H., Rudas, J., Johnson, L., & Bell, J. (1976). Stuttering: Discoordination of phonation with articulation and respiration. *Journal of Speech and Hearing Research*, 19, 509–522.

Peters, H. F. M., & Starkweather, C. W. (1989). Development of stuttering throughout life. *Journal of Fluency Disorders*, 14, 303–321.

Pill, J. (1988). A comparison between two treatment programs for stuttering: A personal account. *Journal of Fluency Disorders*, 13, 385–398.

Pill, J., & St. Louis, K. (1994). Self-help and speech professionals. *Journal of Fluency Disorders*, 19, 200–201.

Polanyi, M. (1967). *The Tacit Dimension*. New York: Doubleday Anchor Books.

Porter, H. K. (1939). Studies in the psychology of stuttering: XIV. Stuttering phenomena in relation to size and personnel of audience. *Journal of Speech Disorders*, 4, 323–333.

Postma, A., & Kolk, H. (1992). Error monitoring in people who stutter: Evidence against auditory feedback deficit theories. *Journal of Speech and Hearing Research*, 35, 1024–1032.

Preus, A. (1981). *Attempts at Identifying Subgroups of Stutterers*. Oslo, Norway: University of Oslo Press.

Prins, D. (1993). Models for treatment efficacy studies of adult stutterers. *Journal of Fluency Disorders*, 18, 333–349.

Prins, D., Hubbard, C. P., & Krause, M. (1991). Syllabic stress and the occurrence of stuttering. *Journal of Speech and Hearing Research*, 34, 1011–1016.

Prins, D., & Lohr, F. (1972). Behavioral dimensions of stuttered speech. *Journal of Speech and Hearing Research*, 15, 61–71.

Rami, M., Kalinowski, J., Stuart, A., & Rastatter, M. (2003). Self-perception of speech language pathologists-in-training before and after pseudostuttering experiences on the telephone. *Disability and Rehabilitation*, 25(9), 491–496.

Ramig, P. R. (1984). Rate changes in the speech of stutterers after therapy. *Journal of Fluency Disorders*, 9, 285–294.

Ramig, P. R., & Wallace, M. L. (1987). Indirect and combined direct-indirect therapy in a dysfluent child. *Journal of Fluency Disorders*, 12, 41–49.

Reardon, N. A., & Reeves, L. (2002). Stuttering therapy in partnership with support groups: The best of both worlds. *Seminars in Speech and Language*, 23(3), 213–218.

Reed, C. G., & Godden, A. L. (1977). An experimental treatment using verbal punishment with two preschool stutterers. *Journal of Fluency Disorders*, 2, 225–233.

Richter, E. (1982). Ein Beitrag zur Atiologie des Stotterns. *Sprachheilarb, 27,* 239–245.

Rieber, R. W. (Ed.) (1977). *The Problem of Stuttering: Theory and Therapy.* New York: Elsevier North-Holland.

Riley, G. D. (1972). A stuttering severity instrument for children and adults. *Journal of Speech and Hearing Disorders, 37,* 314–321.

Riley, G. D. (1984). *Stuttering Prediction Instrument for Young Children.* Austin, TX: PRO-ED.

Riley, G. D., & Riley, J. (1979). A component model for diagnosing and treating children who stutter. *Journal of Fluency Disorders, 4,* 279–293.

Riley, G. D., & Riley, J. (1986). Oral motor discoordination among children who stutter. *Journal of Fluency Disorders, 11,* 335–344.

Riley, G. D., & Riley, J. (1989). Physician's screening procedure for children who may stutter. *Journal of Fluency Disorders, 14,* 57–67.

Roman, K. G. (1959). Handwriting and speech. *Logos, 2,* 29.

Rosenfield, D. B., & Freeman, F. J. (1983). Stuttering onset after laryngectomy. *Journal of Fluency Disorders, 8,* 265–268.

Rosenfield, D. B., Jones, B. P., & Liljestrand, J. S. (1981). Effects of right hemisphere damage in an adult stutterer. *Journal of Fluency Disorders, 6,* 175–179.

Roth, C. R., Aronson, A. E., & Davis Jr., L. J. (1989). Clinical studies in psychogenic stuttering of adult onset. *Journal of Speech and Hearing Disorders, 54,* 634–646.

Rubin, T. I. (1969). *The Angry Book.* New York: Macmillan.

Salamy, J. N., & Sessions, R. B. (1980). Spastic dysphonia. *Journal of Fluency Disorders, 5,* 281–290.

Schloss, P. J., Freeman, C. A., Smith, M. A., & Espin, C. A. (1987). Influence of assertiveness training on the stuttering rates exhibited by three young adults. *Journal of Fluency Disorders, 12,* 333–353.

Schuell, H. (1946). Sex differences in relation to stuttering. Part I. *Journal of Speech Disorders, 11,* 277–298.

Schwartz, H. D. (1994). Transferring fluency: Older children and adolescents. *Journal of Fluency Disorders, 19,* 207.

Schwartz, H. D., Zebrowski, P. M., & Conture, E. G. (1990). Behaviors at the onset of stuttering. *Journal of Fluency Disorders, 15,* 77–86.

Schwartz, M. F. (1976). *Stuttering Solved.* New York: McGraw-Hill.

Schwartz, M. F., & Carter, G. L. (1986). *Stop Stuttering.* New York: Harper & Row.

Scripture, E. W. (1931). *Stuttering, Lisping, and Correction of the Speech of the Deaf.* New York: Macmillian.

Seeman, M. (1934). Uber somatische befunde bei stottern. *Monatschrift fur Ohrenheilkunde, 68,* 895–912.

Seider, R. A., Gladstein, K. L., & Kidd, K. K. (1982). Language onset and concomitant speech and language problems in subgroups of stutterers and their siblings. *Journal of Speech and Hearing Research, 25,* 482–486.

Shames, G. H. (1989). Stuttering: An RFP for a cultural perspective. *Journal of Fluency Disorders, 14,* 67–77.

Shames, G. H., & Florance, C. L. (1980). *Stutter-free Speech: A Goal for Therapy.* Columbus, OH: Charles E. Merrill.

Shames, G. H., & Sherrick, C. E., Jr. (1963). A discussion of nonfluency and stuttering as operant behavior. *Journal of Speech and Hearing Disorders*, 28, 3–18.

Shapiro, A. K. (1964). Factors contributing to the placebo effect: Implications for psychotherapy. *American Journal of Psychotherapy*, 18 (Supplement 1), 73–88.

Sheehan, J. G. (1974). Stuttering behavior: A phonetic analysis. *Journal of Communication Disorders*, 7, 193–212.

Sheehan, J. G., & Martyn, M. M. (1970). Spontaneous recovery from stuttering. *Journal of Speech and Hearing Research*, 13, 279–289.

Sheehan, J. G., & Voas, R. B. (1954). Tension patterns during stuttering in relation to conflict, anxiety-binding, and reinforcement. *Speech Monographs*, 21, 272–279.

Sheehy, G. (1976). *Passages: Predictable Crises of Adult Life*. New York: E. P. Dutton.

Shenker, R. C., Mayberry, R., Scobble, M., Grothe, M., & White, K. (1994). The gesture-speech relationship in stuttering: Results of preliminary findings and applications to treatment. *Journal of Fluency Disorders*, 19, 207.

Shirkey, E. A. (1987). Forensic verification of stuttering. *Journal of Fluency Disorders*, 12, 197–203.

Shklovskii, V. M., Krol, L. M., & Mikhailova, E. L. (1988). The psychotherapy of stuttering: On the model of stuttering patients' psychotherapy group. *Soviet Journal of Psychiatry and Psychology Today*, 1, 130–141.

Shumak, I. C. (1955). A speech situation rating sheet for stutterers. In W. Johnson (Ed.), *Stuttering in Children and Adults: Thirty Years of Research at the University of Iowa*. Minneapolis: University of Minnesota Press, 341–347.

Siegel, G. M. (1970). Punishment, stuttering, and disfluency. *Journal of Speech and Hearing Research*, 13, 677–714.

Siegel, G. M. (1991). Response to Perkins, "What is stuttering?" *Journal of Speech and Hearing Research*, 34, 1081–1083.

Silverman, E.-M. (1972a). Generality of disfluency data collected from preschoolers. *Journal of Speech and Hearing Research*, 14, 84–92.

Silverman, E.-M. (1972b). Preschoolers' speech disfluency: Single syllable word repetition. *Perceptual and Motor Skills*, 35, 1002.

Silverman, F. H. (1960). Forensic therapy. *Quarterly Journal of Speech*, 46, 305–306.

Silverman, F. H. (1970a). Course of nonstutterers disfluency adaptation during 15 consecutive oral readings of the same material. *Journal of Speech and Hearing Research*, 13, 382–386.

Silverman, F. H. (1970b). Concern of elementary-school stutterers about their stuttering. *Journal of Speech and Hearing Disorders*, 35, 361–363.

Silverman, F. H. (1970c). Distribution of instances of disfluency in consecutive readings of different passages by nonstutterers. *Journal of Speech and Hearing Research*, 13, 874–882.

Silverman, F. H. (1970d). A note on the degree of adaptation by stutterers and nonstutterers during oral reading. *Journal of Speech and Hearing Research*, 13, 173–177.

Silverman, F. H. (1971a). The effect of rhythmic auditory stimulation on the disfluency of nonstutterers. *Journal of Speech and Hearing Research*, 14, 350–355.

Silverman, F. H. (1971b). A rationale for the use of the hearing-aid metronome in a program of therapy for stuttering. *Perceptual and Motor Skills*, 32, 34.

Silverman, F. H. (1974). Disfluency behavior of elementary-school stutterers and nonstutterers. *Language, Speech, and Hearing Services in Schools*, 5, 32–37.

Silverman, F. H. (1975). How "typical" is a stutterer's stuttering in a clinical environment! *Perceptual and Motor Skills*, 40, 458.

Silverman, F. H. (1976a). Communicative success: A reinforcer of stuttering. *Perceptual and Motor Skills*, 43, 398.

Silverman, F. H. (1976b). Long-term impact of a miniature metronome on stuttering: An interim report. *Perceptual and Motor Skills*, 42, 1322.

Silverman, F. H. (1980a). Dimensions of improvement in stuttering. *Journal of Speech and Hearing Research*, 23, 137–151.

Silverman, F. H. (1980b). The Stuttering Problem Profile: A task that assists both client and clinician in defining therapy goals. *Journal of Speech and Hearing Disorders*, 45, 119–123.

Silverman, F. H. (1981). Relapse following stuttering therapy. In Norman J. Lass (Ed.), *Speech and Language: Advances in Basic Research and Practice (Vol. 5)*. New York: Academic Press.

Silverman, F. H. (1988a). Impact of a T-shirt message on stutterer stereotypes. *Journal of Fluency Disorders*, 13, 279–281.

Silverman, F. H. (1988b). The Monster Study. *Journal of Fluency Disorders*, 13, 225–231.

Silverman, F. H. (1995). *Speech, Language, and Hearing Disorders*. Needham Heights, MA: Allyn & Bacon.

Silverman, F. H. (1997a). Stuttering in Tin Pan Alley. *Journal of Communication Disorders*, 30, 1–6.

Silverman, F. H. (1997b). Telecommunication relay services: An option for stutterers. *Journal of Fluency Disorders*, 22, 63–64.

Silverman, F. H. (1998). *Research Design and Evaluation in Speech-Language Pathology and Audiology* (4th Ed.). Boston, MA: Allyn & Bacon.

Silverman, F. H. (1999a). *Professional Issues in Speech-Language Pathology and Audiology*. Boston, MA: Allyn & Bacon.

Silverman, F. H. (1999b). *The Telecommunication Relay Service Handbook*. Newport, RI: Aegis Publishing Group.

Silverman, F. H. (2000). *Second Thoughts about Stuttering*. Greendale, WI: CODI Publications.

Silverman, F. H., & Bloom, C. M. (1973). Spontaneous recovery of nonstutterers' disfluency following adaptation. *Journal of Speech and Hearing Research*, 16, 452–455.

Silverman, F. H., & Bohlman, P. (1988). Flute stuttering. *Journal of Fluency Disorders*, 13, 427–428.

Silverman, F. H., Gazzolo, M., & Peterson, Y. (1990). Impact of a T-shirt message on stutterer stereotypes: A systematic replication. *Journal of Fluency Disorders*, 15, 35–37.

Silverman, F. H., & Goodban, M. K. (1972). The effect of auditory masking on the fluency of normal speakers. *Journal of Speech and Hearing Research*, 15, 543–546.

Silverman, F. H., & Hummer, K. (1989). Spastic dysphonia: A fluency disorder? *Journal of Fluency Disorders*, 14, 285–293.

Silverman, F. H., & Paynter, K. K. (1990). Impact of stuttering on perception of occupational competence. *Journal of Fluency Disorders*, 15, 87–91.

Silverman, F. H., & Silverman, E.-M. (1971). Stutter-like behavior in manual communication of the deaf. *Perceptual and Motor Skills*, 33, 45–46.

Silverman, F. H., & Trotter, W. D. (1973a). Bibliography: Literature related to the use of instrumental aids in stuttering therapy. *Perceptual and Motor Skills*, 36, 247–251.

Silverman, F. H., & Trotter, W. D. (1973b). Bibliography related to the use of instrumental aids in stuttering therapy: Supplement 1. *Perceptual and Motor Skills*, 37, 552.

Silverman, F. H., & Trotter, W. D. (1973c). Impact of pacing speech with a miniature electronic metronome on the manner in which a stutterer is perceived. *Behavior Therapy*, 4, 414–419.

Silverman, F. H., & Trotter, W. D. (1974). Bibliography related to the use of instrumental aids in stuttering therapy: Supplement 2. *Perceptual and Motor Skills*, 38, 1329–1330.

Silverman, F. H., & Trotter, W. D. (1975). Bibliography related to the use of instrumental aids in stuttering therapy: Supplement 3. *Perceptual and Motor Skills*, 40, 240.

Silverman, F. H., & Williams, D. E. (1967). Loci of disfluencies in the speech of nonstutterers during oral reading. *Journal of Speech and Hearing Research*, 10, 790–794.

Silverman, F. H., & Williams, D. E. (1972a). Prediction of stuttering by school-age stutterers. *Journal of Speech and Hearing Research*, 15, 189–193.

Silverman, F. H., & Williams, D. E. (1972b). Performance of stutterers on a single-word adaptation task. *Perceptual and Motor Skills*, 34, 565–566.

Silverman, F. H., & Williams, D. E. (1973). Use of revision by elementary-school stutterers and nonstutterers during oral reading. *Journal of Speech and Hearing Research*, 16, 584–585.

Smith, A. (1990a). Factors in the etiology of stuttering. *ASHA Reports* (Number 18), 39–47.

Smith, A. (1990b). Toward a comprehensive theory of stuttering: A commentary. *Journal of Speech and Hearing Disorders*, 55, 398–401.

Snidecor, J. C. (1947). Why the Indian does not stutter. *Quarterly Journal of Speech*, 33, 493–495.

Snidecor, J. C. (1955). Tension and facial appearance in stuttering. In W. Johnson & R. R. Leutenegger (Eds.), *Stuttering in Children and Adults*. Minneapolis: University of Minnesota Press.

St. Louis, K. O. (1999). Person-first labeling and stuttering. *Journal of Fluency Disorders*, 24, 1–24.

St. Louis, K. O., & Hinzman, A. R. (1986). Studies of cluttering: Perceptions of cluttering by speech-language pathologists and educators. *Journal of Fluency Disorders*, 11, 131–149.

St. Louis, K. O., Hinzman, A. R., & Hull, F. M. (1985). Studies of cluttering: Disfluency and language measures in young possible clutterers and stutterers. *Journal of Fluency Disorders*, 10, 151–172.

St. Louis, K. O., & Rustin, L. (1992). Professional awareness of cluttering. In F. Myers & K. O. St. Louis (Eds.), *Cluttering: A Clinical Perspective* Leicester, Great Britain: Far Communications, 23–35.

Stampfl, T., & Levis, D. (1967). Essentials of implosive therapy. *Journal of Abnormal Psychology*, 72, 496–503.

Stansfield, J. (1995). Word-final disfluencies in adults with learning difficulties. *Journal of Fluency Disorders*, 20, 1–10.

Starkweather, C. W. (1987). *Fluency and Stuttering*. Englewood Cliffs, NJ: Prentice-Hall.

Starkweather, C. W. (1993). Issues in the efficacy of treatment for fluency disorders. *Journal of Fluency Disorders*, 18, 151–168.

Starkweather, C. W. (1994). The electronic self-help group. *Journal of Fluency Disorders*, 19, 213.

Starkweather, C. W. (2002). The epigenesis of stuttering. *Journal of Fluency Disorders*, 27(4), 269–287

Starkweather, C. W., Gottwald, S. R., & Halfond, M. M. (1990). *Stuttering Prevention: A Clinical Method*. Englewood Cliffs, NJ: Prentice-Hall.

Stern, E. (1948). A preliminary of bilingualism and stuttering in four Johannesburg schools. *Journal of Logopedics*, 1, 15–25.

Stewart, J. L. (1960). The problem of stuttering in certain North American Indian societies. *Journal of Speech and Hearing Disorders, Monograph 6* (Supplement).

Stewart, J. L. (1985). Stuttering Indians: A reply to Zimmermann et al. *Journal of Speech and Hearing Research*, 28, 313–315.

Stocker, B. (1980). *The Stocker Probe Technique*. Tulsa, OK: Modern Education Corporation.

Stocker, B., & Gerstman, L. J. (1983). A comparison of the probe technique and conventional therapy for young stutterers. *Journal of Fluency Disorders*, 8, 331–339.

Stuart, A., Xia, S., Jiang, Y., Jiang, T., Kalinowski, J., & Rastatter, M. P. (2003). Self-contained in-the-ear device to deliver altered auditory feedback: Applications for stuttering. *Annals of Biomedical Engineering*, 31(2), 233–237.

Tanner, D. C. (1980). Loss and grief: Implications for speech-language pathologists and audiologists. *ASHA*, 22, 916–928.

Tatchell, R. H., Van Den Berg, S., & Lerman, J. W. (1983). Fluency and eye contact as factors influencing observers' perceptions of stutterers. *Journal of Fluency Disorders*, 8, 221–231.

Throneburg, R. N., Yairi, E., & Paden, E. P. (1994). Relation between phonologic difficulty and the occurrence of disfluencies in the early stage of stuttering. *Journal of Speech and Hearing Research*, 37, 504–509.

Tiger, R. J., Irvine, T. L., & Reis, R. P. (1980). Cluttering as a complex of learning disabilities. *Language, Speech, and Hearing Services in Schools*, 11, 3–14.

Tillis, M., & Wager, W. (1984). *Stutterin' Boy*. New York: Rawson Associates.

Tonev, P. (1994). Speech control, correction, and overcoming stuttering: A solution by Perfectly Mastered Breathing (PMB). *Journal of Fluency Disorders*, 19, 216.

Trotter, W. D., & Kools, J. (1955). Listener adaptation to the severity of stuttering. *Journal of Speech and Hearing Disorders*, 20, 385–387.

Trotter, W. D., & Lesch, M. M. (1967). Personal experiences with a stutter-aid. *Journal of Speech and Hearing Disorders*, 32, 270–272.

Trotter, W. D., & Silverman, F. H. (1973). Experiments with the stutter-aid. *Perceptual and Motor Skills*, 36, 1129–1130.

Trotter, W. D., & Silverman, F. H. (1976). The stutterer as a character in contemporary literature: A bibliography. *Journal of Speech and Hearing Disorders*, 41, 553–554.

Tudor, M. (1939). An experimental study of the effect of evaluative labeling on speech fluency. Master's Thesis, University of Iowa.

van Lieshout, P. H. H. M., Peters, H. F. M., Starkweather, C. W., & Hulstijn, W. (1993). Psysiological differences between stutterers and nonstutterers in perceptually fluent speech: EMG amplitude and duration. *Journal of Speech and Hearing Research*, 36, 55–63.

Van Riper, C. (1935). The quantitative measurements of laterality. *Journal of Experimental Psychology*, 18, 372–382.

Van Riper, C. (1936). Study of thoracic breathing of stutterers during expectancy and occurrence of stuttering spasm. *Journal of Speech Disorders*, 1, 61–72.

Van Riper, C. (1973). *The Treatment of Stuttering*. Englewood Cliffs, NJ: Prentice-Hall.

Van Riper, C. (1979). *A Career in Speech Pathology*. Englewood Cliffs, NJ: Prentice-Hall.

Van Riper, C. (1982). *The Nature of Stuttering* (2nd Ed.). Englewood Cliffs, NJ: Prentice-Hall. Reprinted 1992, Pospect Heights, IL: Waveland Press.

Vanryckeghem, M., & Brutten, G. J. (1992). The Communication Attitude Test: A test-retest reliability investigation. *Journal of Fluency Disorders*, 17, 177–190.

Walle, E. L. (1980). Masking devices and the Edinburgh Masker—Clinical applications within a prison setting. *Journal of Fluency Disorders*, 5, 69–74.

Wallen, V. (1961). Primary stuttering in a 28-year-old adult. *Journal of Speech and Hearing Disorders*, 26, 393–395.

Watson, B. C., Freeman, F. J., Chapman, S. B., Miller, S., Finitzo, T., Pool, K. D., & Devous, M. D. (1991). Linguistic performance deficits in stutterers: Relation to Laryngeal Reaction Time profiles. *Journal of Fluency Disorders*, 16, 85–100.

Watson, J. B. (1988). A comparison of stutterers' and nonstutterers' affective, cognitive, and behavioral self-reports. *Journal of Speech and Hearing Research*, 31, 377–385.

Watson, J. B., Gregory, H. H., & Kistler, D. J. (1987). Development and evaluation of an inventory to assess adult stutterers' communication attitudes. *Journal of Fluency Disorders*, 12, 429–450.

Watts, F. (1971). The treatment of stammering by the intensive practice of fluent speech. *British Journal of Disorders of Communication*, 6, 144–147.

Webster, R. L. (1980). Evolution of a target-based behavioral therapy for stuttering. *Journal of Fluency Disorders*, 5, 303–320.

Wedberg, C. F. (1956). *The Stutterer Speaks*. Magnolia, MA: The Expression Company.

Weiss, D. A. (1964). *Cluttering*. Englewood Cliffs, NJ: Prentice-Hall.

Weiss, D. A. (1967). Similarities and differences between cluttering and stuttering. *Folia Phoniatrica*, 19, 98–104.

West, R. (1958). An agnostic's speculations about stuttering. In Jon Eisenson (Ed.), *Stuttering: A Symposium*. New York: Harper & Brothers, pp. 167–222.

West, R., Nelson, S., & Berry, M. (1939). The heredity of stuttering. *Quarterly Journal of Speech*, 25, 23–30.

Wexler, K. B. (1982). Developmental disfluency in 2-, 4-, and 6-year-old boys in neutral and stress situations. *Journal of Speech and Hearing Research*, 25, 229–234.

Whitney, J. L., & Goldstein, H. (1989). Using self-monitoring to reduce disfluencies in speakers with mild aphasia. *Journal of Speech and Hearing Disorders*, 54, 576–586.

Williams, D. E. (1955). Masseter muscle action potentials in stuttered and nonstuttered speech. *Journal of Speech and Hearing Disorders*, 20, 242–261.

Williams, D. E. (1968). Stuttering therapy: An overview. In Hugo H. Gregory (Ed.), *Learning Theory and Stuttering Therapy*. Evanston, IL: Northwestern University Press, pp. 52–66.

Williams, D. E. (1978). The stuttering problem. In Frederic L. Darley & D. C. Spriestersbach (Eds.), *Diagnostic Methods in Speech Pathology*. New York: Harper & Row, 65–72.

Williams, D. E. (1979). A perspective on approaches to stuttering therapy. In Hugo H. Gregory (Ed.), *Controversies about Stuttering Therapy*. Baltimore, MD: University Park Press, pp. 241–268.

Williams, D. E. (1982). Stuttering therapy: Where are we going—and why? *Journal of Fluency Disorders*, 7, 159–170.

Williams, D. E., & Kent, L. R. (1958). Listener evaluations of speech interruptions. *Journal of Speech and Hearing Research*, 1, 124–131.

Williams, D. E., Melrose, B. M., & Woods, C. L. (1969). The relationship between stuttering and academic achievement in children. *Journal of Communication Disorders*, 2, 87–98.

Williams, D. E., Silverman, F. H., & Kools, J. A. (1968). Disfluency behavior of elementary school stutterers and nonstutterers: The adaptation effect. *Journal of Speech and Hearing Research*, 11, 622–630.

Williams, D. E., Silverman, F. H., & Kools, J. A. (1969a). Disfluency behavior of elementary school stutterers and nonstutterers: The Consistency Effect. *Journal of Speech and Hearing Research*, 12, 301–307.

Williams, D. E., Silverman, F. H., & Kools, J. A. (1969b). Disfluency behavior of elementary school stutterers and nonstutterers: Loci of instances of disfluency. *Journal of Speech and Hearing Research*, 12, 308–318.

Wingate, M. E. (1964). A standard definition of stuttering. *Journal of Speech and Hearing Disorders*, 29.

Wingate, M. E. (1976). *Stuttering: Theory and Treatment*. New York: Irvington Publishers.

Wingate, M. E. (1982). Early position and stuttering occurrence. *Journal of Fluency Disorders*, 7, 243–258.

Wolpe, J. (1958). *Psychotherapy by Reciprocal Inhibition*. Stanford, CA: Stanford University Press.

Wolpe, J. (1969). Behavior therapy in stuttering: Deconditioning the emotional factor. In Burl Gray and Gene England (Eds.), *Stuttering and the Conditioning Therapies*. Monterey, CA: The Monterey Institute for Speech and Hearing, pp. 15–27.

Woods, C. L., & Williams, D. E. (1976). Traits attributed to stuttering and normally fluent males. *Journal of Speech and Hearing Research*, 19, 267–278.

World Health Organization (1977). *Manual of the International Statistical Classification of Diseases, Injuries, and Causes of Death* (Vol. 1). Geneva: World Health Organization.

Wyatt, G. L. (1969). *Language Learning and Communication Disorders in Children*. New York: Free Press.

Yairi, E. (1981). Disfluencies of normally speaking two-year-old children. *Journal of Speech and Hearing Research*, 24, 490–495.

Yairi, E. (1982). Longitudinal studies of disfluencies in two-year-old children. *Journal of Speech and Hearing Research*, 25, 155-160.

Yairi, E. (1993). Epidemiologic and other considerations in treatment efficacy research with preschool age children who stutter. *Journal of Fluency Disorders*, 18, 197–219.

Yairi, E., & Ambrose, N. (1992a). A longitudinal study of stuttering in children: A preliminary report. *Journal of Speech and Hearing Research*, 35, 755–760.

Yairi, E., & Ambrose, N. (1992b). Onset of stuttering in preschool children: Selected factors. *Journal of Speech and Hearing Research*, 35, 782–788.

Yairi, E., Ambrose, N., & Niermann, R. (1993). The early months of stuttering: A developmental study. *Journal of Speech and Hearing Research*, 36, 521–528.

Yairi, E., & Lewis, B. (1984). Disfluencies at the onset of stuttering. *Journal of Speech and Hearing Research*, 27, 154–159.

Yaruss, J. S., & Conture, E. G. (1993). F2 transitions during sound/syllable repetitions of children who stutter and predictions of stuttering chronicity. *Journal of Speech and Hearing Research*, 36, 883–896.

Yaruss, J. S., Quesal, R. W., & Murphy, B. (2002). National Stuttering Association members' opinions about stuttering treatment. *Journal of Fluency Disorders*, 27(3), 227–241.

Young, M. A. (1985). Increasing the frequency of stuttering. *Journal of Speech and Hearing Research*, 28, 282–293.

Yovetich, W. S. (1984). Message therapy: Language approach to stuttering therapy with children. *Journal of Fluency Disorders*, 9, 11–20.

Zebrowski, P. M. (1994). Duration of sound prolongation and sound/syllable repetition in children who stutter: Preliminary observations. *Journal of Speech and Hearing Research*, 37, 254–263.

Zebrowski, P. M., & Conture, E. (1989). Judgments of disfluency by mothers of stuttering and normally fluent children. *Journal of Speech and Hearing Research*, 32, 307–317.

Zebrowski, P. M., & Schum, R. L. (1993). Counseling parents of children who stutter. *American Journal of Speech-Language Pathology*, 2(2), 65–73.

Zimmermann, G. N., Liljeblad, S., Frank, A., & Cleeland, C. (1983). The Indians have many terms for it: Stuttering among the Bannock-Shoshoni. *Journal of Speech and Hearing Research*, 26, 315–318.

Name Index

Adamczyk, B., 44
Adams, M. R., 45, 46, 53, 243, 248, 258
Aguirrebengoa, L., 270
Ainsworth, S., 111, 133
Ambrose, N. G., 53, 96, 100, 111, 134
Amman, J. O. C., 128
Amster, B., 112
Anderson, D., 32
Andrews, G., 11, 43, 44, 46, 47, 76, 88, 112, 132, 133, 134, 135, 138, 153, 155, 244, 245, 257
Andy, O. J., 267
Anthony, J. F. K., 264
Appelt, A., 121, 122, 126
Arnold, G. E., 19, 20, 152, 153, 262, 265
Arnott, N., 128
Aronson, A. E., 15, 19, 167
Arthur, B., 225
Atkins, C. P., 14, 54, 83, 102, 103, 160
Attanasio, J. S., 15
Azrin, N. H., 47, 244, 245

Baer, T., 56
Barbara, D. A., 54, 81, 207
Barber, V., 43
Bastijns, P., 267
Baumgartner, J. M., 42, 93

Bayle, C., 123
Bebout, L., 225
Beech, H. R., 70, 133
Bell, A. M., 128
Bell, J., 75
Bellak, L., 191
Benecken, J., 32
Benitez, M., 46
Bennett, S., 142
Berlin, C. I., 102
Berlin, L., 238, 242
Berlin, S., 238, 242
Bernstein-Ratner, N., 46
Berry, M., 153
Bhatnagar, S. C., 267
Blanton, M. G., 124
Blanton, S., 124
Blood, G. W., 88, 142
Blood, I. M., 142
Bloodstein, O., 12, 13, 17, 18, 19, 27, 28, 36, 37, 38, 43, 46, 47, 48, 49, 51, 54, 56, 58, 59, 71, 78, 79, 100, 101, 105, 107, 108, 129, 130, 132, 133, 134, 135, 136, 137, 139, 142, 143, 150, 151, 157, 158, 173, 227, 240, 248, 277
Bloom, C. M., 49, 52
Bloom, L., 143
Bluchard, L., 245
Bluemel, C. S., 104, 105, 107

Boberg, E., 74, 87, 120, 226, 228, 257, 261
Boberg, J. M., 87, 228, 261
Bogue, B. N., 125
Bohlman, P., 17, 163
Bo-Lassen, P., 74
Bond, L., 146
Boome, E. J., 10, 240
Boone, D. R., 19
Borden, G. L., 56, 57
Boves, L., 236, 271
Boyce, W., 29
Bradberry, A., 269
Brady, J. P., 44, 166, 228, 243
Brady, W. A., 112
Braun, A., 248
Brauneis, E., 248
Brewer, D. W., 56
Brill, A. A., 127
Broers, T., 29
Brown, G., 266
Brown, S. F., 39, 40, 41
Brumfitt, S. M., 49
Brutten, G. J., 10, 39, 42, 55, 56, 57, 69, 76, 159, 161, 197, 202, 203, 246
Bryngelson, B., 237
Buffalo, M. D., 63
Burlison, A. E., 218
Burnett, M. L., 91

Cady, B. B., 47
Calver, P., 227, 258
Canter, G., 62
Carlisle, J. A., 45, 78, 80, 87, 235, 243, 269
Carter, G. L., 81, 244
Cash, T. F., 249, 250
Chapman, S. B., 89
Cherry, C., 45
Christensen, L., 16
Cicero, 122
Cleeland, C., 145
Collins, C. R., 88
Commodore, R. W., 46
Conture, E. G., 53, 56, 98, 102, 171, 226, 261
Cooper, C. S., 203

Cooper, E. B., 46, 47, 81, 83, 171, 202, 203, 207, 208, 209, 215, 225, 226, 227, 261, 269
Cordes, A. K., 35, 246
Coriat, I. H., 10, 127, 143
Cote, C., 245
Cox, N., 134
Craig, A. R., 226, 258
Craven, D. C., 46, 197
Cross, D. E., 75
Cudd, P. A., 49
Cullinan, W. L., 266
Culton, G. L., 111
Curlee, R. F., 119, 156, 165, 166

Dailey, D., 80
Daly, D. A., 14, 15, 60, 61, 91, 108, 180, 253, 263, 264, 265
Darley, F. L., 96, 194, 200
Darwin, E., 128
Davis, L. J., 15
de l'Isère, C., 122
De Nil, L., 202
Deal, J. L., 63, 64
Dempsey, G. L., 15
Denhardt, R., 162
Devous, M. D., 89
Devreux, F., 63
Dewar, A. D., 264
Dickson, S., 112
Dieffenbach, J. F., 123
Dietrich, S., viii
Diggs, C. C., 256, 269, 270
DiLollo, D., 258
Donahue-Kilburg, G., 146
Doro, J. M., 64
Drayna, D. T., 131
Drummond, S. S., 63
Duffy, J. K., 152
Duncan, M. H., 155
Dunlap, K., 128, 154
Dyer, J., 148, 149
Edwards, S. G., 78
Eldridge, M., 44, 122, 123, 124, 126, 242
Erickson, J. G., 225
Erickson, R. L., 200
Espin, C. A., 256

Felsenfeld, S., 131
Fenichel, O., 143
Finitzo, T., 89
Finn, P., 271
Fitch, J. L., 16, 17, 164
Flanagan, B., 47
Fletcher, J. M., 71
Florance, C. K., 242, 265
Frank, A., 145
Franken, M. C., 236, 242, 271
Frankl, V. E., 48, 144, 198, 255
Fransella, F., 48, 70, 87, 133
Frantz, S. E., 244
Fraser, J., 261
Fraser-Gruss, J., 111, 133
Freeman, C. A., 256
Freeman, F. J., 16, 57, 89
Freud, S., 127
Freund, H., 28, 58, 61, 63, 127, 157,
     162, 163, 207, 226, 227, 237
Froeschels, E., 238

Gaines, N. D., 40
Galaburda, A. M., 133, 141
Gazzolo, M., 52, 249
Gerstman, L. J., 245
Geschwind, N., 133, 141
Gilman, M., 240
Gladstein, K. L., 111
Glauber, I. P., 131, 142, 143, 158
Goda, S., 153
Godden, A. L., 245
Goldberg, B., 120
Goldiamond, I., 46, 47
Goldstein, H., 266, 267
Goodban, M. K., 45
Gootwald, S. R., 222
Gordon, P. A., 203
Gottwald, S. R., 227, 257
Granich, M., 15
Gregory, H. H., 200, 269
Grothe, M., 39
Guitar, B. E., 47, 146, 226
Gutzmann, H., 152

Haasler, S. K., 49
Haefner, R., 140

Halfond, M. M., 227, 257
Hall, D. E., 112
Hall, N. E., 222
Halvorson, J. A., 47, 149
Ham, R. E., 31, 238, 239, 240, 265
Hammer, C. S., 225
Hamre, C., 150
Harle, M., 154
Haroldson, S. K., 245, 258
Harris, M., 133, 135, 138, 153, 155,
     243
Helm-Estabrooks, N., 15, 62, 93, 267
Herodotus, 121
Hillis, J. W., 271
Hinzman, A. R., 59, 60
Hippocrates, 121, 139
Horsburgh, G., 45, 197
Hotz, G., 15
Howie, P. M., 120, 136, 137, 257
Hubbard, C. P., 41, 42
Hugh-Jones, S., 88
Hulit, L. M., 31, 49
Hull, F. M., 59
Hulstijn, W., 35
Hummer, K., 19
Hunt, H., 122, 123, 128
Hutchinson, J. M., 57

Ingham, J. C., 211
Ingham, R. J., 13, 35, 45, 71, 197,
     240, 242, 243, 246, 258, 271
Irvine, T. L., 264
Irwin, J., 152

Jacobson, E., 49, 240, 246
James, S. E., 49
Jensen, K. H., viii
Jiang, Y., 242
Johnson, L., 75
Johnson, W., ix, 7, 10, 11, 24, 25, 26,
     32, 34, 36, 37, 38, 41, 42, 43, 44,
     46, 49, 52, 55, 57, 78, 81, 82, 85,
     87, 96, 97, 98, 99, 102, 103, 107,
     129, 135, 140, 143, 144, 146,
     147, 148, 153, 173, 175, 190,
     191, 192, 217, 234, 250, 260,
     271, 277
Jones, B. P., 73

Jones, P. K., 73
Juhl, P., 245

Kalinowski, J., 31, 242
Kalinowski, L. S., 202
Kamhi, A. G., 48, 258
Kelly, E. M., 53
Kenney, M. K., 56
Kent, L. R., 102
Kent, R., D., 69, 156, 165, 166
Kidd, K. K., 111
Kistler, D. J., 200
Klencke, H., 126
Knott, J. R., 41, 42, 49, 52, 55, 57
Kolk, H., 142
Kools, J. A., 7, 13, 40, 41, 228
Krause, M., 41
Krol, L. M., 257
Kroll, R. M., 202
Kully, D., 261
Kushner, H. S., 121

Ladouceur, R., 245
Lay, T., 216, 222
Leach, E., 246
Leahy, M. M., 31, 272
Leblond, G., 245
Lebrun, Y., 36, 41, 62, 63, 123, 166
Leith, W. R., 225
Leleux, C., 62, 63
Leney, M., 258
Lerman, J. W., 16, 202
Lesch, M. M., 45, 243
Levis, D., 247
Lewis, B., 99, 146
Liles, B. Z., 16
Liljeblad, S., 145
Liljestrand, J. S., 73
Lincoln, M., 245
Lindsay, J. S., 144
Linebaugh, C. W., 266
Lohr, F., 54
Luchinger, R., 152, 153, 262, 265
Ludlow, C. L., 248
Luper, H. L., 75, 203

Macfarlane, F. K., 240, 241
Maestas, A. G., 225

Maier, S. F., 227
Mallard, A. R., 243
Manders, E., 267
Manning, W. H., 80, 108, 109, 218, 246, 258
Market, K. W., 63, 267
Martin, R. R., 47, 245, 258
Martyn, M. M., 112
Matsuda, M., 225
Mayberry, R., 39
McCall, G. N., 56
McClean, M. D., 35
McDonough, A., 84, 202
McKeehan, A. B., 272
McOsker, T. G., 48
Melrose, B. M., 260
Meltzer, A., 17, 163
Meyer, L. A., 243
Meyers, S. C., 40, 99
Mikhailova, E. L., 257
Miller, D. T., 162
Miller, S., 51, 89
Moeller, D., 129
Montague, J. C., 63
Montgomery, B. M., 16, 17, 164
Moore, J. C., 256
Moore, M. A. S., 45, 243
Moore, W. H., 74
Morgenstern, J. J., 135
Muellerleile, S., 46, 197
Murphy, B., 269
Murphy, W. P., 88
Murray, F. P., 78
Myers, F., 14, 60, 166, 262, 265
Mygind, H., 153

Nadoleczny, M., 163
Nagel, R., 203
Neimeyer, R. A., 258
Nelson, S., 152
Newman, L. L., 149
Niermann, R., 53
Nowack, W. J., 62
Nunn, R. G., 244

Oates, D. W., 140
Ojemann, R. H., 140
Onslow, M., 150, 163, 245, 258

Otsuki, H., 154

Packman, A., 163
Paden, E. P., 41, 127
Paterson, J., 29
Paul-Brown, D., 256
Paynter, K. K., 259
Penfield, W., 72, 73
Perkins, W. H., 11, 12, 13, 75, 88,
    144, 150, 156, 165, 166, 215,
    227, 238, 242, 257
Peters, H. F. M., 35, 108, 236, 271
Peterson, Y., 52, 249
Pill, J., 244, 269, 270
Polanyi, M., 186
Pool, K. D., 89
Porter, H. K., 46, 52
Postma, A., 142
Preus, A., 108
Prins, D., 41, 54, 227
Pruzinsky, T., 249, 250

Quesal, R. W., 84, 88, 202, 269

Rami, M., 31
Ramig, P. R., 46, 238, 242
Rastatter, M., 31
Reardon, N. A., 269
Reed, C. G., 245
Reeves, L., 269
Reis, R. P., 264
Richardson, M. A., 10, 240
Richter, E., 112
Rieber, R. W., 123, 124
Rigo, T. G., 256
Riley, G. D., 75, 171, 195, 211, 254
Riley, J., 75, 171, 254
Robbins, C. J., 47
Roberts, L., 72, 73
Roman, K. G., 91
Rosen, B., 43, 44, 46
Rosenfield, D. B., 16, 73
Roth, C. R., 15, 16, 63, 268
Rousseau, J., 63
Rubin, T. I., 81, 249
Rudas, J., 75
Runyan, C. M., 40, 258
Rustin, L., 14, 225

Ryan, B. P., 46, 197

Salamy, J. N., 19
Sayers, B., 45
Schaefer, H. K., 146
Schloss, P. J., 256
Schopflocher, D., 74
Schuell, H., 133
Schum, R. L., 261
Schwartz, H. D., 98, 257
Schwartz, M. F., 81, 242, 244
Scobble, M., 39
Scripture, E. W., 127
Sears, R. L., 46
Seeman, M., 76
Seider, R. A., 111, 112
Seligman, M. E. P., 227
Sessions, R. B., 19
Shames, G. H., 47, 225, 242, 265
Shapiro, A. K., 224, 241
Shaw, C. K., 246
Sheehan, J. G., 37, 57, 112, 207
Sheehy, G., 108
Shenker, R. C., 39
Sherrick, C. E., 47
Shirkey, E. A., 17, 28, 173
Shklovskii, V. M., 257
Shoemaker, D. J., 10, 39, 55, 56, 57,
    69, 76, 159, 161, 197, 202, 246
Shumak, I. C., 200
Siegel, G. M., 13, 47
Silverman, E.-M., 16, 26, 98, 99, 146,
    164
Silverman, F. H., 7, 11, 13, 16, 17,
    19, 25, 30, 32, 34, 38, 40, 41, 42,
    43, 44, 45, 49, 52, 69, 101, 134,
    147, 149, 150, 159, 163, 164,
    173, 175, 180, 187, 191, 192,
    197, 198, 199, 201, 205, 207,
    222, 226, 227, 228, 235, 242,
    243, 245, 249, 259, 261, 273
Simon, C. A., 265
Simpson, K. C., 142
Sinn, A., 42, 55, 57
Skinner, B. F., 47, 245
Smith, A., 13, 131, 132, 158, 159
Smith, N. A., 256
Smith, P. K., 88

Snidecor, J. C., 58, 145
Solomon, A., 42, 55, 57
Southwood, H., 45, 197
Spriestersbach, D. C., 194, 200
St. Ledger, J., 16
St. Louis, K. O., viii, 14, 59, 60, 166, 265, 269, 270
Stampfl, T., 247
Stansfield, J., 36
Starkweather, C. W., 27, 41, 35, 108, 156, 160, 227, 231, 257, 270
Stern, E., 137
Stewart, J. L., 145
Stocker, B., 193, 245
Stone, R. E., 62
Stuart, A., 31, 242

Tanner, D. C., 81, 103
Tanner, S., 244, 245, 257
Tatchell, R. H., 14
Thaxton, D., 218
Thompson, J. D., 265
Throneburg, R. N., 41
Tiger, R. J., 264
Tillis, M., 32, 44, 86, 235, 269
Tonev, P., 245
Trotter, W. D., 32, 44, 45, 197, 228, 242, 243, 271
Trutna, P. A., 246
Tudor, M., 147, 148, 149, 150, 245
Turnbill, W., 162

Ushijima, T., 57

Van Borsel, J., 36, 41
van Eupen, A-K., 203
van Lieshout, P. H. H. M., 35
Van Riper, C., 10, 11, 27, 36, 37, 38, 42, 44, 48, 50, 51, 53, 55, 57, 58, 69, 72, 85, 86, 87, 97, 98, 100, 101, 102, 104, 108, 109, 110, 128, 129, 133, 134, 135, 137, 140, 143, 150, 151, 154, 155, 157, 158, 159, 172, 174, 194, 195, 196, 198, 207, 208, 211, 222, 226, 227, 229, 233, 235, 237, 238, 239, 240, 244, 248, 255, 263, 268
Vanryckeghem, M., 203
Voas, R. B., 57

Wager, W., 32, 86, 235, 269
Wallace, M. L., 238
Wallace, S., 80
Walle, E. L., 45
Wallen, V., 15
Watkin, K. L., 57
Watson, B. C., 51, 89
Watson, J. B., 79, 200
Watt, J., 202
Watts, F., 242
Webster, M., 42
Webster, R. L., 236, 242, 244, 271
Wedberg, C. F., 78
Weiss, D. A., 14, 28, 60, 61, 90, 113, 262, 263, 265
Wertz, H., 142
West, R., 141, 152
Wexler, K. B., 108
White, K., 39
Whitney, J. L., 266, 267
Williams, D. E., viii, ix, 7, 13, 36, 37, 38, 39, 40, 41, 42, 49, 52, 57, 69, 72, 101, 102, 148, 161, 186, 198, 201, 202, 232, 248, 260
Wingate, M. E., 13, 39, 40, 44, 123, 124, 226, 242
Wolpe, J., 49, 241, 246, 247, 254, 255, 256
Woods, C. L., 202, 260
Woods, L., 120
Wyatt, G. L., 154

Xia, S., 242

Yairi, E., 41, 42, 53, 96, 98, 99, 100, 107, 111, 134, 146
Yaruss, J. S., 171, 240, 269
Yeudall, L. T., 74
Young, M. A., 49, 51, 52
Yovetich, W. S., 253, 257

Zebrowski, P. M., 98, 102, 238, 261
Zimmermann, G. N., 145

Subject Index

Abstracting, 10, 85, 102, 188–189, 228

Acquired stuttering. *See* Neurogenic acquired stuttering; Psychogenic acquired stuttering

Acupuncture, 248

Adaptation effect
cluttering and, 63
repeating a speaking task and, 49
spastic dysphonia and, 19
spontaneous recovery and, 52

Adaptation tasks, as fluency device, 49–50

Adults
development of stuttering in, 108
neurogenic acquired stuttering in, 113–114
onset of stuttering in, 103–104
psychogenic acquired stuttering in, 114

Age
as predisposing factor for stuttering, 134
chronological, as risk factor for fluency disorders, 21
influence on choice of intervention strategy, 233
mental, and language development, 21
middle, decrease in stuttering

severity in, 108
onset of stuttering and, 96
See also Preschool-age children

Agoraphobia, 164

"American Method" for treating stuttering, 122

American Speech-Language-Hearing Association (ASHA), 206, 216, 220

Anger, 80–81, 143, 185, 249

Anoxia, 15

Anticipatory-struggle hypotheses, 17, 131, 143–151, 158–159, 162–163

Anxiety
perception of, preceding stuttering, 58–59
personality trait of, in stutterers, 84
reduction of, 254–256. *See also* Relaxation; Tension
while waiting to speak, 51

Aphasia, 92

Aphonia, 93

Apraxia, 75, 137–138, 183

Articulation
abnormalities in, 57
brain damage and, 92
secondary stuttering and, 105
tactile-kinesthetic perception of stutterers', 58

without phonation, as fluency device, 46
Articulatory musculature, 19, 27, 37, 47, 57, 75, 239–240
Articulatory postures, 98–100
Assertiveness training, 256
Attending speech
cluttering and, 60
stuttering and, 48
Attention span, limited, 89–90
Attributes
of clutterers, physiological and psychological, 89–90
language skills of stutterers, 88–89
of neurogetic acquired stutterers, 92
of psychogenic acquired stutterers, 92–93
physiological, of stutterers, 70–77
psychological, of stutterers, 78–88
Auditory feedback
defects, as stuttering cause, 142
delayed, 31–32, 46, 63, 65, 197, 241–242, 264, 267
Auditory functioning of stutterers, 76
Auditory musculature, tensing of, 39
Auditory tracking, 74
Authority figures, 51–52, 60, 86
Autism, 16
Autonomic nervous system, 56, 69, 76, 121
Autosuggestion, 240
Avoidance of disfluency
Bluemel on, 105
causing worse disfluency, 28, 52, 86, 135–136, 217–218, 248
as defining characteristic of stuttering, 12
diagnosogenic theory and, 144
high price paid for, 80
identifying, 184
level of, 28
in young children, 101, 217
See also Avoidance of stuttering
Avoidance of stuttering
causing increased stuttering, 52
disabilities and handicaps caused by, 35
identifying stuttering mind-set, 184

incomplete phrases and, 37
in Van Riper's "four tracks," 110
in young children, 100, 102
See also Avoidance of disfluency
Awareness of disfluency
body image and, 85
emotional well-being and, 78
in hesitation phenomena, 8–9
in neurogenic acquired stuttering, 92
lack of, 14–15, 22, 59–60, 85, 89–90, 100, 106, 112–113
parental, 102–103, 146, 250–253, 277–278
in young children, 100, 102
See also Perception; Reactions to disfluency

Badge wearing, 272
Behavior modification, 271–272
Behaviors
assessing for progress, 172–173
attempts to modify for evaluation purposes, 197
defining fluency disorders through, 172, 181–186
identifying mind-set of client, 69, 93–94, 170, 172, 181–186, 199, 256
observable, during moments of stuttering, 36–39
observing, for evaluation purposes, 187–188
partial reinforcement schedule of, 159
stuttering as learned, 159–161
Belief systems, modification of client, 241, 250
belle indifférence, la (indifference to stuttering), 63
Bilinguality, and fluency, 46, 137
Biochemical functioning of stutterers, 71
Biochemical imbalance, as stuttering cause, 140–141
Biofeedback, as tension-reducing device, 47, 241
Blockages and blocking, 35, 37–38, 54–55, 58, 98, 104, 183, 238–239, 268

Bloodstein's etiology of stuttering category, 130

Bloodstein's four phases in stuttering development, 105–108

Bluemel's primary and secondary stages of stuttering, 104–105

Body image, 85. *See also* Self-concept

Books, self-help, 270

Bounce, 218, 237, 268

Brain injuries, 137

Brain wave activity, in stutterers, 71, 74

Brain waves. *See* Cerebral lateralization of function

Breakdown hypotheses, 130, 139–140, 157–158

Breathing
  abnormal, during moments of stuttering, 56, 70
  audible irregularities in, 27
  diaphragmatic, 111
  exercises, as stuttering treatment, 124
  perfectly mastered breathing (PMB) program, 245
  reducing abnormalities in, 244–245
  regulated-breathing method, 244–245
  secondary stuttering and, 104
  tense/unfilled pauses and, 9

Broken words, 8, 29, 36–37, 98, 183

Cancellation technique, 238–240

Cardiovascular functioning, 71

Case studies, excerpts from clinicians', 62, 284–292

Causes. *See* Etiology

Causes of stuttering
  categorizing hypotheses about, 129–131
  demand for fluency exceeding capacity, 156
  desiring to avoid disfluency, 28, 52, 86, 217–218, 248
  dyssynchronous speech components, 156–157
  emotional and communicative

conflicts, 154–155
  etiology of vs. moment of, 130.
    See also Stuttering, etiology of
  illness, 152–153
  imitation, 153–154
  physiological vs. psychological, 131–132
  predisposing, 133–138
  reduced ability to generate temporal patterns, 156
  shocks and fright, 151

Central nervous system, 71–75, 121, 156

Cerebral dominance, disturbance in, 71–74, 139–141, 147

Cerebral lateralization of function, 72–75

Cerebral palsy, 137

Certainties, 250, 259–261

Checklists
  Cooper Chronicity Prediction, 323–325
  Daly's, for Possible Cluttering, 325–327
  Southern Illinois University Speech Situation, 318–320
  of stuttering behavior, 195, 315–316

Childhood disfluency, normal.
    See Normal disfluency

Children
  avoidance and prediction of stuttering in, 101
  cluttering, onset and development of, 112
  determining fluency disorders in, 177–178
  developmental characteristics of stuttering in, 104–110
  at high risk of disfluency diagnosis, 21
  normal repetition in, 11, 146.
    See also Normal disfluency, childhood
  onset and development of cluttering in, 113
  onset of stuttering in, 97–102
  parental reaction to onset stuttering in, 102–103, 146

prevention of stuttering in, 276–279

secondary stuttering diagnosed as normal disfluency, 217

self-concepts of, 101–102

See also Normal disfluency, childhood

Children's Apperception Test (CAT), 191

Children's Attitudes about Talking Revised (CAT–R), 322–323

Chorus, reading in, 19, 43–44, 63, 174, 180–181, 187, 195

Chronic perseverative stuttering (CPS) syndrome, 208–209, 269

Circumlocutions, 105, 107, 184, 188, 193–194

Classical vs. instrumental conditioning, 161, 197

Classmates, changing the reactions of, 253

Clinical relationship
characteristics of productive, 223–224
cultural considerations in, 224–225

Clinicians
essential information for, 2–3
goals of, 1
See also Speech-language pathologists

Closet stutterers, 13, 35

Cluttering
characteristics of, 60
defined, 14–15
development of, 113
etiology of, 165–166
genetic predisposition for, 22
language disorders accompanying, 60
language skills and, 90–91
link with stuttering, 113
onset of, 112–113
phonemic foci of, 62
physiological/psychological characteristics of, 89–90
self-concept and, 90
simulation of, 65
speaking rate and, 22

stuttering vs., 59–61, 179–180
symptomatology and phenomenology of, 59–61

Code of ethics, ASHA, 216, 221, 278

Colombat de l'Isère, 122

Commercial stuttering schools, 124–125

Communication
attitude test, 203
conflicts, as stuttering source, 154–155
emphasis over fluency, 184, 257, 278–279
impact of fluency disorders on, 16–17, 29–30
in good therapeutic relationships, 223

Concealing disfluency, 35, 48, 84–85, 88, 172, 178, 184–185, 235, 280–281. See also Stuttering, concealing

Concomitants of moments of stuttering, 57–59

Conditioning, 161, 197, 245–246. See also Learned behavior

Conflicts, as source of stuttering, 154–156

Consistency effect, 41, 160

Consonant contact, "light," 238

Contacts, hard, 58

Continuity hypothesis, 150–151

Contracts, written and oral, 224

Control, loss of, 157, 209

Cooper Chronicity Prediction Checklist, 203, 323–325

Cortical potentials. See Brain waves

Cost, 187

Counseling, family. See Family

Cryosurgery, 15

Cultural considerations
in evaluation, 175–176
factors affecting prognosis, 276
in stuttering prevention, 276
in therapeutic relationships, 224–225

Cultural expectations, 133

Culture, and likelihood of stuttering, 136

Daly's Checklist for Possible Cluttering, 325–327
Data collection, evaluative, 186–203
Delayed auditory feedback, 31–32, 46, 63, 65, 197, 241–242, 264, 267
Demands and capacities model of stuttering, 156
Dementia, 15
Denial, 81, 85, 92, 103
Depression, 81–82
Desensitization, 237, 246–247, 254–255
Development of stuttering
    characteristics of, 110
    middle-age, 108
    stages of, 104–108
Diagnosis
    mistaken, 2, 20, 99, 142, 181. *See also* Diagnosogenic theory
    necessary conditions for, 7–9
Diagnosogenic theory, 23, 28, 135, 143–150, 177, 277
Diarrhea, 164
Dichotic listening, 73–74
Disability(ies)
    fluency disorders as, 29–30
    insufficient focus on clients', 220–221
    preventing stuttering from becoming, 279–280
    reducing extent of client, 228–229
Disabled persons
    stuttering, and central nervous system, 71–72
    stutter-like disfluencies in, 16
Disfluency Descriptor Digest, 202–203, 320–322
Disfluency(ies)
    in clutterers, 60
    fear of. *See* Fear of disfluency
    normal childhood. *See* Normal disfluency, childhood
    See also Fluency disorders, Speech disfluency
Disrhythmic phonations, 8, 36–37
Down syndrome, 137
Drugs, treatment with, 248
Dysarthria, 92, 137, 183, 267
Dysnomia, 137

Dysphonia, 93
Dysrhythmic phonations, 8, 21, 25, 61

Edinburgh masker, 197, 243–244, 264
Electroencephalography, 74
Electroglottography, 56
Electromyographic (EMG) biofeedback, 47, 56, 241
Embarrassment, 12–14, 43, 83, 87, 102–103, 106, 110, 148, 160, 184, 188, 218–219, 228, 249–250, 281
Emotional adjustment, as disfluency factor, 78–79
Emotional conflicts, as stuttering source, 154–155
Emotional states
    flooding (implosive therapy), 247
    and likelihood of successful therapy, 208
    during moments of stuttering, 13–14, 182
    stuttering increase and, 52–53, 106
Empathy, in clinicians, 223
"Emperor's New Clothes" game, 100, 145, 249
Endocrine system, 121
Environment, influence of, on fluency, 46
Epilepsy, 137, 141, 153
Erotic gratification, oral/anal, 142–143
Ethics code, ASHA, 216, 221, 278
Etiology of stuttering category, Bloodstein's, 130
Etiology
    of cluttering, 165–166
    of neurogenic acquired stuttering, 166
    of psychogenic acquired stuttering, 166–167
    of stuttering. *See* Causes of Stuttering
European League of Stuttering Associations (ELSA), 270
Evaluation
    abstracting information, methods of, 188

identifying behaviors defining the disorder, 181–186
case studies, 284–292
communicating results of, 211–212
cultural considerations in, 175–176
expert opinions, 173
improvement potential for fluency, 229
interviewing informants, 175, 189–190
likelihood of fluency disorder, determining, 176–179
motivation assessment, 203–206
observation and data collection, 186–203
onset stuttering, determining presence of, 177–178
overview of process of, 173–175
making a prognosis, 206–209
progress, assessing client, 172–173
of tasks performed by clients, 190–203. *See also* Task analysis
of therapy outcome, 271
type of fluency disorder, determining, 179–181
reasons for, 170–173
reports, writing of, 211–212
when fluency seems normal, 178–179
Evaluative labeling, 147–148
Expectancy (anticipation) phenomenon of stuttering, 42–43
Expectancy neurosis, 162–163, 268
Expert opinions, 173
Expressive language impairments, 91
Extrapyramidal diseases, 15
Eye contact, 14, 54, 64, 83, 93, 102, 110, 145, 159–160, 174, 183–184, 225, 249–250, 287
Family
counseling for client's, 261. *See also* Parental reaction to children's stuttering
predisposition for stuttering, 134–135. *See also* Genetic predisposition

Fear of disfluency
anticipatory-struggle hypothesis and, 158–159
avoidance as a result of, 184
in chronic perseverative stuttering, 209
closet stutterers and, 35
diagnosogenic theory and, 143–150
emotional conflicts and, 154
expectancy neurosis and, 162–163, 268
overlay caused by, 268
in Phase IV stuttering, 107
in stuttering, 13, 35
secondary stuttering and, 217
STUTT-L commentary on, 35
on the telephone, 50
in Van Riper's "four tracks," 109–110
while waiting to speak, 51
See also Avoidance of fluency; Diagnosogenic theory
Feedback. *See* Biofeedback; Delayed auditory feedback
Filled pauses, 38
Finger tapping, 74, 267
Fluency
in clutterers, 60
demand exceeding capacity for, 156
disorders of. *See* Fluency disorders
evaluation of, 170–211
failure to use techniques outside of therapy, 219
maintaining after treatment, 257–258
reducing tendency to overvalue, 184, 257, 279
Fluency disorders
"curing," 226–227
as disabilities, 29–30
evaluation process, overview of, 173–175
degree of tension during, 26–27
faking, 28–29
famous persons with, 30
genetic predisposition for, 22–23, 134–135

as handicaps, 30–31
historical explanations for,
    118–129
identifying behaviors that define,
    181–186
as impairments, 29
literary depiction of, 32
major types of, 2
in manual communication,
    16–17
predisposition to expect, 28
presence or likelihood of, deter-
    mining, 170–171, 176–179
reducing severity of, 227–228
secondary symptoms accompany-
    ing, 27–28
self-help for, 269–270
trauma precipitating, 22
type of, determining, 171–172,
    179–181
variations in, under certain
    conditions, 195–196
Fright, as cause of stuttering,
    151–152

Generality, 187
Genetic predisposition, 275–277
    for cluttering, 166
    delayed language development
        and, 138
    expectancy neurosis and, 163
    within families, 60, 134
    for fluency disorders, 20, 22–23
    for stuttering, 134–135
    in twins, 137
Gestures, 27, 39, 54–55, 156, 160,
    184, 188, 202–203, 320.
    See also Stuttering, physiologi-
    cal events accompanying
"Giant in chains" allegory, 86, 231,
    235, 280
Glottis, spastic, as cause of stutter-
    ing, 123
Goals
    avoiding ambiguity in setting,
        230–231
    client, helping to establish and
        prioritize, 225–226
    of clinicians, 1

general intervention, 226–229
specific intervention, 230–231
Grieving, 81, 92, 103, 206, 220, 268
Grimaces, facial, 137, 154, 159, 194
Guilt, 81–83, 143, 218–219, 251–
    253, 278, 281

Handicaps
    fluency disorders as, 30–31
    insufficient focus on client,
        220–221
    preventing stuttering from
        becoming, 279–280
    reducing extent of client, 228–229,
        258–261
Harm
    avoidance of, as clinician's goal, 1
    ways of causing stutterers,
        216–222
Headaches, 164
Hearing
    abnormal tensing of tympanic
        membrane, 39
    auditory feedback defects as
        cause of stuttering, 142
    auditory function of stuttering, 76
    hearing-impaired persons who
        stutter, 76
    stutterers' auditory perception of
        their stuttering, 57–58
Heredity. *See* Genetic predisposition
Hesitation phenomena
    awareness of and concern about, 27
    categorization of, 7–9
    chronological/mental age and, 21
    duration of, 24–26
    frequency of, 23–24
    identification of, 31
    normal vs. abnormal, 20–21
    onset of, sudden vs. gradual, 97
    in preschoolers, 115
    speaking rate and, 22
    types of, 21
Hieroglyphic symbol for stuttering,
    119
Honesty, in clinicians, 223
Hoover's sign, 64
Hope, engendering in clients, 223
Humor, developing a sense of, 236

Hyperactivity, 89–90
Hypotheses, general themes of,
    130–131. *See also* Anticipatory-
    struggle hypotheses; Break-
    down hypotheses; Diag-
    nosogenic theory; Repressed-
    needs hypotheses

Illness, as cause of stuttering,
    152–153
Imitation, as stuttering cause, 135,
    153–154
Impairments
    expressive language, 91
    fluency disorders as, 29
    receptive language, 90
Incomplete phrases, 8–9, 24, 37
Individualized Training Programs
    (IEPs), 171
Informants, 175, 189–190
Informed consent, 207
Instrumental vs. classical condi-
    tioning, 161
Intelligence, 78
Interactional theory, 144
Interaction-frame model, 234–236,
    248
Interjections (of sounds, syllables,
    words, or phrases), 7–8, 38, 54,
    287
Internal stutterers, 58, 207
International Stuttering Associa-
    tion (ISA), 270
Interpersonal relationships, 184
Intervention strategies
    for cluttering, 262–265
    constraints of economy and time
        on, 232
    counterintuitive, 221
    factors affecting choice of,
        231–233
    humor, developing a sense of, 236
    interaction-frame model,
        234–236
    modifying client and listener
        reactions to disfluency,
        248–257
    modifying stuttering directly,
        236–248
    for neurogenic acquired stutter-
        ing, 266–268
    for psychogenic acquired stutter-
        ing, 268
    reducing stuttering severity,
        233–236
    self-help groups, 269
Introspective concomitants of
    moments of stuttering, 57–59
Inventory of Communication Atti-
    tudes, 200, 306–309
Investment, client. *See* Motivation
Iowa Scale of Severity of Stuttering,
    194–195, 314

Job task, 175, 190
Jokes, telling, 51

Kinesthetic feedback, 77, 265

la belle indifférence, 63
Labeling, evaluative, 147
Language development, delay in, 60,
    113, 138
Language impairments
    expressive, 91
    receptive, 90
Language skills
    of children who stutter, 88–89
    of clutterers, 90–91, 113, 263
    of neurogenic acquired stutterers,
        92
    of psychogenic acquired stutter-
        ers, 93
    of stutterers, 74, 88–89
Larnyx, stuttering caused by mal-
    function of, 75, 122
Laryngeal functioning, reducing
    anomalies in, 244
Laryngectomy, acquired stuttering
    following, 16
Learned behavior
    learned helplessness, 227
    maladjustive, 162
    stuttering as, 128–129,
        159–161
Light consonant contact, 238
Lipped speech, 46
Locus of control, 84, 202

Loudness, abnormal, 38, 54

"Magic" rituals, 54–55
Maintaining cause of stuttering, 129–130
Maintenance programs, fluency, 219, 257–258
Malingering, 17–18, 28–29
Manual communication, stutter-like disfluencies in, 16–17, 163
Masking noise, 45, 63, 196–197, 243, 264
Medical model of stuttering, 125
Mental retardation, 16, 21, 78, 137, 141, 188
Message therapy, 257
Metronome, as fluency device, 44–45, 123, 197, 242, 264, 267
Mimed reading, and psychogenic acquired stuttering, 64
Mind-set
    identifying client, 69, 170, 172, 181–186, 199
    of listener, 115
    of parents of stutterers, 102
    of stutterer, 93–94, 256
    See also Behaviors
Moment of stuttering hypothesis, Bloodstein's, 130
Moments of speech disfluency, 7–9
Monotone speech, 43, 46
Monster study, 147–149
Motivation
    assessment of, 190, 203–206
    causing client guilt for lack of, 218
    increasing client, 229
    level of, influencing intervention strategy, 233
Motor capabilities of stutterers, 75, 157
Muscular tension, 9, 39, 57–58, 240–241, 285. See also Tension; Relaxation
Musical instruments, stutter-like disruptions in playing, 163
Muthonome, 123

Name, saying one's, 19, 51

National Stuttering Association, 257
Nationality, as stuttering risk factor, 136
Neurogenic acquired stuttering
    development of, 114
    distinguishing from other fluency disorders, 180–181
    etiology of, 166
    language skills and, 92
    onset of, 113–114
    physiological and psychological characteristics of, 92
    self-monitoring program for, 266
    symptomatology and phenomenology of, 61–63
    trauma as precipitating, 22
Neuropsycholinguistic function, theory of, 156–157
Nonhabitual manner, speaking in, 22, 43, 54–55, 124, 182, 220, 242, 244
Normal disfluency, childhood
    continuity hypothesis and, 150
    distinguishing from early stuttering, 98–99, 100, 105, 107, 150–151
    misdiagnosing as stuttering, 146, 149–150, 177
    parents' familiarity with, 252
    providing parents with information on, 251–252
    as operant response, 47
    diagnosing secondary stuttering as, 217
    See also Children

Oath of Hippocrates, 216
Observation
    data-gathering through questions and behavior observation, 174
    informal, information obtainable by, 187–189
Onset stuttering
    adult, 103–104
    characteristics of, 109
    parental reaction to children's, 102–103, 146, 252
    symptomatology and phenomenology of, 96–102

Operant conditioning, 245–246
Operant responses, 47
Oral-motor discoordination, 75
Overlays
  caused by fear of disfluency, 280
  determining presence or likeli-
    hood of, 179
  on neurogenic acquired stutter-
    ing, 92, 268
  prevention of, 276, 280–281

Pacing board, 267
Paradoxical intention, 198,
    255–256
Parental reactions to children's stut-
    tering, 102–103, 135–136, 146,
    252–253, 277–278
  modifying, 250–253, 278
Part-word repetitions, 7–8
Pauses, tense and unfilled, 9, 37
Peer evaluation, negative, 87–88
Perception
  of anxiety, before moments of
    stuttering, 58–59
  auditory, of stutterer, 57–58
  impact of others', 87–88, 253
  impact of stutterers' mind-set on
    self, 93–94
  stutterers' expectation of others',
    87–88
  tactile-kinesthetic, 58
Perceptions of Self Semantic Differ-
    ential Task, 202, 317–318
Perfectionism, 81, 112, 185, 208, 230
Perfectly mastered breathing (PMB)
    program, 245
Personality traits
  of clutterers, 90
  and likelihood of successful ther-
    apy, 208
Persons who stutter. See Stutterers
Phenomenology
  of cluttering, 59–61
  of neurogenic acquired stuttering,
    61–63
  of onset of stuttering, 96–102
  of psychogenic acquired stutter-
    ing, 63–64
  of stuttering, 34–59

Phonation, 56–57
  disrhythmic, 8, 21, 25, 61
Phrases, incomplete, 8–9, 24, 37
Physician's Screening Procedure for
    Children Who May Stutter, 171,
    311–312
Physiological causes of stuttering,
    131–132
Physiological events, accompanying
    stuttering, 55–57
Pitch, 38, 43, 46–47, 54, 202, 288
Placebo effect, 204, 224, 241
Predisposing cause of stuttering,
    129–130. See also Diagnosogenic
    theory
Prediction of stuttering, 101, 171,
    184, 197–198
Predisposing factors for stuttering
    likelihood, 132–138
Preparatory-set technique, 238–240
Prevention
  in young children, 276–279
  cultural considerations affecting,
    276
  of overlay stuttering, 280–281
  of stuttering, 275
Problem Profile for Elementary-
    School-Age Children Who Stut-
    ter about Talking, 200–201, 206,
    309–310
Professional organizations, 295
Profile of Stuttering Severity,
    195–196
Prognosis, 69, 172, 206–209, 220,
    241, 258, 265, 276
Progress, assessing, 172–173
Prolongation, 183
  as disrhythmic phonation, 8–9,
    36–37
  in cluttering, 62
  in normal speech, 11
  in stuttering, 9, 11–12, 37, 98,
    100, 183, 242
Psychogenic acquired stuttering, 15
  distinguishing from other fluency
    disorders, 181
  etiology of, 166–167
  history of psychopathology and,
    93

language skills of persons with, 93

onset and development of, 114

physiological characteristics of, 92–93

psychological characteristics of, 93

symptomatology and phenomenology of, 63–64

trauma as precipitating, 22

Psychological causes of stuttering, 131–132

Psychopathology

emotional adjustment of stutterers and, 78

psychogenic stuttering and, 93

stuttering as symptom of, 125–127

Psychotherapy, 79

Public speaking, and increased stuttering, 51–52

Pull-out technique, 238–239

Punishment for sin, as explanation for stuttering, 121, 276

Punishment/reinforcement, response-contingent, 245–246, 248–249

Pyknolepsy, 141

Questionnaires, 198–200, 202–203, 303, 306–309, 318–320, 322–323

Questions

to define fluency disorders, 182–186

evaluative, 186–203

importance of wording specifically, 173

Rate of speaking

abnormal variations in, 22, 38, 54

accelerated (tachylalia), 15

of clutterers, 22, 59, 112–113, 264

reduced, 28, 46, 242, 267

Reactions to disfluency

desensitizing. See Desensitization

modifying, 248, 250–257, 278. See also Parental reactions to children's stuttering

Reading

disorder, in clutterers, 90

identification of hesitation phenomena in, 31

in chorus, 19, 43–44, 180–181, 195

mimed, and psychogenic stuttering, 64

oral samples, 193–194

repetition of same passage, 19, 49, 52

at slower rate than usual, 196

speech sample for task analysis, 190, 193–194

spontaneous recovery and, 53

Receptive language impairments, 90

Reciprocal inhibition principle, 246–247, 254–256

Recovery from stuttering, 111–112, 261–262

Referrals

client reluctance to accept, 229

clinician failure to make, 221

to self-help/support groups, 221

Reinforcement/punishment, response-contingent, 245–246, 248–249

Relapse, 83, 112, 120, 125, 127, 159, 215, 219–220, 226–227, 257–258

Relaxation, 49, 167, 240–241

Reliability, 165, 186–187, 245, 271

Repetition

categorization of, 7–8

in cluttering, 62, 112–113

as defining characteristic of stuttering, 9

in early onset stuttering, 97–99

mental age and, 21

in normal speech, 11, 146

in psychogenic acquired stuttering, 63

in stuttering, 11–12, 36, 106

syllabic. See syllable repetition

types of, 7–8

Repressed-need hypotheses, 131, 142–143, 158–159

Respect, mutual, 223

Respiration, 56, 70. See also Breathing

Response-contingent punishment/reinforcement, 47, 245, 248–249

Responsibility, failing to encourage
  clients to assume, 222
Revisions–incomplete phrases, 8, 38
Rhythm, disturbance of normal, in
  stuttering, 11, 36
Rhythmic speech, metronome-timed,
  242–243
Role playing, as fluency aid, 48
Romantic relationships, 80, 260

Screening, physician's procedure for
  children, 171, 311–312
Secondary symptoms, 13, 27–28,
  53–55
  absence of, in cluttering, 63
  lack of, in psychogenic acquired
    stuttering, 64
Seizures, 141
Self-concept, 84–85, 87–88, 90, 92,
  101–102, 107, 185, 249
Self-help groups, 221, 269–270,
  293–294
Semantics formulations, general, 147
Semantogenic theory, 144
  Set. See Mind-set
Shadowing, as fluency device, 44
Shame, 14, 83, 87, 102, 160, 184,
  188, 218, 249–250, 281
Shocks, as cause of stuttering,
  151–152
Sidedness. See Cerebral lateralization
Sin, punishment for, as explanation
  of stuttering, 121
Singing, 44, 63, 196
Slow, prolonged speech, 241–243
Social status, 85–86
Socioeconomic status, as stuttering
  risk factor, 135
Sounds, repetition and prolongation
  of, 9. See also Prolongation;
  Repetition; Syllable repetition
Southern Illinois University Speech
  Situation Checklist, 202,
  318–320
Spastic dysphonia, 18–20
Speaking rate. See Rate of speaking
Speech
  anxiety about, 84
  articulating without phonating, 46

to large audience, 52
disfluency of. See Speech disfluency
dyssynchronous components of,
  as cause of stuttering, 156–157
fluency increase with slower rate
  of, 196
locus-of-control orientation for, 84
masking noise accompanying, 45,
  196–197, 243
metronome-timed, 197, 242–243
monotone, 43, 46
nonhabitual manner of, 43, 218,
  220, 242
oral reading samples, 193–194
rate of. See rate of speaking
repetition and prolongation of.
  See Prolongation; Repetition;
  Syllable repetition
rhythmic, 243
self-monitoring of, in clutterers,
  262–263
shadowing of, 44
spontaneous samples, 190–193
syllable-timed, 243
on the telephone, 49–50, 197
waiting to respond, 51
Speech disfluency
  abnormality of, judging, 7
  desire to avoid, 28
  hesitation phenomena, types of,
    7–9
  moments of, as fluency disorder
    symptoms, 20–29
Speech disorders
  cluttering, 14–15
  laryngectomy, stuttering follow-
    ing, 16
  neurogenic acquired stuttering, 15
  psychogenic acquired stuttering,
    15–16
  stuttering, 9–14
  with stuttering-like symptoms,
    16–20
Speech fluency. See Fluency
Speech Foundation of America, 270
Speech Locus of Control Scale, 202
Speech mechanism
  defects in structure or function of,
    121–125

motor capabilities of, 75
oral-motor coordination differ-
    ences in, 75
seizures affecting, 141
stuttering as disruption of, 161
tensing musculature of, 239–240.
    See also Articulatory musculature
Speech-language functioning in clut-
    terers, 263
Speech-language pathologists
    attending self-help groups, 269
    establishing therapeutic relation-
        ships with clients, 222–224
    failing to make referrals, 221
    helping clients establish goals,
        225–229
    providing post-treatment mainte-
        nance, 257–258
    reasons for evaluating speech flu-
        ency, 170–173
    reasons for not scheduling ther-
        apy, 209–211
    selecting and implementing inter-
        vention strategies, 231–257
    shortcomings in serving clients,
        216–222
    working with classroom teachers,
        253
    See also Clinicians
Spontaneous recovery, 52–53
S-Scale, 199–200, 299–300
Stammering, 9–10
Starters, 38, 54, 105, 160, 184, 188,
    287
Stocker Probe Technique, 193
Stress, as cause of stuttering, 141–142
Stutterer's Self-Ratings of Reac-
    tions to Speech Situations, 200,
    301–303
Stutterers
    locus-of-control orientation of, 84
    others' perception of, 87–88
    personality traits of, 79–80
    physiological characteristics of,
        70–77
    psychological characteristics of,
        78–89
    restricted social relationships of, 80
    self-concept of, 84–85, 87–88

social status and, 85–86
visual functioning of, 77
Stutter-Free Speech Program, use
    with clutterers, 265
Stuttering
    anticipatory-struggle hypotheses
        of, 143–151, 161–164
    anxiety, perception of, preceding,
        58–59
    as expectancy neurosis, 162
    as learned behavior, 159–161
    as part of a class of disorders, 164
    at-risk factors for, 132–138
    auditory perception of, 57–58
    avoidance/fear of, Bloodstein's
        four phases of development,
        105–107
    Bluemel's primary and secondary
        stages of, 104–105
    breakdown hypotheses of,
        139–142
    bringing out into the open, 52,
        185, 188, 190, 226, 232, 235,
        239, 249
    childhood disfluency vs., 98–99.
        See also Normal disfluency;
        Preschool-age children
    cluttering vs., 59–61, 179–180
    concealing, 35, 48, 84–85, 88, 172,
        178, 184–185, 235, 281
    continuation of, reasons for,
        157–159
    decrease in, conditions for, 43–49
    defined, 9–14, 35
    deliberate, and paradoxical inten-
        tion, 198
    development of, 104–112
    devices that initially reduce, 54–55
    diagnosogenic theory of, 23, 28,
        135, 143–150, 177, 277
    disrhythmic phonations in, 36
    distribution of, in speech
        sequence, 39–42
    duration of moments of, 35
    early (primary) speech character-
        istics of, 97
    early theorizing about, 122
    embarrassment of, 12
    encouraging avoidance of, 218

etiology of, 118, 130–132, 165–166.
See also Causes of stuttering
expectancy (anticipation) phenomenon of, 42–43
family predisposition for, 134–135
fear of, 12
in hearing-impaired persons, 76
history of diagnosis and treatment of, 122–124
increase in, conditions for,
49–53
involuntary nature of, 12
inward vs. outward, 13
language skills and, 88
link with cluttering, 113
malingered, 17–18
in middle age and beyond, 108
misconceptions/false certainties
about, 259–261
moments of, defined, 35
neurogenic acquired, 61–63, 91–92,
113–114, 166
non-speech-related physiological
factors causing, 121
not desiring to conceal/avoid, as
fluency aid, 48
observable behaviors during,
36–39
onset of, 96, 103–104
parental reaction to children's,
102–103, 135, 146, 252
perspectives of stutterer vs. listener, 12
physiological vs. psychological
cause of, 131, 139
physiological events accompanying, 55–57, 98
precipitating causes of, 138–140,
142–143
predicting moments of, 197–198
predisposing factors for, 163
prevention of, 275–281
psychogenic acquired, 15, 63–64,
92–93, 114, 166–167
psychological concomitants of,
57–59
recovery from, 111–112, 261–262
reduced amount observed in therapy room, 101

repetitions of sound, syllable and
word in, 36
repressed-need hypotheses of,
142–143
response-contingent stimulation
of, 47
secondary symptoms accompanying, 53–55
as self-defining, 82
self-help for, 269–270
sex of child and, 133
simulation exercise, 31
situational variation in, 101
spastic dysphonia, 18–20
speaking anxiety and, 84
speech loci of moments of, 39–42
stammering vs., 9–10
stress-decreasing strategies for, 85
symptomatology and phenomenology of, 34–59
tactile-kinesthetic perception of,
58
testing theories about, 165–166
Van Riper's four tracks of stuttering development, 108–110
voluntary, 236–237
wind instrument playing and, 17
Stuttering Prediction Instrument for
Young Children (SPI), 171
Stuttering Problem Profile, 199, 271,
303–306
Stuttering Severity Instrument
(SSI), 194–195, 313
STUTT-L participants
on fear and avoidance of stuttering, 35
on importance of stutterer's perspective, 13
on inexpert speech-language
practitioners, 6
on inward vs. outward stuttering, 13
on stutterers being blamed for
stuttering, 216
on word substitution, 42
Success, and good therapeutic relationships, 223
Suggestion
power of, on stuttering, 48–49

waking and hypnotic, as tension
    reducer, 240
Support groups
    anxiety reduction through, 256
    failing to make referrals to, 221
    reciprocal inhibition principle
        and, 247
Surgery, 16, 73, 123
Syllabic stress, 41
Syllable repetition
    abnormal vs. normal, 99–100
    as diagnostic tool, 2
    as hesitation phenomenon, 7–8
    as speech characteristic of early
        stuttering, 97
    as symptom of abnormal disflu-
        ency behavior, 183
    awareness of and concern about,
        27
    in early (primary) stuttering, 97,
        99
    language development and, 21–22
    mental and chronological age
        and, 21
    muscular tension and, 27
    neurogenic acquired stuttering
        and, 62
    of beginning clutterers, 113
Syllable-timed speech, 243
Symptomatology
    of cluttering, 59–61
    of neurogenic acquired stuttering,
        61–63
    of onset of stuttering, 96–102
    of psychogenic acquired stutter-
        ing, 63–64
    of stuttering, 34–59
Symptoms, secondary, 13, 27–28,
    53–55
Systematic desensitization, 246–247,
    255

Tachistoscopic viewing procedure,
    74
Tachylalia, 15
Tachyphemia, 14, 22
Tacit knowing, 186
Tactile-kinesthetic feedback/func-
    tioning, 77, 265

Task analysis, 174
    as data-gathering tool, 174
    case study, 287–288
    Checklist of Stuttering Behavior,
        315–316
    Disfluency Descriptor Digest,
        320–322
    evaluative, 190–203
    Iowa Scale of Severity of Stutter-
        ing, 314
    passages for client oral reading,
        298
    Perceptions of Self Semantic
        Differential Task, 317–318
    Problem Profile for Elementary-
        School-Age Children Who
        Stutter about Talking,
        309–310
    sentence repetition, 299
    S-Scale, 299
    Stutterer's Self-ratings of Reac-
        tions to Speech Situations,
        301– 303
    Stuttering Problem Profile,
        304–306
    Stuttering Severity Instrument
        (SSI), 313
    tools of, 190, 199–203
    See also Evaluation
Teacher reactions to children's dis-
    fluencies, 253
Telephone, talking on, 49–50, 80,
    197
Temporal patterns, reduced ability
    to generate, 156
Tense pauses, 9, 13, 21, 37
Tension
    biofeedback monitoring of, 47, 241
    communicated to listeners, 14
    continuity hypothesis and,
        150–151
    degree of, while being disfluent,
        26–27
    intervention strategies for reduc-
        ing, 240–241
    muscular, 9, 39, 57–58, 240–241,
        285
    observable, during moments of
        stuttering, 38–39

signs of, in onset stuttering, 98
Tenuous fluency, 258
Test taking, as evaluation tool, 203
Thalamic stimulation electrode implant, 267
Thematic Apperception Test (TAT), 191–192
Therapeutic relationships. *See* Clinical relationship; Clinicians
Therapy
    assessing motivation for, 204–206
    factors influencing success of, 207–208
    failure to consult clients in goal setting, 217
    guilt following relapse after, 83
    implosive (emotional flooding), 247
    ineffective or harmful, 1
    influence of past attempts on success of present, 204
    outcome of, assessing and documenting, 271
    past attempts influencing success of present, 207, 210
    to improve self-concept, 85
    when not to schedule, 209–211
"Three wishes" task, 201, 205–206
Time
    clinicians wasting clients', 222
    stutterers' fear of taking excessive amounts of others', 83
Tongue, as cause of stuttering, 122
Trauma
    as cause of stuttering, 151–152
    precipitating a fluency disorder, 22
    psychogenic acquired stuttering and, 93
Tremors, 57
Trust, in therapeutic relationships, 223
Twins, stuttering in, 136–137

Tympanic membrane, 39

Unfilled pauses, 9
Units of repetition, 36, 99, 183

Validity, 165, 186–187
Van Riper's "four tracks" of stuttering development, 108–110
Ventriloquism speech, 238
Vicious circle/spiral of stuttering, 144–145, 162–164. *See also* Expectancy neurosis
Visual functioning of stutterers, 77
Vocations, avoidance of, by persons with fluency disorders, 30, 80, 185
Voice, abnormal pitch and loudness of, 38, 288
Voluntary stuttering, 233, 236–237, 247, 254–255

Wada Test, 73
Waiting to speak, and fear of disfluency, 51
Web sites, 295
Wind instrument stuttering, 17
Words
    consistency of, 41
    grammatical function and length of, 40
    initial phoneme of, 40–41
    length of, 40
    position of, in utterances, 39–40
    repetitions of, 8
    retrieval deficits, 266
    speaker's degree of familiarity with, 41
    substitution of, 35, 42, 84, 102, 107, 184, 188–189, 193–194
    syllabic location of stuttering within, 41
World Health Organization (WHO), 12, 29